Additional Praise for
Prevent, Halt & Reverse Heart Disease

"I was skeptical: Why one more cardiac self-help book? But then I started reading—till the very end. I could not put it down: well-written, little med-speak and entirely up-to-date and accurate. This is something I can recommend to all my patients."
—V.F. FROELICHER, M.D.,
Professor of Medicine, Stanford University

"Whether you're trying to prevent that first heart attack or reduce your risk of a second one, this is the book to read. It tells you what you need to know about exercise, nutrition and handling stress—all in terms you can understand and apply in your daily life."
—REDFORD WILLIAMS, M.D.,
Director, Behavioral Medicine, Duke University Medical Center

"Joe Piscatella and Dr. Barry Franklin have made an important contribution to the heart health of the nation. This eminently readable book combines medical information and suggestions for self-help."
—NANETTE K. WENGER, M.D.,
Professor of Medicine (Cardiology), Emory University School of Medicine

"*Prevent, Halt & Reverse Heart Disease* is superb—an outstanding book by two of the foremost experts on lifestyle modification and heart disease prevention. It is must reading for anyone who wants to prevent a heart attack or avoid another if they have already had one."
—NEIL F. GORDON, M.D., PH.D., M.P.H.,
Chief Medical and Science Officer, Nationwide Better Health

"A must-read for anyone who wants a science-based, comprehensive and sensible approach for reducing their risk of heart disease. It offers the gold-standard dietary recommendations, as well as the new discoveries in nutrition to promote health, all in 'how-to' examples that readers will value."
—PENNY KRIS-ETHERTON, PH.D., R.D.,
Distinguished Professor of Nutrition, Penn State University

"This easy-to-read book takes the mystery out of heart disease and translates the latest science into a remarkable 'how-to' manual of prevention. Reliable, current and practical advice for anyone who has a beating heart!"
—GARY J. BALADY, M.D.,
Director of Preventive Cardiology, Boston Medical Center,
Boston University School of Medicine

"A comprehensive guide for anyone concerned about heart disease. It's filled with practical advice and cutting-edge information. Read it today!"
—WAYNE M. SOTILE, PH.D.,
Director of Psychological Services,
Wake Forest University Healthy Exercise and Lifestyle Programs

"A sensible, clear and comprehensive approach to improving heart health. It highlights the latest findings in cardiovascular research and provides useful tools for putting our current prevention and treatment guidelines into practice."
—RONALD M. KRAUSS, M.D.,
Children's Hospital Senior Scientist, Oakland Research Institute

"A well-written treasure trove of information. Utilized properly, this book can add a significant dimension to our overall educational effort to positively influence and improve the cardiovascular health of our society."
—GERALD F. FLETCHER, M.D.,
Mayo Clinic Jacksonville

"This is an excellent, easily readable book, which is loaded with information and should be of great value to all who want to take the best possible steps to prevent heart disease."
—SIDNEY C. SMITH JR., M.D.,
Professor of Medicine, Director, Center for Cardiovascular Science and Medicine,
University of North Carolina School of Medicine

"Take a short cut to a long life with a few hours of entertaining reading."
—GERALD C. TIMMIS, M.D.,
Medical Director Emeritus, Clinical Research, William Beaumont Hospital

Prevent, Halt & Reverse Heart Disease

109 Things You Can Do

Prevent, Halt & Reverse Heart Disease

BY JOSEPH C. PISCATELLA
& BARRY A. FRANKLIN, Ph.D.

WORKMAN PUBLISHING • NEW YORK

The material in this book is provided for information only and should not be construed as medical advice or instruction. Always consult with your physician or other appropriate health professionals before making any changes in diet, physical activity and/or drug therapy.

Library of Congress Cataloging-in-Publication Data is available.
ISBN 978-0-7611-6073-1

Originally published as *Take a Load Off Your Heart*, now revised and updated

Book design by Yin Ling Wong
Cover illustration by Eric Palma

Workman books are available at special discounts when purchased in bulk for premiums and sales promotions as well as for fund-raising or educational use. Special editions or book excerpts can also be created to specification. For details, contact the Special Sales Director at the address below or send an e-mail to specialsales@workman.com.

Workman Publishing Company, Inc.
225 Varick Street
New York, NY 10014-4381
www.workman.com

Printed in the U.S.A.
First printing February 2011
10 9 8 7 6 5 4 3 2 1

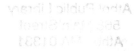

To my wife, Bernie, my most constructive critic,
ardent supporter and best friend.
The journey with her has been a gift from God.
—J.C.P.

To Lynn Strong, lover of books, editor extraordinaire, friend.
Her fingerprints are all over this book.
—J.C.P.

To my wife, Linda, for her love, patience,
understanding, encouragement and support.
She has helped, in so many ways,
to turn my dreams into reality.
—B.A.F.

Acknowledgments

I T TAKES A TEAM OF DEDICATED PEOPLE to put a book together. In particular, we are grateful to the medical professionals who gave of their time and expertise, providing information and insight and offering valuable suggestions. These include William C. Roberts, M.D., and Beverly Utt, R.D., M.P.H.

The book would not be possible without our respective staff support, particularly Brenda White at William Beaumont Hospital and Sue Tomaszycki, who helped with the graphics.

And finally, the dedication and expertise at Workman Publishing have been instrumental. Our thanks to Peter Workman for his faith in our work, to Susan Bolotin and Lynn Strong for their masterful editorial touch, and to the entire Workman team—especially Jenny Mandel, Selina Meere, Beth Wareham, Walter Weintz, Page Edmunds, David Matt, Janet Vicario and Yin Ling Wong—for their dedicated support.

Contents

Prescriptions,
Procedures and Programs.............307

Appendix:
Sources, Credits and Websites...............345

Before We Start . . .

WE KNOW FROM OUR OWN EXPERIENCE that when questions of health are pressing, many of us want quick answers even before we know exactly what to ask. Since the two of us have counseled literally thousands of patients, we've gotten pretty good at guessing what's on people's minds. We hope you'll find the answers you're looking for on these pages.

What does a heart attack feel like?
Everyone—not just cardiac patients—needs to know the answer to this one. Among the most common heart attack symptoms are pain, pressure or a sense of fullness under the breastbone that lasts two minutes or more.

Men often say the pain feels like "having an elephant on my chest"; women typically experience a milder chest pain. The sensation may radiate to the shoulders, neck, jaw, back or arms. (Or it may not.) Women generally experience the radiating pain throughout the neck, jaw, shoulders, arms, back or abdomen; in general, their symptoms are more subtle. Men tend to have sharp pain in their arms and shoulders. Dizziness, sweating, nausea, heart rhythm irregularities and shortness of breath may also occur. Nevertheless, some heart attacks are "silent" and occur with few or no symptoms.

Should I call 911 even if I don't have all these symptoms?
Not all symptoms may be present. If you think you might be having a heart attack, seek medical help immediately.

Is there anything I should do while I'm waiting for EMS to arrive?
Chew and swallow one regular uncoated adult aspirin (325 mg). According to the latest science, it has been estimated that this recommendation alone, if widely adopted, could save an additional 5,000 to 10,000 lives in the United States each year!

What if I'm wrong? I'd feel like an idiot if I got to the hospital and they told me I had indigestion!

This is not the time for foolish pride. Balloon angioplasty and new clot-busting drugs can literally halt heart attacks in progress—or at least minimize the damage—if administered soon after the onset of symptoms. Unfortunately, the majority of heart attack victims wait several hours before seeking medical attention. By that time, irreversible heart muscle damage—or even death—can occur. Remember: Time is muscle.

Is there a particular time of day—or day of the week—when the risk of heart attack is greatest?

You bet. Between six A.M. and noon is the riskiest time of day, perhaps because morning increases in hormone levels, blood pressure and artery stiffness heighten the possibility of clot formation. And more heart attacks happen on Monday than on other days of the week— a phenomenon scientists refer to as "Blue Monday." Why Monday? Many believe that the stress of a frenetic work environment, especially after a relaxing weekend, may be the cause.

How big a problem is cardiovascular disease in the United States?

Cardiovascular disease afflicts about half the adult population. Indeed, coronary artery disease and stroke are the number one and number three killers of adults, respectively. And one person dies from cardiovascular disease every 37 seconds. This means that by the time the 11 o'clock news has ended, the death toll each day stands at 2,335—equivalent to the number of people lost on 9/11!

But what are my own odds of dying from heart disease?

Let's try to put this in a comparative setting. Your odds of being hit by a wayward asteroid are one in 500,000. Your chance of being murdered is one in 10,000. But your risk of dying from cardiovascular disease is one in three.

I always thought heart disease was a "man's problem," but over the past year three female friends of mine have been diagnosed with serious heart trouble. Are they the exception?

The truth is that heart disease is an equal opportunity affliction. It has been diagnosed in almost as many women as men, but it's the leading cause of death among American women. In the United States, more than 38 million women are living with cardiovascular disease, and the population at risk is even larger. According to Dr. Lori Mosca of Columbia University, "In many countries, including the United States, more women than men die every year of cardiovascular disease." Fortunately, says Dr. Mosca, "Most cardiovascular disease in women is preventable. With few exceptions, recommendations to prevent cardiovascular disease in women do not differ from those for men."

Some gender differences do exist. Men may develop the first signs of heart disease at ages 35 to 40. Men aged 30 to 49 are 6.5 times more likely to have a heart attack than women in that age group. The condition doesn't usually affect women until a decade or more later. Between ages 45 to 64, one out of nine women has heart disease. Over age 65, the ratio is one out of three—about the same as men.

Are there any differences between men's and women's chances of surviving a heart attack?

Women stand a greater chance of dying within a year of their first heart attack. Moreover, there is evidence that women are traditionally less likely to get state-of-the-art diagnostic cardiac studies and treatments. And when they do get treatment, their disease is generally more advanced. Women are also more likely to die during heart surgery. These findings led to major funding for the groundbreaking Women's Health Initiative, commissioned by the National Institutes of Health.

I have heart disease, and I'm concerned about my children and grandchildren. At what age should doctors look for a problem?

According to the American Heart Association, screening patients for heart disease risk should start as early as age 20. In particular, people 40 or older, or anyone who has two or more risk factors, should know their chances of developing heart disease. The Framingham Risk Score, discussed later in this book, allows one to estimate his or her risk of having a heart attack in the next decade.

....

What is angina?

There are often no warning signs in the early stages of coronary heart disease. But as the coronary arteries become gradually narrowed and compromised, many people experience angina, or angina pectoris, which in Latin means "pain in the chest." This is a temporary chest pain caused by the heart muscle receiving insufficient oxygen to maintain its workload. Generally interpreted as a certain indicator of significant coronary artery blockage, angina affects over six million Americans. More women than men experience angina.

Can you tell me more about what it feels like?

Typically, angina comes on as a sharp, sudden pain often described as a tightness behind the breastbone, heaviness, squeezing, numbness, burning or pressure. It may be confused with heartburn. And the pain may radiate into the arms (generally, the left arm), neck, jaw, back and shoulder. Men usually experience angina more intensely than women.

Is all angina the same?

No. Stable angina, which most often occurs during or soon after physical exertion, eating a heavy meal, going out in very cold or hot weather or as a reaction to emotional stress, will usually force you to stop what you're doing until the pain subsides. Unstable angina, often a symptom of an impending heart attack, produces escalating pain even at rest. The pain may become more frequent, more intense, or both.

How long does an angina attack last?

It can vary from 30 seconds to several minutes, but most attacks last only a few minutes. Your doctor will likely prescribe an appropriate drug and encourage you to stop smoking and eat a low-fat diet.

But I'm on angina medication and I still get pain.
If rest in combination with drugs (many experts consider three consecutive nitroglycerin tablets a rule of thumb) doesn't bring relief, seek medical assistance NOW. This would suggest an impending heart attack.

What is a heart attack?
A heart attack, also called a myocardial infarction (MI), takes place when blood flow to a portion of the heart is completely stopped. Caused by an abrupt blockage in a coronary artery, usually resulting from the rupture of unstable plaque and a blood clot that seals off the artery, a heart attack produces permanent damage to the cardiac muscle. New research has shown that most MIs occur from modestly blocked (less than 50%) coronary arteries. One study found that in cases of sudden cardiac death, 76% were attributed to plaque rupture.

How do doctors know if a heart attack is mild or severe?
The percentage of blood that is pumped out of the left ventricle with each beat of the heart is called the ejection fraction. Under normal circumstances, half or more of the volume of blood is pumped out, so a normal ejection fraction ranges from 50% to 65%. A mild heart attack could result in an ejection fraction of 45%. A major heart attack may cause the ejection fraction to drop to 25% or even lower.

What is cardiac arrest?
Almost everyone has heard of someone who suddenly collapsed and died of a heart problem without having had any known risks or warning signs. Most likely that person experienced cardiac arrest, or sudden cardiac death (SCD). About 350,000 Americans die of SCD each year.

Cardiac arrest is not the same as a heart attack. Instead, this event is related to problems with the heart's electrical conduction system. The most common cause is ventricular fibrillation, a condition that may result in the heart beating chaotically. This causes an inadequate blood supply to all the organs, including the heart and brain. In some cases, however, a heart attack can lead to these chaotic electrical rhythms, which can cause SCD.

Is there anything that can be done for someone in cardiac arrest?
Move quickly! Immediate CPR can save a life. A doctor, nurse or trained paramedic can use an automated external defibrillator (AED) to electrically shock the heart back to a normal rhythm. These days, you'll even find easy-to-operate AEDs in major airports, shopping malls and sports stadiums. If defibrillation occurs within the first minute of collapse, the survival rate can be as high as 90%. For every minute of ventricular fibrillation, the likelihood of survival drops by 10% or more.

Surely there must be some warning!
Some survivors have mentioned lightheadedness, palpitations, or extremely fast or irregular heart rhythms. If you feel those symptoms, you should seek immediate medical attention. Unfortunately, in 16% of all cases, SCD is the first symptom.

....

Three months ago, our neighbor had an exercise stress test; the doctors told him he was fine. Yesterday, he had a heart attack! What happened?
No medical test can accurately predict future heart attacks 100% of the time. A stress test is often able to detect major coronary blockages (i.e., greater than 70% obstruction) that result in severe deprivation of blood flow to areas of the heart muscle during exercise. But a patient may have several blockages between 30% and 60% and still achieve normal results if no single lesion causes reduced blood flow to register. It is often these more modest lesions that rupture suddenly, causing a heart attack.

Can air pollution trigger heart attacks and other cardiac problems?
High levels of air pollution have been linked to heart attacks. The particles found in air pollution can cause vasoconstriction, transiently

elevating blood pressure and triggering heart rhythm irregularities; moreover, pollution can increase the likelihood of blood clotting. Although these individual effects may be modest, collectively they can cause serious problems, especially in diseased or damaged hearts. It's unfortunate that we can't do much to decrease the risk from air pollution, other than supporting environmental regulations to reduce it.

Is there a relationship between snoring and heart disease?
Yes. A disorder called obstructive sleep apnea has been shown to have major cardiovascular consequences. This form of apnea, or the cessation of breathing during sleep, is caused by a temporary obstruction of the throat. Although this condition traditionally affects obese people, it can occur in anyone. As the throat relaxes, snoring occurs and then the cessation of breathing. After a pause, there is an arousal response that may be associated with gasping. The altered breathing pattern results in a decrease in oxygen and an increase in carbon dioxide in the blood, an adrenaline response by the body and a marked increase in blood pressure and lung pressure. This cycle repeats, causing a disruption in the sleep pattern and daytime drowsiness.

Obstructive sleep apnea stresses the entire cardiovascular system. It can contribute to heart attack, stroke, congestive heart failure, life-threatening heart rhythm disorders, high blood pressure and thickening as well as weakening of the heart muscle. Also, pulmonary problems may develop, straining the heart.

A polysomnograph, which measures oxygen, brain waves and heart rhythm during sleep, can be used to diagnose the condition. A CPAP (continuous positive airway pressure) device, which lightly blows air into the throat to keep the airway open, may solve the problem. A recent study demonstrated improvement of heart structure and function after only six months of treatment with CPAP.

My husband had his heart attack just 20 minutes after a terrible argument with his boss. Could the argument have triggered his cardiac event?
Yes. The combination of underlying heart disease and the physiologic responses that can occur with anger or rage can, without question,

increase the likelihood of threatening heart rhythms, plaque rupture and thrombosis (blood clotting). In a classic study at Harvard, researchers reported that the probability of suffering a heart attack in the two hours after an episode of anger increased two- to threefold!

I'm following my doctor's advice to reduce my fat intake. Will this prevent a worsening of my heart disease?
Quite possibly. According to Dr. William C. Roberts, editor of the *American Journal of Cardiology*, "Our excessive intake of meat is killing us. We fatten our cows and pigs, kill them, eat them, and then they kill us!" One landmark study showed that heart patients who consumed 23% or less of their total calories from fat showed little or no progression in their heart disease. While it is critical to cut fat (which helps to reduce calories) for weight control, reducing saturated fat and trans fat is more directly connected to lowering cholesterol.

If I do regular exercise, do I also need to change my diet if I want to improve my blood lipid profile?
Yes. Exercise alone results in only *modest* changes in blood lipids and lipoproteins. If you really want to improve your cholesterol and triglyceride levels, you must improve your dietary habits.

Can exercise trigger a cardiac event?
Although considerable evidence suggests that regular exercise may help protect against heart disease, unconventionally vigorous physical exertion and other stressors such as emotional upsets can also trigger cardiovascular complications. Consequently, cardiac patients should stop exercising and seek medical help if any of the following symptoms persist despite rest and medication:

- Chest pain or pressure
- Rapid or irregular heartbeat
- Extreme shortness of breath
- Dizziness

Indeed, Dr. Paul Thompson, director of Preventive Cardiology at Hartford Hospital in Connecticut, tells his patients: "Vigorous physical activity both protects against and provokes acute cardiac events. Any discomfort from your earlobes to your belly button that comes on with exercise and goes away with rest could be angina." If the discomfort persists, get help.

Can brisk walking reverse some of the deleterious effects commonly attributed to aging?
Yes. After age 20, aerobic fitness typically declines by approximately 1% per year. A three-month exercise program can lead to a 15% to 20% increase in your heart-lung fitness (or MET capacity), which transforms to a 15-to-20-year functional rejuvenation. The moral of the story? Ponce de León sailed in search of the Fountain of Youth. He should have stayed on land and walked.

I understand that being obese and having a potbelly is bad for my heart. My waist circumference is 43 inches and my body mass index is 34. What does all this mean?
The pattern of body-fat distribution is recognized as an important predictor of the health risks of obesity. Individuals with more fat on the trunk, especially abdominal fat, are at increased risk of hypertension, diabetes, elevated blood cholesterol, coronary artery disease and premature death as compared with those who are equally fat but have more of their fat on the hips and extremities. The former group are commonly referred to as "apples," and the latter are called "pears." Thus waist circumference can be used alone as an indicator of health risk because abdominal obesity is the issue. A waist circumference greater than 40 inches in men and 35 inches in women is associated with increased health risks.

The body mass index (BMI) is used to assess weight relative to height. For most people, obesity-related health problems increase beyond a BMI value of 25. A BMI of 25.0 to 29.9 is considered overweight, whereas a BMI greater than or equal to 30.0 signifies obesity. Recently, researchers examined the association between BMI and acute coronary events in more than 54,000 middle-aged men and women who were followed for nearly eight years. After adjustments for numerous lifestyle factors, each unit of BMI was associated with a 7% and 5% higher risk of coronary events in men and women, respectively. An accompanying editorial concluded, "Even if you are doing everything right, extra weight carries an excess risk of acute coronary events."

My husband recently had a heart attack, and now he wants to take up scuba diving. This sounds like a bad idea to me, but he says I'm being a worrywart. Who's right?
Death rates from scuba diving are similar to those associated with skydiving and professional car racing, in part because it places considerable strain on the heart—much more than regular swimming does. So, we're siding with you on this one.

Does regular exercise make the heart more efficient?
Definitely. On average, a regular endurance exercise program will decrease a person's heart rate by more than three million beats per year. That's efficiency!

If the object of an exercise program is to increase heart rate to a certain level and hold it there for 30 minutes or more, can't I just sit in the steam room or sauna to raise my heart rate?
Ah, if only you could. But contrary to popular belief, it is not an increased heart rate per se that causes the body to become physically fit. The actual training stimulus is increased body metabolism or oxygen consumption. If you become extremely anxious, for example, your heart rate may transiently skyrocket, yet you're not really getting the equivalent of a workout. If it worked that way, high-strung, nervous types would be the most physically fit people in the world!

Because of my beta-blocker therapy, my resting heart rate is in the 50s and my exercise heart rate is generally in the low 80s. Can I still improve my aerobic fitness with such low training heart rates?
Absolutely! Numerous studies have shown that patients taking beta-blockers can still achieve substantial improvements in aerobic fitness with a regular exercise program, despite a reduced training heart rate.

Again, an increase in heart rate alone does not cause your body to become physically fit. The key to improved aerobic fitness is the rise in total body oxygen consumption, which still occurs in exercisers who are taking cardiac medications, including beta-blockers.

How much exercise would I have to do to halt or even reverse coronary heart disease?

The optimal amount of exercise for such cardioprotective benefits remains controversial. However, one major study, which included a low-fat, low-cholesterol diet, showed that burning a minimum of 1,600 calories per week may halt the progression of heart disease, while expending 2,200 calories per week may even lead to a slight regression in heart disease. For many people, this would translate into walking 15 and 20 miles per week, respectively. Further support for this recommendation comes from the American Heart Association, which suggests that the maximum benefits of exercise can be achieved with five to six hours per week of physical activity.

Is sexual activity strenuous enough to cause a heart attack or even sudden cardiac death?

This question is a favorite among middle-aged and older patients with a history of heart problems, so here's what we know. According to research conducted at Harvard Medical School and the Harvard School of Public Health, sexual activity is a probable contributor to heart attacks in fewer than 1% of patients. (Another interesting finding was that the risk of a heart attack during or immediately after sexual activity was lower in patients who engaged in vigorous physical exertion at least three days per week.)

In truth, sexual activity is just not that strenuous for most of us. One of the earliest studies of heart disease and sexual activity found that the average maximal heart rate during sexual intercourse was 117 beats per minute and that systolic blood pressure generally increased by only 30 to 40 millimeters of mercury. Achieving similar increases in heart rate and blood pressure during an exercise stress test would require an energy output equivalent to walking on level ground at a pace of approximately three miles per hour.

In addition, even if your heart rate rises to fairly high levels during sexual activity, this increase does not necessarily mean that you're expending considerable energy. Emotional stress—and excitement—can also increase nervous system activity and elevate your heart rate.

But is there anything I should be doing to make sex "safer"?

Years ago, a widely cited study showed that 80% of deaths precipitated by sexual intercourse occurred in hotel rooms "in relations with lovers" rather than with wives, and most of the victims had been eating and drinking heavily. The actual energy expenditure during intercourse is relatively low, equivalent to walking on level ground at a pace of three miles per hour. Recent research suggests that sexual activity is a probable contributor to heart attack in less than 1% of all cases; the absolute risk appears to be extremely low (one chance in a million). Regular exercisers (three or more times per week) have a significantly lower risk of experiencing a cardiac event during or immediately after sexual activity, as compared with their habitually sedentary counterparts.

Is it possible that my medication is having an effect on my sex life?

Yes. Medications people take after a heart attack or coronary intervention to reduce the workload on the heart or control arrhythmias (irregular heartbeats), as well as drugs commonly prescribed to relieve anxiety or depression, can have adverse side effects, most notably impotence in men and diminished sex drive in both men and women. On the other hand, some medications, such as beta-blockers and nitroglycerin, may enhance sexual activity by alleviating angina during exertion. Indeed, some patients may be advised to take such drugs prophylactically, that is, before sexual activity.

Can I take Viagra?

Since the approval by the FDA for the treatment of erectile dysfunction (ED), millions of prescriptions (legal and illegal) for sildenafil citrate

(Viagra), vardenifil (Levitra) and tadalafil (Cialis) have been filled. Reported adverse complications associated with the use of sildenafil include infrequent heart attacks, threatening heart rhythm irregularities, plummeting blood pressure and, in rare instances, death, especially in patients with heart disease who were simultaneously taking nitrates. In another study of carefully selected men with ED and known or probable heart disease, sildenafil administered one hour before maximal exercise testing was well tolerated and did not worsen the cardiovascular and electrocardiographic responses to exercise. If you're considering drug therapy to treat ED, check with your doctor.

So let's cut to the chase. Can I have sex?

In general, you can resume sexual activity within a few weeks of a heart attack or coronary artery bypass surgery and within a few days of a balloon angioplasty procedure. As we've said, having sex is comparable to walking at a pace of about three miles per hour, so anyone who can do that without abnormal signs or symptoms can probably have sex. Here are some specific concerns:

■ If you're taking an antianginal medication such as nitroglycerin, you might want to ask your doctor about taking it prior to sex. In addition, you should avoid sexual activity after heavy meals and drinking alcohol, when you're excessively fatigued or you find yourself in too hot or cold an environment.

■ If you want to have better sex with less anxiety, you should exercise regularly, eat a low-fat diet, lose weight if necessary, not smoke and not drink more than a moderate amount of alcohol.

■ Experiment to see if you prefer the on-top or the on-the-bottom position. While the cardiovascular response is the same, the on-the-bottom spot may slightly reduce cardiac cost, eliminating isometric support of the body weight by the arms.

■ As mentioned above, some medications, by easing the symptoms of angina, may decrease anxiety and enhance sexual activity. On the other hand, men whose cardiovascular medications cause problems such as impotence should never abruptly stop using these drugs without their physician's approval, especially if they're taking beta-blockers such as propranolol (Inderal), atenolol (Tenormin), metoprolol (Lopressor) or nadolol (Corgard). Often a change in or gradual tapering of medication can solve the problem, or various other treatments for impotence may be prescribed.

....

Are there safe cigarettes?

According to a recent landmark study of more than 34,000 male British doctors, men who smoked only cigarettes and continued smoking died on average about 10 years younger than lifelong nonsmokers. Cessation at age 60, 50, 40 or 30 gained, respectively, about 3, 6, 9 or 10 years of life expectancy. Another report found that men who smoked cigarettes with reduced levels of tar and nicotine did not have a lower risk of heart attack than those who smoked regular brands—perhaps because they inhaled more deeply than smokers of other types of cigarettes. If you smoke, you must stop.

But I'm afraid I'll gain weight if I stop smoking.

It's very likely that you will. Smoking 24 cigarettes over a 24-hour period increases daily caloric expenditure by about 10%. If you don't want to gain weight, you'll have to reduce your caloric intake, increase your exercise, or both.

....

I recently had a heart attack. When can I return to work?

For young and middle-aged cardiac patients, returning to work is a particularly important objective. Nearly two decades ago, researchers at Stanford University demonstrated that an occupational work evaluation (treadmill testing and counseling) could accelerate return-to-work rates among heart attack patients by reassuring them, their spouses and their doctors that the demands of their job could be safely tolerated.

Today, heart attack victims can often return to their jobs, at least on a part-time basis, within two to six weeks, especially if the work does not involve strenuous physical labor. Patients who have undergone coronary artery bypass surgery may take a bit longer, whereas those undergoing balloon angioplasty generally return within a week. Economic conditions, the patient's state of mind, employer stereotypes and the availability of pension benefits can make going back to work seem less appealing, but we agree with the assessment presented by Sterling B. Brinkley of the former Department of Health, Education and Welfare: "Work is an essential ingredient for quality of living. We have seen too many people quit too soon, sitting on porches, watching cars go by. I have also been impressed by the numbers who die within a year or two after retirement. I have wondered if the stimulus of work did not, in fact, give life itself."

Do white-collar workers have any advantage over blue-collar workers when it comes to death from heart disease?

Blue-collar workers are 43% more likely to die of heart disease than white-collar workers, even after differences in risk have been considered. But it remains unclear whether other influences—diet, medical care or socioeconomic status—may play an even greater role than the jobs performed. For example, a recent study found that four measures of socioeconomic status (income, education, housing and occupation) were associated with a reduced treadmill exercise capacity and adverse cardiovascular outcomes in adults with heart disease. Differences in conventional cardiac risk factors and health behaviors did not explain these negative associations.

Where do heart surgeons get the blood vessels that they use for bypass grafts during surgery?

Bypass grafts for people with clogged coronary arteries may be constructed using an "extra" vein removed from the leg (a saphenous vein) or an artery that lies inside the chest wall (an internal mammary artery). Research indicates that artery grafts have a far better long-term patency rate (the percentage of grafts that remain open).

....

My husband survived a major heart attack. Because of serious heart rhythm problems, he recently received an implantable defibrillator. In addition to supporting his efforts at major lifestyle changes, what can I do?

Learn basic cardiopulmonary resuscitation (CPR). Reversal of sudden cardiac death can be brought about not only by trained physicians, nurses and paramedics, but by any of us, anywhere, using no tools except our hands, our lungs and our brains. To enroll in a CPR course, contact your local office of the American Heart Association, the American Red Cross, a hospital or a local high school that offers community courses. It may be the most valuable course you'll ever take.

Also, consider purchasing an automated external defibrillator for your home. These devices can deliver shocks (if necessary) to restore a normal heart rhythm. The machines, which cost about $1,500, are so simple to use that even young children can use them correctly.

My father had a heart attack last summer, but now he insists that he can shovel snow this winter. Do you agree?

No, we don't agree. Snow shoveling puts a tremendous workload on the heart, and cold temperatures can add to the stress. Several years ago, Dr. Barry Franklin and associates at William Beaumont Hospital in Royal Oak, Michigan, studied the physical demands of snow shoveling on healthy but inactive men. After only 10 minutes, the blood pressure and heart rate of the subjects rose to dangerously high levels, equaling or exceeding the maximum responses of the same subjects during exhaustive treadmill testing. Among people with heart disease, such high numbers can lead to inadequate oxygen supply to the heart muscle, anginal chest pain and potentially fatal heart rhythm disturbances. Furthermore, the marked increases in heart rate and blood pressure that accompany snow shoveling may cause greater than usual flows that dislodge plaque and other fragments from blood vessel walls. The result: a heart attack or sudden cardiac death.

A more recent study by these investigators reported 36 sudden deaths (33 men, 3 women) in the greater metropolitan Detroit area that were attributed to snow removal after heavy snowfalls. Four of the victims were using a snowblower at the time!

It may be best for middle-aged and older persons at risk for heart disease to hire a snowplow service to clear the driveway. We'd certainly recommend this approach in your father's case. As a reminder for him, we suggest making a copy of this label and pasting it on your snow shovel:

> # WARNING
> Use of this instrument for snow removal may be hazardous to your health!

A friend who just had coronary artery bypass surgery seems to be very forgetful these days. Is it my imagination, or is there a connection?
Memory problems are a relatively common side effect of coronary bypass surgery. Fortunately, for almost all patients, the lapses usually disappear within a few months.

Folk wisdom says, "Laughter is the best medicine." Is there any truth to the notion?
Laughter is actually very strong medicine. Dr. William Fry Jr., professor emeritus at Stanford University and a pioneer in laughter research, believes that even the physical act of laughing is good for you. But the most astonishing evidence of the healing power of laughter comes from a 1997 study of 48 heart attack patients. Half the patients watched comedic films for 30 minutes every day; the other half served as controls. After a year, patients in the control group had a greater number of recurrent heart attacks. Indeed, other researchers suggest that laughter is a powerful antidote to stress, reducing hormone levels that can trigger dangerous heart rhythms, blood clotting, or both.

A coworker recently suffered a heart attack. His doctor told him he had already had a heart attack sometime earlier but was unaware of it. Is that possible?

Yes. Believe it or not, approximately one in four heart attacks go unrecognized. In other words, they occur without severe chest pain and other ominous symptoms. Oftentimes (and more frequently among women than men), mild chest discomfort may be denied or simply considered "heartburn."

What is acute congestive heart failure? It sounds scary.

Generally not as ominous as it sounds, congestive heart failure can occur after a heart attack or whenever the pumping capacity of the heart is significantly compromised. Symptoms include unusual fatigue (especially after mild exertion), shortness of breath, sudden weight gain and swelling in the ankles. Contact your doctor if you have any of these symptoms.

On the other hand, chronic congestive heart failure is the most frequent diagnosis among the growing geriatric population. It occurs when the left ventricle has been permanently weakened, decreasing the heart's ability to pump blood properly. Because of the associated poor prognosis, young and middle-aged individuals with this condition are sometimes considered candidates for a heart transplant.

Why is congestive heart failure more common after a heart attack?

When heart muscle dies and is replaced by scar tissue, which does not have the ability to contract and expand, the heart loses some of its effectiveness as a pump. This is particularly true if scarring has occurred in the left ventricle, the principal pumping chamber of the heart. If the left ventricle is no longer able to pump enough blood to the body but the right ventricle continues to pump normally, the difference may cause blood to back up in the lungs and in the large leg veins. This disrupts the circulatory flow and causes distention of the tissues and a leaking of fluid into the abdomen and extremities.

Is that why people with chronic congestive heart failure often have swelling in their ankles and feet?
Yes, and it also explains why they frequently gain weight from fluid buildup, called edema. Fluid that backs up into the lungs can cause pulmonary edema—and extreme shortness of breath. If that happens to you, you may have to adjust your sleep position.

Wow, this is pretty depressing.
It's not fun, but your doctor has lots of ways to make you more comfortable. Commonly prescribed medications include digoxin, diuretics, ACE inhibitors and beta-blockers. In some cases, angioplasty or bypass surgery may be beneficial for patients with congestive heart failure. Moreover, moderate-intensity exercise using interval training (a work-rest approach) is increasingly recommended for those with congestive heart failure.

I've had angina for 12 years. Unfortunately, medications, angioplasty and bypass surgery failed to give me any lasting relief. Now my doctor has recommended EECP. What can you tell me about this treatment?
Enhanced external counterpulsation (EECP) is a noninvasive outpatient treatment that may be helpful in relieving or eliminating your symptoms. Patients typically attend one-hour treatment sessions once a day, five days a week for seven weeks. While you lie on a padded table in a treatment room, a therapist will wrap a set of inflatable cuffs around your calves, thighs and buttocks. The system compresses your lower limbs and, through heartbeat-synchronized inflation and deflation, rhythmically increases blood flow toward your heart. Studies suggest that EECP can improve exercise capacity and reduce anginal symptoms, possibly by increasing blood flow to the heart, enhancing coronary artery function and augmenting the heart's pumping performance.

What is your opinion of chelation therapy? A local clinic provides this treatment option, but my health insurance doesn't cover it.
Chelation therapy purports to clean out blocked arteries without surgery. The process involves introducing an amino acid called ethylenediamine

tetraacetic acid (EDTA) into the veins. Normally used to treat mercury or lead poisoning, since it causes heavy metals to be excreted in the urine, this chemical is believed to help reduce damage to artery walls and remove calcium, a key component of plaque, from the bloodstream. Supposedly, it causes potentially harmful heavy-metal molecules (such as calcium, lead, zinc or iron) to be bound with other chemicals and eliminated from the body. A single treatment takes about two hours and costs about $50 to $100 (usually not covered by insurance). A normal treatment schedule calls for 30 treatments. About 2,500 doctors in the United States offer chelation therapy.

The American Heart Association and the American College of Cardiology do not recognize chelation therapy as an effective method for treating heart disease; in fact, they cite possible adverse side effects such as kidney damage, decreased bone density and heart rhythm irregularities. A widely cited study of 84 patients, 41 of whom had undergone an extended series of chelation treatments, concluded that there was no benefit when compared with placebo. Moreover, a review of the topic published in *Circulation* in 1997 found that only 4 of 50 studies surveyed met the criteria for sound science—and none of those 4 studies showed that chelation therapy worked in treating heart disease. In support of this conclusion, a more recent study conducted by doctors from the University of Calgary found no benefit from the therapy. Says Dr. D. George Wise, one of the authors of the study, "My advice to patients is there is no evidence that chelation works."

....

I recently had a heart attack and usually get only about five hours of sleep a night. My wife read that sleep deprivation may contribute to heart problems. Is this so?

Yes. According to Dr. Mehmet Oz, professor and vice chairman of surgery at Columbia University, people who are sleep-deprived are at increased risk for a heart attack, although he readily admits, "We're not entirely sure why." Recent research studies suggest that people who get five or fewer hours of sleep a night double their risk of developing high blood pressure, as compared with those who sleep seven or eight hours. Researchers also note that sleep deprivation is associated with overweight/obesity and diabetes. In addition, Dr. Oz emphasizes that poor sleep impairs the body's production of growth hormone, which is essential for coping with stress as well as exposure to toxins. Others contend that the disturbed sleep patterns associated with obstructive sleep apnea can have an adverse impact on heart health. For these reasons, and more, it's helpful to get your zzz's.

People say you can avoid heart trouble by taking an aspirin once a day. Is this true?

The answer largely depends on your specific medical history. If you're healthy and without major risk factors for heart disease, the negatives associated with regular aspirin use (stomach bleeding and an increased incidence of stroke) probably outweigh the positives (decreased incidence of cardiac events). However, if you have one or more major risk factors for heart disease, especially if you're over 40 years of age and you're a cigarette smoker and/or you have an elevated blood cholesterol, aspirin may be helpful. In fact, a recent review and analysis of studies to date suggest two baby aspirin (160 mg per day) for patients with coronary and other atherosclerotic vascular disease and for those with a 10% or higher risk of developing heart disease within 10 years, using the Framingham Risk Score. Exceptions, of course, include those with aspirin intolerance and those at increased risk for gastrointestinal bleeding and hemorrhagic stroke.

- The Harvard Nurses' Health Study showed a 30% reduction in heart attacks among women aged 50 and older who took aspirin daily, compared with a similar group of women who did not.

- A study of 4,500 Italian men and women aged 50 and older found that one aspirin per day cut the risk of dying from heart attack or stroke by 50%. This group was followed for 3.6 years before the trial was stopped prematurely due to the clear benefit of aspirin.

- The ongoing Harvard Physicians' Health Study involved more than 22,000 male doctors, all of whom were in apparently good health. Half the group took a buffered, or coated, aspirin every day;

the other half received a look-alike placebo. For the study subjects who took aspirin, the risk of heart attack was cut by 47%. In this case, the beneficial effect of aspirin was so apparent that the doctors who monitored the trial felt ethically compelled to recommend that it be stopped and that those volunteers who were getting the placebo be informed so they, too, could take aspirin.

In 2009, the U.S. Preventive Services Task Force updated its recommendations on the benefits of aspirin therapy to decrease the risk of initial heart attacks and stroke in persons with one or more major risk factors (such as elevated cholesterol, high blood pressure, cigarette smoking, obesity and diabetes). In particular, men between the ages of 45 and 79 were encouraged to take aspirin to reduce heart attack risk, while women between the ages of 55 and 79 were encouraged to do the same to reduce stroke risk.

The bottom line is that aspirin therapy is generally underutilized in this country, especially in emergency settings and in preventing recurrent heart problems. But it's not for everyone. Any benefit in heart attack and stroke reduction may be offset, for instance, in people at risk of major gastrointestinal bleeding complications. If you're not taking aspirin regularly and think you should be, or if you're taking it and wondering if you shouldn't be, check with your doctor.

ASPIRIN BENEFITS FOR MEN AND WOMEN

A DAILY ASPIRIN (80 TO 160 MG) CAN:	MEN (ALL AGES)	WOMEN UNDER AGE 65	WOMEN 65 OR OLDER
Prevent a first stroke		x	x
Prevent a first heart attack	x		x
Reduce risk of heart disease	x	x	x
Reduce risk of a second heart attack	x	x	x

I've heard that alcohol can worsen heart disease, but I've also heard that alcohol can prevent it. Which is it?
Drinking alcohol in excessive amounts over many years can lead to alcoholic cardiomyopathy, a weakening of the heart muscle. (Fortunately, complete abstinence from alcohol may often resolve the condition.) In addition, drinking too much can not only lead to cirrhosis of the liver, weight gain and an increased risk for mouth and throat cancer, but also raise the level of triglycerides. On the other hand, moderate alcohol intake has been associated with reduced cardiovascular events in many populations. Still, we do not recommend that anyone *start* drinking alcohol to prevent heart disease. The risks are too great.

Well, I already drink. Can I keep on drinking?
If you do drink, you should limit your alcohol consumption to no more than one drink per day for women and two drinks per day for men, ideally with meals. Whether white or red wine is more protective than beer or liquor remains unclear.

I enjoy grapefruit juice, but my cardiologist told me I shouldn't drink it because I'm taking a cholesterol-lowering statin. What's the connection?
Several of the statin drugs are adversely affected by grapefruit juice, which increases their levels in the bloodstream and any toxic symptoms that may occur. These symptoms include headache, gastrointestinal symptoms and muscle pain or tenderness. One study showed that one glass of grapefruit juice a day for three consecutive days doubled blood levels of lovastatin (Mevacor). Other statins that are likely to interact adversely with grapefruit juice are simvastatin (Zocor) and possibly atorvastatin (Lipitor). On the other hand, such an interaction is unlikely with pravastatin (Pravachol), fluvastatin (Lescol) or rosuvastatin (Crestor).

....

Although I have a "normal" blood pressure, my doctor says I have a heart rhythm abnormality that puts me at risk for a stroke. The whole thing has me confused.

Patients with a heart rhythm disturbance called atrial fibrillation (AF) are clearly at increased risk for a stroke. The good news is that a procedure called cardioversion (during which a synchronized direct current shocks the heart) can often normalize AF. Alternatively, your doctor may perform an invasive ablation procedure to abolish the AF using a special catheter. In addition, you may be prescribed an anticoagulant such as Coumadin to decrease the likelihood of blood clot formation. Other medications like beta-blockers, digoxin and calcium channel blockers are frequently used to control the fast heart rate.

Is a stroke related to a heart attack?
Atherosclerosis, the underlying condition that leads to coronary heart disease, can also cause stroke. In the case of stroke, however, blockages stop blood flow to the brain, not the heart.

Is stroke common?
A stroke occurs every 45 seconds in the United States. Each year, about 700,000 people suffer a stroke and 164,000 of them die.

What are the warning signs of stroke?
Feeling sudden weakness in an arm, hand or leg, or not feeling one side of the face or body are common precursors of stroke. Other symptoms include:

- Suddenly not being able to see out of one eye
- Suddenly having difficulty talking
- Not being able to understand what someone is saying
- Feeling dizzy or losing balance
- Having the worst headache of your life

If you have one or more stroke symptoms for more than a few minutes, call 911.

I had a heart attack five years ago. What's my risk of future cardiac problems?

Doctors rarely talk explicitly to their heart patients about the risk of future cardiac events. Consequently, their patients assume the worst when, in fact, most do just fine.

Years ago, researchers at Stanford University asked a group of patients soon after their heart attacks to rate their likelihood of having another major cardiac problem (fatal or nonfatal) over the next year. Almost uniformly, the interviewees vastly overestimated their subsequent cardiac risk—suggesting that they anticipated an unfavorable prognosis. Yet the annual rate of death in these same patients was actually 1.5%, and only 2% had recurrent nonfatal heart attacks!

The good news? Between 1980 and 2000, death rates from coronary heart disease fell by more than 40%. Why? Recently, researchers developed a model that attributed more than 90% of the observed decrease in deaths from heart disease to reductions in major risk factors and the widespread implementation of effective medical therapies. The latter include initial treatments for heart attacks, an expanding array of cardioprotective drugs and the proven benefits of cardiac rehabilitation programs. In contrast, coronary artery bypass surgery and angioplasty accounted for only 7% of the mortality reduction. The authors concluded that future strategies should actively promote population-based prevention by reducing risk factors via drug therapy and healthy lifestyle modification.

Today, increasing numbers of heart patients are entering their seventies, eighties and nineties, often outliving their counterparts without heart disease. In our experience, these tend to be patients who take care of themselves and develop the *mind-set* necessary to deal with the challenges of heart disease. There is mounting evidence to suggest we get what we expect and attract what we fear. Invariably, those patients who not only survive but thrive believe they can achieve longevity and a high quality of life.

My doctor said I had a heart attack, but my recent cardiac catheterization was perfectly normal (i.e., no blockage). What could have caused the heart attack?
Coronary spasm. Approximately 5% to 10% of patients with anginal chest pain have a transient constriction of a portion of an artery feeding

the heart muscle. Oftentimes, the area of the coronary artery that goes into spasm had no visible cholesterol blockage or plaque. Nevertheless, a sustained coronary spasm can deprive the heart muscle of oxygen (a condition called ischemia) and cause a heart attack.

Coronary spasm can be diagnosed by an electrocardiogram during symptoms or sometimes by cardiac catheterization. The likelihood of future coronary spasm can be diminished by chronic drug therapy, usually with a calcium channel blocker (such as nifedipine, verapamil, diltiazem or amlodipine).

I understand that there's a new method for performing cardiopulmonary resuscitation? Please explain.
Traditional methods of cardiopulmonary resuscitation (CPR) called for chest compressions combined with mouth-to-mouth breathing. The latter, however, discourage many bystanders from participating due to the fear of contagious diseases. A study published in *Lancet* in 2007 evaluated the use of a new form of CPR (using chest compressions only) as compared with conventional methods. Relative to ultimate outcomes, there was no evidence of a benefit from the addition of mouth-to-mouth breathing. The authors concluded that CPR involving only chest compression should be considered the method of choice. For witnessed cardiac arrest, this method was also recently endorsed by the American Heart Association.

The new motto for CPR is *Push hard, push fast.* For adults, the compression rate and depth should be 100 per minute and one and a half to two inches, respectively. (To get the correct rhythm going, sing the Bee Gees hit "Stayin' Alive" from *Saturday Night Fever*. The song's beat is exactly right for CPR.) Providers should allow full chest recoil between compressions and minimize interruptions in chest compressions.

Introduction

I T'S NOT YOUR FATHER'S HEART DISEASE ANYMORE. For many years, doctors focused on cholesterol as the single most important risk factor for coronary heart disease. The connection was simple: the more cholesterol in the bloodstream, the greater the risk of a heart attack. Sure, smoking mattered, as did high blood pressure. But as Dr. Robert Levy, former director of the National Heart, Lung and Blood Institute, once stated, elevated cholesterol was the "chief factor of a heart attack."

Soon after this connection was made, interest in managing blood cholesterol bordered on obsession. Virtually overnight, "low-cholesterol" foods appeared in grocery stores, cooking shows featured heart-healthy recipes and "What's your number?" became a popular topic at cocktail parties. And although the recommendation was a kind of one-size-fits-all approach (get your cholesterol under 200 by eating a low-fat diet, exercising regularly and taking medication if necessary), it seemed to work. Average American cholesterol levels fell in the 1980s and '90s. So did heart attack rates.

But the advice didn't work for everyone. Diagnosed with high cholesterol, a friend changed his lifestyle dramatically. He cut down on red meat and fast foods, ate more fruits and vegetables, and began exercising regularly. His total cholesterol dropped from 220 to around 180 . . . just before he had a massive heart attack.

He was not alone. About half of all heart attacks in the United States occur in people who do not have high cholesterol. Indeed, Dr. Thomas Yannios, author of *The Heart Disease Breakthrough,* reported that about 80% of people who get heart disease have the same total cholesterol levels as those who don't.

A New Perspective

C utting-edge science calls for new thinking about heart disease and its treatment. The most recent findings suggest that cholesterol, while important, is only part of the story, one of multiple factors that in combination can cause a heart attack. Other markers—such as the degree to which the artery wall is injured and inflamed, and how easily your blood clots—are now seen as critical.

In addition, we all know that a balanced diet and sufficient exercise are essential for achieving cardiac health. But such knowledge has not led to healthy action. Why? Are we lazy or just plain stupid? Again, research has the answer. It's chronic stress that keeps many people from shaping a diet and exercise plan. People under stress tend to eat unwisely and to skip exercise. But once stress is managed, healthy dietary and exercise actions are more likely to follow.

These changes in medical thinking lay behind my decision to write this book originally—and to revise it now—but it's a decision consistent with my mission as a writer over the past three decades: to teach people how to apply the most up-to-date science to their everyday lives, all with the goal of achieving better cardiac health. If my readers are heart patients, I want them to have the tools to stabilize and reverse their disease; if they do not as yet have heart disease, I want them to have a manual for prevention. That's the "why" of the book. The "how" takes a little more explanation.

Looking Back

The seeds of this book were planted on July 16, 1977, the day I was diagnosed with advanced coronary disease. Four days later, I had bypass surgery. *I was 32 years old!* My mother had often told me, "Life is what happens while you're making plans," but still, this was more than a little bit of a surprise. While I was aware that our family had a tendency toward high cholesterol and heart disease, I had never thought about my own risk.

My obliviousness is fairly typical. As Dr. William B. Kannel, former director of the long-running Framingham Heart Study in Massachusetts, has said, "If you don't know that you're free of heart disease, don't assume that you are." His studies found that 16% of the time people with heart disease experience sudden cardiac death as the first, last and only symptom of their problem.

So, in a way, I was lucky.

Here's my story. For about a month, I had noticed a shortness of breath and pressure in my chest while warming up to play tennis. After about 10 minutes, these feelings would go away. The pain was not sharp—more like an uncomfortable fullness behind my breastbone. It was certainly not of sufficient concern to stop the match. I recall telling myself, "It's probably a touch of bronchitis."

After waiting a few weeks to see if these feelings would clear up on their own, I made an appointment with our family doctor. He had given me a complete physical exam just four months earlier. There were no problems then, and I didn't expect him to find any now. Just a quick look at my lungs, a prescription, and I'd be on my way home.

I was wrong. The doctor was concerned about the "uncomfortable fullness" and the irregular results of a resting electrocardiogram, and he sent me that very day to a cardiologist. One test led to another, culminating in a cardiac catheterization to X-ray my coronary arteries. The diagnosis changed my life forever: "Joe, you have coronary heart disease, a buildup of blockages in the coronary arteries," he said. "You have two blockages better than 50% and one that has closed about 95% of the artery. This is life-threatening. I recommend bypass surgery within the next few days. You are a heart attack waiting to happen."

I heard his words, but I had difficulty personalizing the diagnosis. Like most people, I knew that heart disease was a major health issue, perhaps the greatest in the western world. But my appreciation was an arm's length away. What did blocked arteries or heart attacks have to do with me, a 32-year-old guy in the prime of his life?

I would soon learn that heart disease was no longer just facts, figures and other people's families. We were now talking about *my* heart, *my* health, and the impact on *my* family. Looking back on the moment my doctor recommended immediate coronary bypass surgery, I recall the words of the famous Spanish matador El Cordobés, who once said that his interest in the bullfight increased in direct ratio to the closeness of the bull's horns. My interest was suddenly very great indeed.

After the six-hour operation, in which a piece of vein taken from my leg was used to create a new coronary artery that went around the blockage, I was euphoric, thinking myself "cured." But a postoperative consultation with my cardiologist was sobering. "Let's be straight on what was accomplished," he said. "The surgery reduced the immediate risk of a life-threatening heart attack, and it took away the pain. But you still have coronary heart disease. You had it the day before surgery, you had it the day after surgery and you have it now. The immediate problem has been solved, but the underlying condition remains. You need to assess the risk factors that got you to this point and change those things that can be changed. The way you choose to live is the key to your cardiac future. Things like what you eat and how you exercise will dictate whether or not the disease progresses. It's in your own hands, Joe."

The time following surgery was very traumatic for my family. My wife, Bernie, and I had been married less than 10 years. Our children, Anne and Joe, were six and four. Instead of the "normal" concerns of a young family—picking the best school for the kids, choosing a vacation spot, scheduling soccer car pools—our focus was on living with heart disease. And there was some question even about that.

In an effort to get educated, I met with a lipids specialist at a major university near my home. He talked to me about cholesterol and blood pressure, diet and medications, and a course of action. His information was helpful, but he'd failed to address the question that was most important to me. "Will I live?" I asked him. "Will I have a normal life span or not?"

Perhaps he was having a bad day, possibly he was being brutally honest, or maybe he just had a terrible bedside manner, but this was his never-to-be-forgotten answer: "You probably won't live to see age 40," he said. "I'd be very surprised if you're at your kids' high school graduation."

I left his office shocked and angry. But I was also scared. The specialist's "opinion" created so much stress for me that I could hardly function. For about a month I moped around home, depressed, anxious and unable to focus on anything. I had always been actively engaged with life; now I had become a passive observer—except when it came to my heart. In that regard I was ever vigilant, always on guard for something terrible about to happen. One day, on a short walk down the road to our mailbox, I felt a pain in my side and was gripped by panic. It turned out to be nothing more than a muscle cramp, but I believed death was imminent. Afterwards, I realized I had become immobilized by stress and fear.

Bernie put the situation into perspective: "Joe, you can't change the cards you were dealt. But you can change the way you play those cards." She was supported by my doctor, who told me, "When General Patton was asked how he would respond to an enemy attack, he replied with one word: *Counterattack*. When the enemy is heart disease, the strategy is the same. Heart disease is not a death sentence. The key to long-term success is to learn about the disease, reduce your risk factors with healthy lifestyle changes, take your medications, get regular checkups and heed warning symptoms immediately."

I knew they were right. I couldn't change my genetic heritage. Besides, as I soon learned, lifestyle habits can offset and counteract "bad genes." Ten percent of the population will get up in the morning, run five miles and still have a heart attack because of bad genes. Ten percent will have cream for breakfast, avoid exercise and yet never have a heart attack because they're protected by good genes. But for the remaining 80%, lifestyle habits are the greatest determinant of cardiac health. Dr. William C. Roberts, editor of the *American Journal of Cardiology*, put it this way: "For every person with coronary heart disease because of family genes, there are 499 people who have it because of lifestyle decisions."

Hope and optimism became my allies, education my friend. I made a commitment to learn all that I could about the disease and about the mitigating effect of lifestyle habits, and to do everything possible to overcome my genetic baggage. The starting point was learning what I could control. It was pretty clear that certain lifestyle habits—eating well, exercising regularly, not smoking and managing stress better—were key to my long-term health. But I needed to make a plan, and I didn't know what to do. I was confused.

- **Confused about diet.** What was a healthy diet, anyway? Information and advice changed so rapidly that I called them studies du jour. One day, eggs were considered breakfast-table suicide; the next day, a new study said they were acceptable. Some experts touted margarine as better; others sided with butter. One day, low fat was in, high protein (really, high fat) was out; the next day, it was reversed. The dueling science left me bewildered.

- **Confused about exercise.** Some experts counseled slow and steady exercise. Others advised kicking up the pace to "go for the burn" and warned of "no pain, no gain." As a heart patient, could I lift weights? Some doctors said yes, some said no. Not knowing who was right made me fearful.

- **Confused about smoking.** I didn't smoke, but I lived for 18 years with parents who did. In college, my roommates smoked; at my office, many coworkers smoked. "You've actually been smoking from two to seven cigarettes a day for a number of years," a pulmonary doctor told me. "You just never bought a pack yourself." How could I avoid being harmed by secondhand cigarette smoke in the future?

- **Confused about stress.** Not much was known in those days about the role of stress, but intuitively I knew that getting all worked up, frequently over minor things, could not be good for my health. I was already feeling "out of time" before I had heart disease. How could I keep the disease from increasing my stress, which in turn would exacerbate my disease?

My need for accurate information and usable advice culminated in my first book, *Don't Eat Your Heart Out*. Over the last three decades, I've continued to pay close attention to the progress in cardiac medicine and treatment. And with the help of dedicated health professionals and the support of my family, I've sorted out how the lifestyle pieces fit together for better cardiac health. More important, I've developed a methodology for putting information into action to achieve long-term lifestyle habits. This approach involves making changes through a sequence of events that promotes adherence. It also utilizes a number of practical tips for heart-healthy living, which I call Heart Savers.

The creation of this approach was not an academic exercise. It was a course of action for living long and well despite having heart disease. And it has worked:

- Critical markers such as weight, cholesterol and blood pressure show that I'm in better health now than I was in 1977.

- Tests show not only that my heart disease has been stabilized, but also that I actually have less disease today than in 1977, a condition called coronary regression.

- I recently celebrated my 33rd anniversary of bypass surgery, making me one of the oldest bypass survivors (number of years post-bypass) in the United States. And that lipids specialist? He's no longer practicing, but every time I have a birthday I send *him* a card to let him know I'm still around. (He has never responded!) I've also derived great satisfaction from keeping him apprised of the many graduation ceremonies I've attended—high school, college, graduate school and law school.

Speaking of those kids whose graduations I was never supposed to see, they're now adults and neither of them demonstrates high cholesterol or other cardiac risk factors. The life skills I learned for rehabilitation, they use for prevention. To a certain extent, that has allowed them to offset any genetic predisposition to heart disease.

Looking Forward

This updated and revised book, a manual for preventing, stabilizing and reversing heart disease, is perhaps my most important. What was known about heart disease and heart-healthy living in 1977 and what is known today are worlds apart. In addition, I've had 33 years of experience in making lifestyle changes, enough time to sort out what is effective and what is not, what is a fad and what is trusted information, what works on paper but breaks down in practical application. Such experience is invaluable. As *Cuckoo's Egg* author Clifford Stoll has written, "Data is not information any more than 50 tons of cement is a skyscraper."

But just to be sure I had the clinical data *and* practical information I needed, I asked Barry A. Franklin, Ph.D., a highly respected national authority on cardiac rehabilitation and a good friend, to collaborate on the project. Since 1985, Barry has served as the director of the cardiac rehabilitation program and exercise laboratories at William Beaumont Hospital in Royal Oak, Michigan. He is an expert on cardiac science, the former editor in chief of the *Journal of Cardiopulmonary Rehabilitation* and past president of both the American Association of Cardiovascular and Pulmonary Rehabilitation and the American College of Sports Medicine. His experience running one of the largest and most successful cardiac rehabilitation programs in the country has given him valuable insight into the human process of making healthy lifestyle changes.

Former New York governor Mario Cuomo once said that his mother gave him two principles for success: 1) Figure out exactly what it is you want to do, and 2) Do it. My approach to healthy living operates on those principles. It turns information into action, telling you how to bring about healthy habits once and for all.

■ **Step 1: Assess your cardiac risk.** The 10 critical markers in the next section of the book will give you a global view of your cardiac risk. Some markers, such as LDL cholesterol, blood pressure and smoking, are well established. Others, such as C-reactive protein, clotting factors and personality/behavior have only begun to emerge.

Each marker is independently important to your cardiac risk. That's why, wherever possible, numeric values have been included as a means of estimating your own risk. For instance, the recommended HDL cholesterol level is 40 or above for men and 50 or above for women. An HDL level of 60 or above suggests a reduced risk; however, if it's only 31, you know you're at risk and you need to take action. By comparing your markers to established norms, you'll have a more accurate picture of where you stand. You can assess some markers using self-scoring testing; for others, you'll need to include them in a blood test as part of your annual physical exam.

■ **Step 2: Manage daily stress.** Unfortunately, we can't eliminate stress from our lives. Stress is a natural by-product of change, and change is constant. There is birth; there is death. The market goes up; the market comes down. But we can learn to handle stress more effectively. People who cope well with stress are in a better position to institute and maintain healthy exercise and eating habits. Read the section on stress and use the Heart Savers to put stress management techniques into practice.

■ **Step 3: Make exercise a habit.** We suggest exercise before dietary change because regular, moderate exercise is easier to achieve. Building up to at least a 30-minute walk five or more times a week is easier than giving up your morning doughnut. Making exercise a regular part of your life causes an improvement in outlook. That's because exercise is positive; it's *doing* something. Dietary change, on the other hand, is often seen as negative; it's about what you can't have. By starting and sticking with an exercise program, you create a platform of success—one that carries over to healthy eating. In addition, exercise has a positive impact on stress management. Read the section on effective exercise and use the Heart Savers to make it a regular part of your life.

■ **Step 4: Balance your diet.** It's important not to base your dietary decisions on pop science or the latest fad. This step lays out accepted, credible science for heart-healthy eating. It's also important to recognize that eating is a quality-of-life issue. That's why our recommendations are not extremely high or extremely low in fat; instead, they call for balance and moderation.

There are a number of simple actions you can take to improve your diet, control weight and reduce cardiac risk. The diet section will provide you with the principles of the smartest way to eat; the Heart Savers will give you the ability to put those principles into action.

In addition, there is a section on critical drug therapy, from aspirin to beta-blockers, which can enhance lifestyle improvements to benefit cardiac health.

Our intent is to provide straight information based on the latest science tempered by experience and common sense. The result, we hope, is usable advice that will help those with heart disease stabilize and even reverse their disease, and those without heart disease to prevent it. Barry and I have updated and revised *Take a Load off Your Heart* with the sincere hope that it can make a difference. It will, if you let it.

Joseph C. Piscatella
Institute for Fitness & Health
Gig Harbor, Washington

STEP 1

Assess Your Risk

10 Critical Cardiac Markers

MOST HEALTH PROFESSIONALS ONCE AGREED that heart disease was basically a problem of blocked pipes. The plumbing analogy is easy to understand, which may explain its popularity among doctors. As one cardiologist put it, "I describe heart disease to my patients as akin to rust accumulating over the years in an old water pipe. Pretty soon the pipe is blocked and there's no water at the tap. When the coronary arteries get blocked by cholesterol buildup, or plaque, there's no blood for the heart. Then the person suffers a heart attack. It's a concept patients can easily grasp."

Unfortunately, this isn't a full and accurate description of how heart disease progresses or how a heart attack takes place. "We now know that the 'rusty pipe' theory is far too simple a notion," says Dr. Ronald Krauss, past chairman of the American Heart Association's Council on Nutrition, Physical Activity and Metabolism. "Elevated cholesterol *is* important, but it's only part of the story." New studies suggest that coronary artery injury, inflammation and blood clotting are involved in the triggering of heart attacks.

Arterial injury is part of the human condition. Each time the heart beats, it pumps 5% of the body's blood back to itself via the coronary arteries. And with each beat, more than 100,000 times a day, these arteries twist and turn with such force that, over time, small tears appear on their inner walls. Elevated levels of LDL cholesterol, hypertension and diabetes may also cause inflammation and injury. Excessive stress hormones and carbon monoxide from cigarette smoke are likewise potentially injurious.

Whatever the cause, the body rushes specialized blood cells to the wound site whenever injury occurs. Cholesterol mixed in with the blood cells is deposited at the site. As it accumulates, plaque is formed. The more cholesterol, the greater the opportunity for plaque to take hold, but it is *injury to the artery wall* that provides the place for cholesterol to collect.

Wherever injury occurs, inflammation naturally follows as part of the body's repair process. Unfortunately, however, inflammation can cause a rupture in the thin, fibrous cap that covers some plaque. When that happens, cholesterol is exposed to the bloodstream and a dangerous blood clot is formed. The clot closes off the artery channel, denies blood to the heart and is the actual trigger for most heart attacks. It's no wonder, then, that an individual whose blood clots easily has an increased risk of heart attack.

Today, cholesterol is only one in a group of interrelated risk factors that together play a causal role in a heart attack. In other words, you should know your cholesterol numbers. But if that's *all* you know, you may be woefully short of information needed to gauge your true cardiac risk. In fact, scientists have identified more than 250 risk factors for the disease. That's a daunting number, to be sure, but easier to live with when you remember that not all markers are created equal. For instance, studies done several years ago suggested that a diagonal earlobe crease or going bald may be an indicator of heart disease. Worrying about

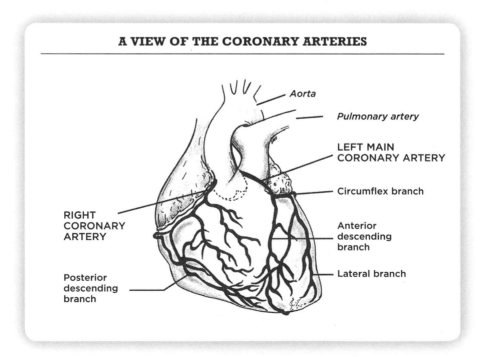

A VIEW OF THE CORONARY ARTERIES

Aorta

Pulmonary artery

LEFT MAIN CORONARY ARTERY

Circumflex branch

RIGHT CORONARY ARTERY

Anterior descending branch

Lateral branch

Posterior descending branch

such characteristics when you ought to be lowering your high blood pressure would be pretty silly.

At the same time, you should know that cardiac markers tend to cluster and may "feed" on one other. According to the Framingham Heart Study, if you *only* smoke or *only* have high cholesterol or *only* have high blood pressure, you have twice the risk of heart disease as someone who has none of these markers. But if you have two of the three markers, your risk goes up four times. And if you have all three, your risk is eight times greater. Moreover, recent studies suggest that the absence of established risk factors at 50 years of age is associated with a very low lifetime risk for developing cardiovascular disease. These findings should promote efforts aimed at preventing development of risk factors in young individuals.

WOMEN AND HEART DISEASE

In the United States alone, more than 500,000 women die of cardiovascular disease each year, exceeding the number of deaths in men and the next seven causes of death in women combined. This translates into approximately one death per minute!

Listed below are 10 of the most important cardiac markers, selected not only because of their direct links to heart health but also because each one of them can largely be controlled by making the right lifestyle changes.

1. Cholesterol and other lipids
2. Coronary inflammation
3. Blood clotting
4. Weight
5. Blood pressure
6. Diabetes
7. Metabolic syndrome
8. Aerobic capacity
9. Smoking
10. Personality

And if you have any doubts about the preeminent role of lifestyle, consider the following facts. Italians do not have high rates of heart disease. Nor do Africans or the people of Japan. But Italian Americans do, as do African Americans and Japanese Americans. Was there a change in the genetic makeup of their families when they arrived in the United States? Not likely. What changed was their lifestyle.

PREDICTING THE FUTURE

Markers for coronary heart disease are extremely predictive. In one of the most comprehensive studies of its type, researchers at Northwestern University Medical School and at the Medical College of Wisconsin spent 20 years looking at the cardiac risk factors of more than 11,000 men aged 18 to 39 and about 9,000 men aged 40 to 59. What they found was that the same factors in older men could be used to predict the future risk of heart disease in younger men.

Based on these findings, researchers concluded that critical cardiac markers, when seen in young men, have a powerful effect on long-term risk for death from coronary disease.

Here's what we can say about Americans today:

- The fat and caloric content of our diet is too high.
- Half the population has high cholesterol.
- Approximately two-thirds of the population is overweight or obese; indeed, obesity in adults has increased by 60% over the last 20 years.
- The incidence of diabetes is skyrocketing.
- Cigarette smoking remains prevalent among younger females, minorities and blue-collar workers.
- Stress is a chronic problem.
- Adults and children are leading increasingly sedentary, inactive lives.

But we *can* change the trend. Harvard's Dr. JoAnn Manson studied nearly 86,000 women and found that heart-healthy habits, rather than medical interventions, accounted for most of a 31% drop in heart disease over a 14-year period. And, more importantly, she discovered that moderate changes in one marker produced multiple risk reductions. For instance, many of the women who started an exercise program also succeeded in elevating their HDL cholesterol levels, lowering their blood pressure, losing weight and reducing blood sugar. The findings were so clear that Dr. Manson was able to chart the reduction in heart attack risk from positive behavior changes.

BEHAVIOR	REDUCTION IN HEART ATTACK RISK
Stop smoking	50% to 70% lower risk within 5 years of quitting
Reduce blood cholesterol	1% reduction in cholesterol produces a 2% to 3% drop in risk
Manage high blood pressure	1 mm Hg reduction in diastolic pressure produces a 2% to 3% drop in risk
Exercise regularly	Active lifestyle reduces risk by up to 45%
Maintain ideal weight	Results in a 35% to 55% lower risk, compared with those who are obese

Seattle cardiologist Steve Yarnall explains the situation this way: "You don't have to be a scientist to understand that the grease you sandblast from your oven and soak off your dishes isn't something you want in your arteries. You don't have to be a physiologist to understand that regular, moderate physical activity is preferable to no exercise. And you don't have to be a genius to figure out that setting fire to tobacco leaves and inhaling the smoke doesn't make a whole lot of sense." Fortunately, by using the Heart Savers listed throughout this book, you *can* eat a healthier diet, exercise regularly and manage stress.

SPEAKING FROM EXPERIENCE

What's the secret of success in making healthy lifestyle changes? In a word, persistence. Many people try for a while, but results come so slowly that they quit and go looking for something easier. What they don't realize is that, if they'd managed to hang on just a little bit longer, they could have achieved an improved coronary risk factor profile.

Heart health is a marathon, not a sprint. In other words, it's what you do over the long term that really counts. Don't worry about one particular point in the race when you may not have stayed the course. Just get back on track and keep going. **—B.F.**

1. Cholesterol and Other Lipids

NOTHING IS MORE CLOSELY IDENTIFIED WITH HEART DISEASE AND heart attacks than cholesterol. And rightly so. Too much cholesterol in the blood tends to deposit in the inner walls of coronary arteries, combining with fibrous tissue to form sludge-like bumps that thicken artery walls and increase the likelihood of a heart attack. Still, cholesterol is not the be-all and end-all of heart disease. Nor is it toxic. It occurs naturally as a soft, waxy substance in all cells and in limited amounts (the approximately 1,000 milligrams the average body makes per day) is necessary for good health. Only when it is *excessive,* a condition called hypercholesterolemia, do we have a problem.

Total Cholesterol

In 1981, the *New England Journal of Medicine* published a classic study wherein rhesus monkeys, which have a basic metabolism not unlike ours, were fed a typical high-fat American diet. The animals showed a significant rise in blood cholesterol; after two and a half years, a number of them suffered heart attacks and died (something that would be unlikely in the wild). Autopsies showed that multiple coronary artery blockages had developed, similar to those in humans with severe coronary artery disease. Researchers concluded that as cholesterol rose, so did the likelihood of arterial plaque.

More recent studies involving humans suggest the same conclusion. The Framingham Heart Study, one of the world's largest and most widely cited cardiovascular studies, has evaluated thousands of men and women since 1948. Its data show that the higher the total cholesterol, the greater the risk of heart attack. The Multiple Risk Factor Intervention Trial (MRFIT), which included more than 350,000 men aged 35 to 57, also found a correlation between cholesterol level and death rate. The risk of a fatal heart attack rose gradually at a level of 150 milligrams per deciliter of blood, increased more steeply after 200 and began to soar at 230.

But just as increased cholesterol predicts increased heart attack risk, decreased levels forecast a reduction in risk. The Scandinavian Simvastatin

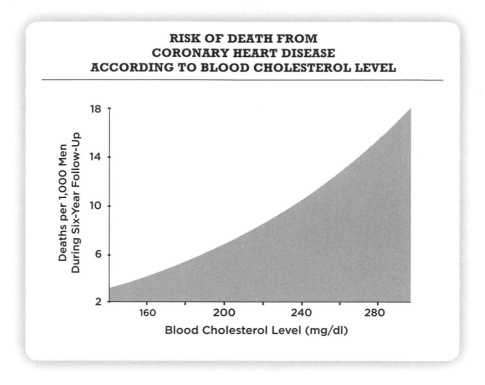

**RISK OF DEATH FROM
CORONARY HEART DISEASE
ACCORDING TO BLOOD CHOLESTEROL LEVEL**

Survival Study (4S) found that lowering cholesterol can prevent heart attacks and reduce death in men and women who already have heart disease and high cholesterol. In this study, more than 4,400 patients were divided into two groups. One group took a cholesterol-lowering drug; the other group, a look-alike placebo. The group using drug therapy reduced their total cholesterol by 25% and their LDL cholesterol by 35%; cholesterol in the second group remained unchanged. After a five-year follow-up, 622 patients in the placebo group had suffered at least one heart attack versus only 431 of the group with lowered cholesterol—a difference of more than 30%. Moreover, treated patients were much less likely to need bypass surgery or angioplasty. This was also the first trial to show that lowering cholesterol reduces major coronary events in women.

Other studies, including the West of Scotland Coronary Prevention Study and the Air Force/Texas Coronary Atherosclerosis Prevention Study, concluded that lowering cholesterol produces similar benefits for people without heart disease, greatly reducing the risk that they

CHOLESTEROL AND ALZHEIMER'S DISEASE

Recently, researchers from The Netherlands studied nearly 7,000 people aged 55 and older. Those who regularly took a cholesterol-lowering statin drug had a 43% lower risk of developing Alzheimer's disease than those who didn't take the drug. Another just-published study found that the degree of memory loss was linked to low levels of HDL cholesterol (below 40 mg/dl). To boost HDL, get regular aerobic exercise, maintain a normal body weight, limit intake of saturated fat, don't smoke and consider niacin therapy.

will develop coronary heart disease. More recently, the JUPITER Trial investigated the effects of statin therapy on almost 18,000 patients with LDL cholesterol levels below 130 but elevated levels of C-reactive protein, a marker for inflammation. Subjects were divided into two groups, one receiving a placebo and the other a statin. After observing the study population for just 1.9 years, researchers found that the combined risk of cardiovascular events in the treated group fell by 44%, and the study was prematurely stopped. In addition, angiographic studies on humans suggest that a reversal (albeit small) in the disease process is possible when cholesterol drops significantly, often causing plaque to shrink at the rate of 1% to 2% per year.

At first glance, these numbers may not seem significant. But the disease may progress at the rate of 2% to 4% a year when cholesterol stays high, so the net gain from lowering cholesterol may be as much as 6% a year. Furthermore, once plaque begins to shrink, the tendency toward inflammation and clotting seems to be much less. The heart attack rate is then diminished even before much reversal has been demonstrated.

Numerous trials have examined the link between cholesterol reduction and disease reversal. Dr. David Blankenhorn at the University of Southern California and Dr. Greg Brown at the University of Washington directed two of the most important. Each trial used a combination of low-fat eating and drug therapy to reduce cholesterol. In both trials, the majority of patients with lowered cholesterol showed a slowing of disease progression. Less cholesterol in the blood simply meant less cholesterol available for plaque to build and the disease to progress. But a more important finding was that when cholesterol subfractions improved (LDL fell to below 100 and HDL rose to 45 or more) coronary regression was achieved in 16% to 30% of patients.

Trials involving intensive dietary and lifestyle changes alone, without drug therapy, have produced similar results. Dr. Dean Ornish at the Preventive Medicine Research Institute conducted one notable study in which 48 men and women, all with coronary arteries between 40% and 100% clogged, were counseled to quit smoking, exercise aerobically for 30 minutes three times a week and use stress dissipation techniques. Twenty-six members of the group followed the American Heart Association's recommended diet, in which 30% of their calories came from fat. The other 22 people ate a strict vegetarian diet with only 8% of calories from fat, exercised moderately for at least three hours a week, meditated regularly for stress management and met twice weekly in support group sessions. When coronary arteries were evaluated after a year, the first group showed a drop in cholesterol of only 13 points, with their disease staying the same or worsening. But the second group experienced an average drop of 55 points, with the vast majority showing less disease. More importantly, 17 of the 22 people in this group demonstrated angiographic evidence of regression. Again, a significant lowering of cholesterol resulted in a shrinkage of plaque.

Newer studies have concentrated on the effect of lowered cholesterol on *plaque stabilization*. In the modern view of heart disease, this may be of even greater importance than regression, since we now know that the nature of the plaque—is it stable or unstable?—has more to do with heart attacks than its size. Almost 70% of heart attacks occur from clots at relatively mild-to-moderate obstructions (less than 50%), not from narrowing of the arteries. Similarly, in cases of sudden cardiac death, 76% involve rupture-prone plaque. "Lowering cholesterol tends to stabilize the plaque," says Dr. John LaRosa, formerly at George Washington University. "So, even though the opening hasn't changed that much, the plaque is no longer susceptible to clotting, spasm and hemorrhaging—the things that cause the closing off of the blood vessel and trigger the heart attack."

Whether you're hoping to prevent heart disease or to stabilize or reverse the disease, medical experts agree that for every 1% decrease in total cholesterol, your chance of having a heart attack decreases 2% to 3%.

But you must realize that the reverse is also true. If your blood cholesterol rises 1%, the frequency of heart attack increases similarly. According to Dr. William C. Roberts, whatever your total cholesterol is, reducing that number by about 40 points cuts your risk of a first or subsequent heart attack *in half.*

TOTAL CHOLESTEROL: KNOW YOUR NUMBER, KNOW YOUR RISK

You and your doctor can't determine your cardiac risk or formulate a response strategy unless you know your cholesterol number. The amount of cholesterol you have in your bloodstream is expressed as the number of milligrams (mg) of cholesterol in one deciliter (dl) of blood. For example, a person with 210 milligrams of cholesterol in a deciliter of blood has a cholesterol level of 210 mg/dl, popularly expressed as a cholesterol "count" of 210. But as we'll discuss later, you really need to know more than that, which is why you should request a standard lipid profile that includes triglycerides, LDL cholesterol and HDL cholesterol. In general, all adults over age 20 should have a lipid profile done at least once every five years. If parents, grandparents or siblings had heart disease before age 55, testing at a younger age may be appropriate. Also, if you have heart disease, or if you have two or more major cardiac markers (smoking, high blood pressure, obesity, diabetes, sedentary lifestyle), you should be retested annually.

While the nonfasting "finger stick" cholesterol test typically used at shopping malls and health fairs is a practical way to screen large numbers of people, readings can vary considerably from the gold-standard fasting laboratory test. In general, if you have a "finger stick" reading above 200, have your doctor check it against a fasting laboratory test.

It's important to use a laboratory that your physician trusts to give reliable measurements. Not all laboratories are standardized or well regulated, and test results can vary. In addition, certain factors can affect your cholesterol number:

- Smoking before a test may cause higher readings.
- Not fasting for 12 hours before a test may cause elevated readings.
- Morning levels are usually higher than those measured later in the day.

- Exercise, stress, dieting, body weight change, medications and phases of a woman's menstrual cycle can affect readings.

This is why a single cholesterol reading is not the whole story—and why you should have a second measurement done within eight weeks of the first. If the second reading is within 30 points of the first, use the average of the two values. Otherwise, have a third test performed and use the average of all three tests.

The National Cholesterol Education Program, in collaboration with the American Heart Association and other medical authorities, has issued guidelines for total cholesterol:

TOTAL CHOLESTEROL	RISK CLASSIFICATION
Below 200*	Desirable
200 to 239	Borderline high
240 and above	High
Your number: _____	Your risk: _____

*In particular, heart patients and those who have two or more risk factors should strive for a level no higher than 200, preferably in the 150-to-160 range.

If your total cholesterol is above 200, you are not alone. The American Heart Association estimates that 105 million Americans are at increased risk for coronary heart disease because of high cholesterol. In fact, about 48% of all Americans over 20 years of age have a cholesterol count above 200, putting them at increased risk for heart attack. By comparison, the average adult in China has a total cholesterol level of 125.

LDL Cholesterol

In the case of cholesterol, the whole is less important than the sum of its major parts (LDL and HDL). For example, take two women, both 50 years of age and both of whom have an identical total cholesterol value of 210. The first woman has an LDL of 105, whereas the second has an

LDL of 155. Provided that all other cardiac risk factors are equal, the second woman is clearly at greater risk of developing heart disease, even though their total cholesterol value is the same.

Just like oil in water, waxy cholesterol is insoluble in blood. In order to be transported, it must first be combined with fat and protein molecules. The resulting chemical package, called a lipoprotein, is nature's vehicle for moving cholesterol throughout the body. Most lipoproteins contain cholesterol and triglycerides in their core, with protein and fat forming an outer coat. Various types of lipoproteins have different sizes, shapes and functions, contain different amounts of cholesterol, triglycerides and protein, and are usually classified on the basis of their density or compactness. One of the most important is low-density lipoprotein, or LDL cholesterol.

LDL CHOLESTEROL RECOMMENDATIONS

For people at "moderate risk" (such as a postmenopausal woman with high blood pressure), the LDL goal is below 130.

For people at "high risk" (such as those with diabetes or multiple risk factors), the LDL goal is below 100.

For patients with established coronary heart disease and/or people at "very high risk" (such as those with metabolic syndrome), the LDL goal is below 70.

Predominantly made of fat and very little protein, LDL transports about 60% to 80% of the body's cholesterol through the bloodstream. Circulating in the blood for several days after its creation, LDL is taken up by body cells as building blocks for hormones and cell parts. But the cells may not require all the cholesterol that is delivered. The excess floats in the blood, collects on artery walls, causes inflammation and produces plaque. Much of the problem stems from the fact that LDL is an unstable chemical package that comes apart quite easily. Should it penetrate an artery wall and "unravel," unused cholesterol can be released and deposited in susceptible blood vessels. LDL is commonly called "bad" cholesterol because of its major role in atherosclerotic cardiovascular disease.

Since many experts believe that LDL is a more accurate marker of cardiac risk than total cholesterol alone, LDL is now viewed as an independent risk factor: the higher your LDL, the greater your risk for arterial buildup. Or, put another way, for every increase of one milligram of LDL per decaliter, the risk of heart attack increases by 2%. For people with cardiovascular disease, the American Heart Association and the American College of Cardiology now recommend lowering LDL cholesterol to below 100 (and perhaps below 70 for very high-risk patients) as *the number one goal* in lipid management. Indeed, a landmark study published in the *New England Journal of Medicine* showed that in patients with stable coronary disease, aggressive LDL lowering (via statin drug therapy) was at least as effective as angioplasty and usual care in reducing the incidence of subsequent cardiac problems. According to Dr. Claude Lenfant, former director of the National Heart, Lung and Blood Institute, lowering the level of LDL can reduce the short-term risk for heart disease by as much as 40%.

LDL CHOLESTEROL: KNOW YOUR NUMBER, KNOW YOUR RISK

The National Cholesterol Education Program created the following scale to assess cardiac risk from LDL cholesterol:

LDL CHOLESTEROL	RISK CLASSIFICATION
Below 100*	Optimal
100 to 129	Near optimal
130 to 159	Borderline high
160 to 189	High
190 and above	Very high
Your number: _____	Your risk: _____

*Heart patients and those with other forms of cardiovascular disease (such as carotid artery disease or peripheral arterial disease), diabetes and/or multiple risk factors should strive for this level; even lower (below 70) for very high-risk patients.

Some authorities suggest that an LDL cholesterol goal of less than 100 for everyone, regardless of other risk factors, would simplify the guidelines and dramatically improve our health. But here's the bottom line: the more LDL cholesterol in your blood, the greater your risk of coronary heart disease. And if your LDL is 130 or greater, you have a cardiac marker that raises heart disease risk, no matter what your total cholesterol may be.

LIPOPROTEIN(A)

As testing has become more sophisticated, subcomponents of LDL are being identified as cardiac markers in their own right. One, lipoprotein(a), or Lp(a), may be an underlying cause in a quarter of premature heart attacks; it is the most common family lipid disorder in people who develop heart disease younger than 60 years of age. Studies by Stanford University and the Jewish Hospital of Cincinnati showed that elevated levels of Lp(a) enhance the oxidation of LDL, thereby promoting the entry of this harmful form of cholesterol into the artery walls. In addition, Lp(a) seems to increase inflammation and clotting, thus dealing heart health a double whammy.

Lp(a) is genetically determined and can vary in individuals by a factor of 1,000. But as Dr. Ronald Krauss says, "It's clear that at high levels— starting at 30—Lp(a) is associated with heart disease and stroke." In studies involving 5,200 people, researchers found that those with the highest levels of Lp(a) had a 70% greater risk of having a heart attack over 10 years than those with the lowest levels. And the Heart and Estrogen/Progestin Replacement Study (HERS) found that women with the highest Lp(a) levels had 54% greater risk of heart problems than those at the lowest levels.

See your doctor to find out if an Lp(a) blood test is advisable. Certainly people with known heart disease, a strong family history and/or multiple risk factors should consider doing so as a preventive effort. You can get it done as part of your lipid profile testing.

Your number: _____   Below 30 (desirable)*

                                       Above 30 (higher risk)

---

*Many experts recommend a level no higher than 20.

As of now, dietary modifications do little to lower Lp(a), although some studies suggest that eating fish frequently may help. If your Lp(a) is over 30, your doctor may advise drug therapy. Niacin or a fibric acid derivative such as gemfibrozil (Lopid) can effectively reduce Lp(a).

Also, reducing LDL cholesterol to below 100 (usually with a statin drug) may get Lp(a) down. Most doctors believe the best treatment for this marker is a heart-healthy lifestyle: control cholesterol, triglycerides, blood pressure, diabetes and weight with a low-fat diet and exercise; don't smoke; and dissipate your stress.

APOLIPOPROTEIN B

Apolipoprotein B is another LDL component now considered a cardiac marker. Apo B, the protein part of a low-density lipoprotein, transfers cholesterol from the lipoprotein to the cells for use or to the liver for excretion. If the amount of Apo B matches up to the amount needed by the cells, there is no health issue. However, if the balance is incorrect, any excess Apo B will circulate in the bloodstream and deposit cholesterol in artery walls. Says Dr. Arthur Moss of the University of Rochester Medical Center in New York, "The cholesterol itself is an innocent passenger. It's Apo B that determines whether cholesterol is used correctly, is eliminated or ends up as plaque."

Early research shows that Apo B may predict heart risk better than LDL level, but much more exploration is needed. Talk with your doctor to determine if it may be a concern for you. Your level can be measured with an Apo B test, which requires a blood draw. A risk classification has been established for men and women in milligrams per deciliter (mg/dl):

MEN	RISK CLASSIFICATION	WOMEN
Below 52	Desirable	Below 49
52 to 109	Normal	49 to 103
110 and above	High	104 and above

Your number: _____   Your risk: _____

Apo B is in large part genetically determined, so taking control of your manageable lifestyle factors becomes even more important.

PATTERN B PARTICLES

A new breed of cholesterol test, the advanced lipid test, has uncovered another cardiac marker: the size and number of LDL particles.

It turns out that smaller LDL particles, called Pattern B, tend to adhere more easily to blood vessel walls and produce blockages. This makes them more dangerous than larger particles, called Pattern A. It is estimated that Pattern B is found in about 30% of the American public, particularly in families with a history of heart disease.

Depending on the particle types that make up their LDL, two people with the same count could have different risks. Take two men, both of whom have an LDL of 130. One has normal LDL particles, Pattern A. The other has small LDL particles, Pattern B, and a lot of them. Although their LDL is the same, the man with the smaller particles would have a greater cardiac risk than the man with the larger particles.

The size of LDL particles is, to a large extent, genetically determined, so there may not be much that can be done about them. Nonetheless, recent research suggests that the appropriate treatment is exercise, reduction of body weight and fat stores, niacin and fibrates—four of the least expensive therapies for heart disease. One widely cited study reported that a high amount of vigorous exercise (walking about 20 miles each week) produced the most beneficial (cardioprotective) changes in the size and number of LDL particles, as compared with a more moderate exercise regimen.

In summary, individuals with small, dense LDL are at a threefold increased risk of developing heart disease. However, affected individuals often have many other metabolic abnormalities (such as high triglycerides, obesity, insulin resistance, diabetes, low HDL cholesterol); therefore, this association cannot be used as conclusive evidence that Pattern B itself increases the risk of heart disease.

As of this writing, Pattern B is not routinely tested. Some experts believe that in the future such testing may be beneficial for those people with "borderline" lipid levels, who need to know whether or not they should get further medical help. As a general rule, triglyceride levels higher than 200 are indicative of Pattern B; if triglycerides are below 100, Pattern B is unlikely.

HDL Cholesterol

High-density lipoprotein, called HDL, is known as "good" cholesterol. Made up of protein and very little fat, HDL forms a stable package; since it does not unravel when it comes in contact with an artery wall, the cholesterol it carries does not become available for deposit.

Furthermore, HDL actually assists in undoing the damage wrought by LDL. It acts as a scavenger, picking up excessive LDL from artery walls and transporting it back to the liver for removal from the body. Because HDL helps to prevent cholesterol from building up on the walls of the arteries, a high HDL level is considered cardioprotective.

While HDL averages only about 25% of total cholesterol, it is critically important as a cardiac marker. Low HDL, defined as below 40 for men and 50 for women, is considered a predictive risk factor. A high level of HDL, defined as 60 or higher, is associated with lower risk. It is estimated that for every one milligram increase in HDL, there is a 4% decrease in cardiac risk.

HDL Cholesterol: Know Your Number, Know Your Risk

The National Cholesterol Education Program proposes the following scale of HDL cholesterol to approximate cardiac risk:

HDL CHOLESTEROL	RISK CLASSIFICATION
60 and above*	Low
40 to 59	Moderate
Below 40	High
Your number: _____	Your risk: _____

*According to the National Cholesterol Education Program, an HDL level of 60 or above is cardioprotective.

Average HDL levels are 45 for men and 55 for women. Female sex hormones, particularly estrogen, tend to raise HDL levels, a difference that in part explains the lower rates of heart disease in women of child-bearing age. However, as women enter menopause and estrogen plummets, so does protective HDL. A low level of HDL cholesterol is taking on growing importance as a risk factor, especially if it's under 40.

KNOW YOUR RATIO

While HDL and LDL are independent markers for heart disease, the ratio of total cholesterol to HDL can be helpful in estimating cardiac risk. To calculate your HDL ratio, divide your total cholesterol by your HDL number. For example, someone with a total cholesterol of 250 and an HDL of 50 has an HDL ratio of 5. According to the American Heart Association, the following chart illustrates the relationship between ratio and risk:

HDL RATIO	RISK CLASSIFICATION
Below 3.5*	Optimal
3.5 to 5.0	Average
5.1 to 6.0	Borderline high
Above 6.0	High
Your ratio: _____	Your risk: _____

*HDL ratio for men should not be above 4.5; for women, not above 4.0.

The latest Adult Treatment Panel III Guidelines suggest that the non-HDL cholesterol value, an additional risk marker, should also be calculated according to this formula: non-HDL cholesterol equals total cholesterol minus HDL cholesterol. For individuals at low, moderate, moderately high, and high risk, the non-HDL cholesterol goals should be below 190, 160, 160 (ideally 130) and 130 (ideally 100), respectively.

Triglycerides

Most of your body's fat is in the form of triglycerides. Almost all is stored in fat tissue for energy, but a small portion is found in the bloodstream as a component of lipoproteins. Like cholesterol, at normal levels triglycerides play a positive role in good health. But numerous studies have shown that elevated triglycerides are a predictor of coronary heart disease, stroke and a high rate of heart attack, particularly in women who are also overweight, hypertensive and diabetic. In addition, high triglycerides are often accompanied by other risk factors, such as high blood pressure and low HDL. The bundling of these factors is reflected in a cardiac marker dubbed metabolic syndrome (see pages 46–48).

Triglycerides, measured by a blood test, are expressed as the number of milligrams in one deciliter of blood. The normal triglyceride range is 50 to 150, depending on age and sex, but obesity and overweight, physical inactivity, smoking, excess alcohol intake, high-carb diets (greater than 60% of calories), several diseases (such as type 2 diabetes), certain drugs (such as higher doses of beta-blockers), various genetic disorders, and liver and kidney disease all contribute to higher triglyceride numbers.

Triglycerides: Know Your Number, Know Your Risk

The American Heart Association recommends keeping your triglycerides below 150 milligrams per deciliter (mg/dl) and, if possible, under 100. The Adult Treatment Panel III Guidelines suggest these risk classifications:

TRIGLYCERIDES	RISK CLASSIFICATION
Below 150	Desirable
150 to 199	Borderline high
200 to 499	High
500 and above	Very high
Your number: _____	Your risk: _____

2. Coronary Inflammation

REMEMBER THE SKINNED KNEE YOU HAD AS A CHILD? REMEMBER how it turned red and felt hot to the touch? That's because white blood cells congregated at the site of the wound. The proteins that were then released, which enabled the wound to heal, produced inflammation that lasted until healing was under way.

It's the same with injuries to the coronary arteries. These arteries flex and twist each time the heart beats, causing minute fissures in the artery lining; since the heart beats more than 100,000 times a day, there is nothing we can do about these wear-and-tear injuries, all of which may cause inflammation. Other variables can also produce arterial injuries; for example, some people have high levels of inflammatory markers in their blood, which, in excess, can damage artery walls. And finally, certain risk factors (hypertension, elevated LDL cholesterol, diabetes) and lifestyle habits promote arterial inflammation. Each time a smoker inhales, carbon monoxide is released into the bloodstream, irritating the artery walls. Stress, which causes cortisone and other powerful hormones to race through the blood vessel system, can also cause injury.

The danger here is that chronic inflammation destabilizes plaque, which makes it easier for the thin protective cap to rupture, releasing cholesterol into the bloodstream. Then a blood clot is formed, which can stanch blood flow to the heart or brain. As Harvard Medical School researcher Dr. Paul Ridker says, "We have learned that coronary heart disease is very much an inflammatory disease, the same way that arthritis and lupus are inflammatory diseases." The implications of this are enormous. Dr. Ridker estimates that between 25 and 35 million healthy middle-aged Americans have normal cholesterol but above-average inflammation, putting them at risk of heart attacks and strokes.

C-Reactive Protein

Produced by the liver and present in the blood during episodes of acute artery inflammation, high-sensitivity C-reactive protein (CRP) is another important marker for heart attack and stroke.

A number of studies confirm its significance:

■ The Harvard Physicians' Health Study found that high CRP levels predicted a first heart attack in healthy men six to eight years in advance; those with the highest level of CRP in their blood had three times the risk of a heart attack compared with those with lower levels. In the Nurses' Health Study, those with the highest levels of CRP had more than four times the risk of heart attack or stroke even if they were nonsmokers with normal cholesterol and no family history.

■ A study reported in the *New England Journal of Medicine* found that the risk of heart attack rises in people as their cholesterol or CRP climbs, but is highest in those who have both high cholesterol and elevated CRP. Out of 12 risk factors studied, CRP was the strongest predictor of future cardiovascular events.

C-REACTIVE PROTEIN: KNOW YOUR NUMBER, KNOW YOUR RISK

Heart attack risk begins to rise with CRP levels such as 0.55 to 0.99 milligrams per deciliter (mg/dl). Levels above 2.5 are associated with a two-to-fourfold increase in cardiac risk. Your doctor may use your test results to check further for coronary heart disease, particularly if your cholesterol is also elevated.

According to a study published in the *New England Journal of Medicine*, the following is a risk guideline for CRP:

TOTAL CRP	RISK CLASSIFICATION
Below 0.70	Lowest
0.70 to 1.1	Low
1.2 to 1.9	Average
2.0 to 3.8	Higher
3.9 to 15.0	Highest
Your number: _____	Your risk: _____

PSORIASIS AND HEART DISEASE

A study published in the *American Journal of Cardiology* suggests a link between psoriasis and coronary artery disease. The most likely cause, said the study, is inflammation.

Testing for CRP as part of your lipid profile is especially appropriate if you have multiple cardiac risk factors, an indication of early heart disease or a strong family history. Ask your doctor to order a high-sensitivity CRP (hs-CRP) test as opposed to the standard CRP test used for arthritis. An hs-CRP test is relatively inexpensive and widely available, but many physicians may not automatically include it in their blood test order. This may change in the future.

Lipoprotein-Associated Phospholipase A_2

Manufactured by macrophages (a type of white blood cell), an enzyme called lipoprotein-associated phospholipase A_2 (PLAC) is released into the blood in response to localized inflammation. The PLAC test, which measures serum levels of the enzyme, is not intended to replace existing lipid/lipoprotein measures; it simply adds complementary information. Studies of the PLAC test have shown it to be most useful in patients who have relatively low levels of LDL cholesterol, that is, less than 130 milligrams per deciliter.

According to Dr. Michael Davidson at the University of Chicago, PLAC is directly involved in the formulation and development of atherosclerotic plaque progression and may not only be a biomarker for risk prediction, but also may represent a novel therapeutic target to reduce the disease process. Numerous risk factors, including LDL cholesterol, diabetes, high blood pressure, obesity and cigarette smoking, have adverse chronic effects on blood vessel walls, which may become inflamed. PLAC is produced in response to this inflammation. Researchers now believe that a high amount of PLAC may indicate that the plaque is more likely to rupture through the inside lining of the artery into the bloodstream, potentially triggering a heart attack or stroke. Think of a canary in a coal mine.

There are other blood tests that measure inflammation, such as high-sensitivity C-reactive protein, or hs-CRP. However, C-reactive protein is not as sensitive to inflammation of the artery walls because it can be affected by other variables, such as obesity. In contrast, elevations in PLAC are independent of traditional risk factors such as body weight and body fat. Thus, for patients at intermediate to high risk for coronary heart disease or ischemic stroke, the PLAC test provides additional information to guide treatment or establish risk.

Elevated PLAC is consistently associated with a doubling of risk for cardiovascular events. Numerous studies now support this relationship:

- In a study from the Mayo Clinic, 95% of patients who had PLAC levels below 200 nanograms per milliliter did not have either a heart attack or stroke over a four-year period, despite the majority having cardiovascular disease at baseline.

- A large study of over 1,300 patients without documented coronary heart disease, sponsored by the National Heart, Lung and Blood Institute, followed the development of heart disease in the group for nine years. A two-to-threefold increased risk was found in subjects with the highest PLAC test results, despite LDL cholesterol levels lower than 130 milligrams per deciliter.

- In the Atherosclerosis Risk in Communities (ARIC) study, patients with elevated PLAC and borderline high systolic blood pressure (greater than 130 mm Hg) had nearly seven times the risk for experiencing ischemic stroke.

- In a substudy of the Pravastatin or Atorvastatin Evaluation and Infection Therapy—Thrombolysis in Myocardial Infarction (PROVE IT-TIMI 22) trial, investigators analyzed serum PLAC levels in more than 3,600 subjects at the onset of their acute cardiovascular event and approximately 30 days later. When participants were divided into five equal-size groups based on PLAC, those in the group with the highest levels of PLAC were found to be at significantly higher risk of experiencing nonfatal or fatal cardiovascular events compared with participants with the lowest PLAC levels. PLAC in the highest group remained an independent predictor of death or recurrent cardiovascular events after the data had been adjusted for numerous potential confounding variables. The study also demonstrated lowering of PLAC with intensive statin therapy, confirming previous smaller reports.

PLAC:
Know Your Number, Know Your Risk

In 2003, the Food and Drug Administration approved the PLAC test to help identify patients at increased risk of cardiovascular events. Today, many health plans and Medicare reimburse for the test, if clinically warranted.

No preparation is needed before a PLAC test. You don't need to be fasting, and you can take your medications as directed. The test simply requires the drawing of a tube of blood. Test results are expressed as nanograms per milliliter (ng/ml) and categorized into progressive levels of cardiovascular risk, as shown below. According to one report, if your PLAC test reveals a level below 160, you have a less than 1% annual risk of a cardiovascular event.

PLAC LEVEL	RISK CLASSIFICATION
Below 160	Very low
160 to 199	Low
200 to 235	Moderate
Above 235	High
Your number: _____	Your risk: _____

3. Blood Clotting

SOON AFTER ELEVATED CHOLESTEROL SETS THE STAGE FOR HEART disease by forming artery-clogging plaque, inflammation moves in to destabilize the plaque, causing its cap to rupture and exposing the soft cholesterol to the bloodstream. Then the third player enters: blood clotting.

The exposed cholesterol causes a blood clot, or thrombosis, to form on the plaque. This combination of clot and plaque seals off the artery opening, choking off the blood supply and causing a heart attack. According to cardiovascular disease expert Dr. Scott Goodnight, "The actual heart attack is caused by a blood clot more than 95% of the time."

A HEART DISEASE BUG?

Researchers are finding that coronary inflammation, much like stomach ulcers, can result from low-grade bacterial or viral infections such as gingivitis and herpes. These infections can trigger the body's immune system response, which causes inflammation to take place as part of the natural healing process, thereby accelerating atherosclerosis.

Nearly two decades ago, researchers reported that traces of *Chlamydia pneumoniae* were often found in cholesterol-clogging deposits within the arteries. They were unable to determine whether this bacterium existed there as an innocent bystander or was produced by inflammation within the artery, but a number of studies have supported the latter theory. For example, rabbits that were fed a high-fat, high-cholesterol diet and infected with chlamydia showed worse plaques than animals merely fed the unhealthy diet.

In another study, frequent users of certain antibiotics (tetracycline or quinolones) showed a reduced risk (30% to 55%) of heart attack when compared with people who didn't use these drugs. The researchers cautioned, however, that their study did not prove that taking the drugs caused the reduced risk.

Coagulation occurs when the small blood cell fragments called platelets come together to form a clot or clots. The more these cells aggregate, the greater the number of blood clots and the larger they become. Therefore, a tendency for blood to clot easily is an important cardiac marker.

How do you know whether or not your blood coagulates easily? Some experts recommend screening for fibrinogen, a protein in the blood that promotes clotting and inflammation. High levels of fibrinogen are often accompanied by other risk factors such as overweight, high triglyceride levels and diabetes, and several studies now suggest that increased fibrinogen is an independent risk factor for heart disease. (Conversely, people with low levels of this clotting factor are known to have a reduced risk of cardiac problems.)

One relevant investigation, based on a follow-up of 2,600 individuals from the Framingham Offspring Study, reported that participants with the highest levels of fibrinogen had more than twice the risk of coronary

ALCOHOL AND INFLAMMATION

A study in Germany reported that both heavy drinkers and nondrinkers had higher concentrations of C-reactive protein and other inflammatory markers than did moderate alcohol consumers, who had the most appropriate levels of the markers.

In addition to inhibiting inflammation, moderate alcohol consumption may lower blood concentrations of fibrinogen, which promotes blood clots.

heart disease and heart attacks as participants with the lowest levels of fibrinogen. The researchers who carried out the study suggested that fibrinogen's function in helping to form blood clots after an injury may be similar to the clotting that occurs in coronary arteries, leading to heart attacks.

Excess fibrinogen is often found among the constellation of metabolic abnormalities that characterize metabolic syndrome (see pages 46–48). Some researchers speculate that elevated fibrinogen may be the lethal link that makes other risk factors so dangerous to heart health. For these reasons, antiplatelet agents/anticoagulants, including aspirin and Plavix, have become increasingly embraced by contemporary guidelines for the primary and secondary prevention of atherosclerotic vascular disease.

BLOOD CLOTTING: KNOW YOUR NUMBER, KNOW YOUR RISK

As with the tests for cholesterol and other lipids, blood is drawn and evaluated to test fibrinogen levels. The following scale approximates relative clotting risk in milligrams of fibrinogen per deciliter of blood (mg/dl):

FIBRINOGEN	RISK CLASSIFICATION
Below 200	Desirable
200 to 400*	Borderline high
Above 400	High
Your number: _____	Your risk: _____

*This is considered a "normal" range.

4. Weight

NO NATION IN THE HISTORY OF THE WORLD HAS EXPERIENCED THE obesity problem that we now have in the United States. Compared with people of normal weight, obese people have a 50% to 100% greater risk of premature death, and yet the American waistline continues to expand. Nearly 70% of our adult population is either overweight or obese. Indeed, the typical man weighs 20 to 30-plus pounds too much and the typical woman is overweight by 15 to 30-plus pounds. In addition, between 1986 and 2000, the number of super-obese individuals (body mass index value greater than 50) quintupled in the United States.

To make matters worse, surveys show that nearly 82% of Americans gain weight each year. The average weight gain in the adult population is nearly two pounds per year.

It's tempting to blame these staggering numbers on genetics, but research suggests that what we weigh is largely determined by our environment and how we live. Ours is a fast-food, couch-potato culture that makes it all too easy to put on extra pounds.

A Dangerous Lifestyle

First and foremost, we eat too much and exercise too little. "The most likely explanation for the current obesity epidemic is a continued decline in energy expenditure that has not been matched by an equivalent reduction in energy intake," says Dr. James Hill, an obesity expert at the University of Colorado. In addition, many people concerned about fat in their diet are overeating fat-free and low-fat foods. And finally, the American sweet tooth now gets to taste 34 teaspoons of sugar a day from food and beverages, especially soda. This has contributed to an average daily calorie consumption of 2,475 in men and 1,833 in women.

The second problem is that we don't get enough exercise. Everyone from the surgeon general on down recognizes regular physical activity as necessary for weight loss, but less than one-third of Americans follow suit.

The bottom line is that the pathways to better health do not generally depend on better health care or, for that matter, genetic predisposition

PORKY PETS

The next time you think about tossing Fido a piece of steak, think again. About 60 million dogs and cats in the United states are overweight. "Our pets often reflect our lifestyles," says veterinarian Kimberly Rudloff. "If we're couch potatoes, so are they."

or social circumstances. Behavioral causes represent the number one determinant of premature death in our society. Obesity, physical inactivity and cigarette smoking cost an estimated 800,000 lives every year!

The prevalence of overweight and obesity in the United States has increased dramatically over the past two decades, with one in three adults currently obese. Eighty-two percent of all adults gain weight annually, averaging nearly two pounds per year. Even more striking is the disproportionate increase in those with morbid obesity (BMI greater than 40) and super obesity (BMI greater than 50), which have quadrupled and quintupled over the last two decades. Collectively, these numbers present a tremendous health care challenge in the treatment of the numerous health problems associated with excess body weight.

Consider the following:

- Experts warn that obesity and physical inactivity may soon surpass smoking as the nation's principal cause of preventable death.

- Actuarial studies have found that the death rate from all causes increases as weight rises, and this risk becomes substantial for people who are obese, defined as weighing 30% or more above ideal weight.

- "Five of the 10 leading causes of death in the United States are linked to weight," says cardiologist Dr. Charles H. Hennekens of the University of Miami Medical School.

SPEAKING FROM EXPERIENCE

A popular Pennsylvania restaurant, Denny's Beer Barrel Pub, is now known for the world's largest burger. Weighing in at nine pounds, it costs $23.95 and comes with all the fixins: 2 tomatoes; half a head of lettuce; 12 slices of American cheese; full cup of peppers; 2 onions; plus a river of mayonnaise, mustard and ketchup and a topping of pickles! Word is, an even larger burger is planned. —B.F.

■ The overweight condition of Americans increases the risk of kidney disorders, gout, gallstones, osteoporosis, arthritis, breathing problems, back pain, certain cancers and—no surprise, you knew we'd get there—heart disease.

The Cardiac Risk

Weight problems and obesity in particular are directly linked to high blood pressure, increased cholesterol and triglycerides, lower HDL cholesterol and their consequences: heart disease and stroke. Over the past year, two landmark studies have confirmed this relationship. The first study examined the association between body mass index (BMI) values and coronary events in more than 54,000 apparently healthy adults. The average follow-up was nearly eight years. After adjusting for numerous lifestyle factors, each unit of BMI (above 25) was associated with a 7% and 5% higher risk of coronary events in men and women, respectively. The second study reported that the age at which a first heart attack occurred was inversely related to BMI. On average, the most obese individuals experienced their heart attack 12 years earlier than the leanest.

Obese people, as compared with their leaner counterparts, have higher levels of plasminogen activator inhibitor 1, a substance that can cause artery-blocking blood clots. Obesity also may heighten inflammation in the arteries, thus increasing the risk for clotting. Says Dr. Paul Ridker, an expert on C-reactive protein, "Overweight and obese people tend to have higher levels of C-reactive protein than people of normal weight. Even an extra 10 or 20 pounds can raise CRP and contribute to a heart attack."

And finally, excessive fatty acids released into the blood by fat stored in the body may trigger irregular heartbeats, which in extreme cases can lead to sudden cardiac death.

Abdominal Obesity

The link between overweight and heart disease is particularly strong if the excess weight is carried around the middle. Says Dr. William Castelli, former director of the Framingham Heart Study, "People with

A woman's size 8 today was, on her mother and grandmother, a size 10. That's because clothing designers now use dress size as a marketing tool, knowing that women are more likely to buy clothing for their size 10 (or 12) body if it says size 8.

wide hips and flat bellies may be over-weight, but the extra weight does not seem to increase their cardiac risk as much as that of people with narrow hips and potbellies. Abdominal obesity, which is more of a male problem, is predictive of coronary disease."

Potbellies make many men appear "apple-shaped," while many more women could be described as "pear-shaped." Perhaps because abdominal fat is more metabolically active than fat stored in thighs, hips and buttocks, "apples" are three to five times more likely than "pears" to suffer heart attacks. Potbelly fat is a strong predictor and reason enough to determine if it's penalizing your cardiac health. "You can do this simply by measuring your waist," says Dr. Scott Grundy of the University of Texas Southwestern Medical Center. "Position a soft tape measure around your waist, just above the navel. The American Heart Association defines a high-risk waistline as 35 inches or more for women and 40 inches or more for men. Studies have shown that people with these measurements are three times more likely to have high blood cholesterol levels, four times more likely to be in poor physical condition and seven times more likely to be diabetic than people with smaller waists."

WEIGHT:
KNOW YOUR NUMBER, KNOW YOUR RISK

The National Institutes of Health recommends using the body mass index (BMI) to assess your susceptibility to disease. BMI describes body weight relative to height and is equal to weight in kilograms divided by height in meters squared. Alternatively, you can estimate BMI from pounds and inches. Simply multiply your weight in pounds by 703 and divide the number by your height in inches squared.

The body mass index table on pages 34 and 35 can save you some time. To use the table, find your approximate height in the left-hand column labeled "Height." Move across to your weight. The number at the top of the column is the BMI value for your height and weight.

It is recommended that all adults have their BMI determined and assessed in light of the following guidelines:

BMI*	CONDITION	RISK
19 to 24.9	Healthy weight	Desirable
25 to 29.9	Overweight	Borderline high
30 to 39.9	Obese	High
40 or above	Very obese	Very high

Your BMI: _____   Your risk: _____

*BMI usually correlates well with body fat, although very muscular people may have a high BMI without excess body fat. In that case, there is little or no added health risk.

WHERE YOU LIVE MATTERS

A recent report from the Centers for Disease Control and Prevention listed the percentage of obese adults living in each state. Beautiful Colorado, where so many engage in winter sports, topped the "leanest" list; Mississippi was ranked the "fattest."

SOME OF THE LEANEST	SOME OF THE FATTEST
Colorado	Mississippi
Montana	Louisiana
Vermont	Alabama
Massachusetts	Kentucky
Rhode Island	South Carolina
Hawaii	West Virginia
Connecticut	Arkansas
Arizona	Tennessee

BODY MASS INDEX TABLE

	HEALTHY WEIGHT						OVERWEIGHT					OBESE					
BMI	19	20	21	22	23	24	25	26	27	28	29	30	31	32	33	34	35
Height (feet/ inches) Body Weight (pounds)																	
4'10"	91	96	100	105	110	115	119	124	129	134	138	143	148	153	158	162	167
4'11"	94	99	104	109	114	119	124	128	133	138	143	148	153	158	163	168	173
5'0"	97	102	107	112	118	123	128	133	138	143	148	153	158	163	168	174	179
5'1"	100	106	111	116	122	127	132	137	143	148	153	158	164	169	174	180	185
5'2"	104	109	115	120	126	131	136	142	147	153	158	164	169	175	180	186	191
5'3"	107	113	118	124	130	135	141	146	152	158	163	169	175	180	186	191	197
5'4"	110	116	122	128	134	140	145	151	157	163	169	174	180	186	192	197	204
5'5"	114	120	126	132	138	144	150	156	162	168	174	180	186	192	198	204	210
5'6"	118	124	130	136	142	148	155	161	167	173	179	186	192	198	204	210	216
5'7"	121	127	134	140	146	153	159	166	172	178	185	191	198	204	211	217	223
5'8"	125	131	138	144	151	158	164	171	177	184	190	197	203	210	216	223	230
5'9"	128	135	142	149	155	162	169	176	182	189	196	203	209	216	223	230	236
5'10"	132	139	146	153	160	167	174	181	188	195	202	209	216	222	229	236	243
5'11"	136	143	150	157	165	172	179	186	193	200	208	215	222	229	236	243	250
6'0"	140	147	154	162	169	177	184	191	199	206	213	221	228	235	242	250	258
6'1"	144	151	159	166	174	182	189	197	204	212	219	227	235	242	250	257	265
6'2"	148	155	163	171	179	186	194	202	210	218	225	233	241	249	256	264	272
6'3"	152	160	168	176	184	192	200	208	216	224	232	240	248	256	264	272	279
6'4"	156	164	172	180	189	197	205	213	221	230	238	246	254	263	271	279	287

				VERY OBESE														
36	37	38	39	40	41	42	43	44	45	46	47	48	49	50	51	52	53	54
172	177	181	186	191	196	201	205	210	215	220	224	229	234	239	244	248	253	258
178	183	188	193	198	203	208	212	217	222	227	232	237	242	247	252	257	262	267
184	189	194	199	204	209	215	220	225	230	235	240	245	250	255	261	266	271	276
190	195	201	206	211	217	222	227	232	238	243	248	254	259	264	269	275	280	285
196	202	207	213	218	224	229	235	240	246	251	256	262	267	273	278	284	289	295
203	208	214	220	225	231	237	242	248	254	259	265	270	278	282	287	293	299	304
209	215	221	227	232	238	244	250	256	262	267	273	279	285	291	296	302	308	314
216	222	228	234	240	246	252	258	264	270	276	282	288	294	300	306	312	318	324
223	229	235	241	247	253	260	266	272	278	284	291	297	303	309	315	322	328	334
230	236	242	249	255	261	266	274	280	287	293	299	306	312	319	325	331	338	344
236	243	249	256	262	269	276	282	289	295	302	308	315	322	328	335	341	348	354
243	250	257	263	270	277	284	291	297	304	311	318	324	331	338	345	351	358	365
250	257	264	271	278	285	292	299	306	313	320	327	334	341	348	355	362	369	376
257	265	272	279	286	293	301	308	315	322	329	338	343	351	358	365	373	379	386
265	272	279	287	294	302	309	316	324	331	338	346	353	361	368	375	383	390	397
272	280	288	295	302	310	318	325	333	340	348	355	363	371	378	386	393	401	408
280	287	295	303	311	319	326	334	342	350	358	365	373	381	289	396	404	412	420
287	295	303	311	319	327	335	343	351	359	367	375	383	391	399	407	415	423	431
295	304	312	320	328	336	344	353	361	369	377	385	394	402	410	418	426	435	443

5. Blood Pressure

BLOOD PRESSURE, THE FORCE NEEDED TO MOVE BLOOD THROUGH the vascular system against the resistance of the artery walls, is often compared to the pressure inside an ordinary garden hose. When the nozzle of the hose is opened, the water pressure in the hose decreases. But if the nozzle is tightened or more water is added, the pressure increases.

High blood pressure is usually attributed to a narrowing of arteries and their smaller vessels (the arterioles), to a loss of elasticity, or to both. Resistance creates pressure, causing the heart to work harder just to keep the blood moving. This added stress, both on the heart and on the vascular system, can lead to the bulging and rupture of an artery (called an aneurysm), hardening of the arteries, stroke, heart attack, kidney failure, congestive heart failure and death. Constant high blood pressure affects the artery linings, causing sufficient trauma to create arterial injury and inflammation. This circumstance in turn causes even more narrowing of artery openings, so the heart is less likely to receive an adequate supply of blood. Then it has to expend more energy, which means it needs more oxygen, resulting in a no-win situation.

Afflicting about 72 million Americans (and more common in African Americans than in Caucasians), high blood pressure represents a major public health threat. One study done at the Boston University School of Medicine estimated that 9 out of 10 middle-aged Americans will, at some point, develop high blood pressure.

High blood pressure is a predictive, primary risk factor for heart disease and stroke. People with high blood pressure are up to five times more likely to have a heart attack and more than twice as likely to have a stroke than people with normal blood pressure. Yet, according to Dr. Sidney Smith, past president of the American Heart Association, many hypertensive patients do not receive adequate treatment. Recent studies indicate that of those with hypertension, 30% don't know they have it, 34% are on medication and have it controlled, 25% are on medication but don't have their hypertension under control and 11% are not on medication.

Like coronary heart disease itself, high blood pressure progresses silently, increasing year after year with no overt symptoms other than, perhaps, some nonspecific complaints: dizzy spells, chest pains, swelling in ankles and feet, headaches, changes in vision, leg cramps, loss of concentration. Then quite suddenly, typically in middle age, hypertension appears. By this time, however, it's usually too late to repair the damage done. Chronic illness and death may ultimately occur.

In addition, people with high blood pressure are twice as likely to develop type 2 (non-insulin-dependent) diabetes as compared with those with normal blood pressure. Forty percent of all those with high blood pressure also have an abnormal blood lipid profile. High blood pressure is also linked to age-related macular degeneration, a progressive loss of vision due to the deterioration of nerve tissue in the retina.

BLOOD PRESSURE: KNOW YOUR NUMBERS, KNOW YOUR RISK

Blood pressure is expressed as two numbers representing millimeters of mercury (mm Hg). The top number represents *systolic pressure,* which is taken when the heart beats—at that moment when blood is pumped out of the heart in one big burst of peak pressure and the aorta expands to

---

THE POWER OF INTIMACY

A study at the State University of New York at Oswego found that spending a little quality time with your significant other, regardless of what you do together, seems to have a calming influence on a person's blood pressure. Researchers theorize that the familiarity of an intimate relationship sends out a "safety signal" that lowers blood pressure.

"This does not mean that single people are doomed to high blood pressure," said lead study author Dr. Brooks Gump. "Rather, the findings suggest that comfortable relationships—close friends included—have a soothing effect on blood pressure." While it is unclear what such a short-term change in blood pressure means to health, we do know that temporary flare-ups in blood pressure can take a cardiovascular toll. It may well be that the calming influence of a spouse or partner acts as a counterbalance and eventually benefits the heart.

HYPERTENSION AND MEMORY LOSS

If left untreated, high blood pressure in midlife can cause memory loss later in life. The Framingham Heart Study found that for every increase of 10 points of systolic pressure in middle age, there was a 7% or greater risk of impaired cognitive skills 20 years later.

handle the flow. The bottom number is the *diastolic pressure*, registered between heartbeats when the pressure falls to its lowest point as the heart relaxes to normal and refills with blood. Normal systolic pressure is below 120 mm Hg and normal diastolic pressure is below 80 mm Hg, typically expressed in figures as 120/80 and verbally as "120 over 80."

Blood pressure, however, varies naturally with weight, activity, body position, age and even time of day. Because of such fluctuations, you would not be considered to have high blood pressure unless you had three elevated readings in a row. Furthermore, if you're anxious about having your blood pressure taken, you may have what's called "white-coat hypertension"—a temporary condition responsible for elevated readings. That's why some doctors use ambulatory blood pressure monitoring, in which the patient wears a blood pressure cuff that inflates periodically over a 24-hour period; a small recorder attached to the cuff stores the readings as they're taken. This technique is also useful for evaluating the effectiveness of blood pressure medications, as well as the relationship between blood pressure and abnormal symptoms (such as dizziness) during the day.

So, let's say you're tested and your doctor tells you that you have high blood pressure, or hypertension. What does this mean? Only that the pressure in your arteries is consistently above the goal range—generally agreed to be less than 140/90. (If you have diabetes, another important cardiac marker, even lower blood pressure is recommended, ideally less than 130/80.) The higher your numbers, the greater the risk.

For many years, it was thought that the bottom number (diastolic pressure) was more important. Doctors suggested that this number reflected the minimum pressure to which the arteries are constantly exposed and found it to be less variable than the top number (systolic pressure), so systolic hypertension was often undertreated. But study after study now shows that the percentage of people who experience heart attacks or strokes increases with both elevated systolic and diastolic pressure. Which of these two numbers should be used to diagnose the presence and severity of hypertension? The commonsense answer is, of course, both.

The following standards have been established by the National Institutes of Health for assessing high blood pressure:

BLOOD PRESSURE READING

SYSTOLIC		DIASTOLIC	RISK
Below 120	and	Below 80	Normal
120 to 139	or	80 to 89	Prehypertension
140 to 159	or	90 to 99	Stage 1 hypertension
160 and above	or	100 and above	Stage 2 hypertension

Your systolic pressure: _____   Your diastolic pressure: _____

The ranges above are used so that you can determine whether or not this marker is a cardiac risk for you. Obviously, risk is more easily estimated at the extremes. A person with a systolic pressure of less than 120 has a lower risk, while one who has a reading higher than 160 is already showing advanced hypertension. But what about borderline risk? Is someone with a systolic pressure of 139 "safe" while a person with a systolic pressure of 141 is "at high risk"? The line is not that clear. Ask your doctor for more specific information on your numbers and your risk.

Also, it's important to understand that just because your blood pressure isn't high, this doesn't mean it's low enough. High blood pressure doesn't suddenly occur at 140/90. The fact is, the risk for heart disease rises along a continuum as blood pressure increases. Researchers examining records of 7,000 people in the Framingham Heart Study found that over a 10-year period those with prehypertension were about twice as likely to suffer a heart attack as compared with people with optimal blood pressure.

RECOMMENDED ACTIONS

For healthy people over 18 years of age, the following actions are recommended, based on an initial blood pressure check:

BLOOD PRESSURE READING

SYSTOLIC	DIASTOLIC	WHAT TO DO
Below 120	Below 80	Recheck in 2 years
120 to 139	or 80 to 89	Recheck in 1 year
140 to 159	or 90 to 99	Confirm within 2 months
160 and above	or 100 and above	See your doctor immediately

If your systolic and diastolic readings cross categories, follow the recommendations for the shorter follow-up time. If you have questions or concerns, talk with your doctor.

It's important to have your blood pressure checked regularly. If your readings are usually within normal range, keep on doing what you're doing to avoid an upward climb. But if they're consistently elevated, talk with your doctor about methods to control your blood pressure. This is crucial. According to the Framingham Heart Study, a man in his thirties with a diastolic pressure between 85 and 94 has a five times greater risk of a heart attack than a man with a diastolic pressure below 70. But the opposite is also true. For every one-point drop in diastolic blood pressure, there is a 2% to 3% drop in heart attack risk. Therefore, aggressive management of blood pressure is a prudent measure. As blood pressure expert Dr. Sheldon G. Sheps has observed, "You shouldn't be satisfied unless your blood pressure is controlled."

Numerous major trials have examined the effects of aggressive blood pressure treatment in persons aged 60 and older with isolated systolic hypertension. Subjects were randomly assigned to drug treatment with antihypertensive medications or to a placebo group that received a look-alike (but inactive) pill. Those in the treatment group had markedly fewer cardiovascular events over the follow-up periods.

6. Diabetes

ABOUT 24 MILLION AMERICANS, NEARLY 8% OF THE POPULATION, have diabetes, a condition that disrupts the way the body uses glucose, a sugar molecule that comes from the food we eat. For the body to absorb glucose, the hormone insulin, which is produced by the pancreas, is necessary. But in people with diabetes the pancreas does not produce insulin (or produces too little of it) or the body does not properly use the insulin that is produced. As a consequence, glucose builds up in the blood and eventually begins to appear in the urine. Over time, high glucose levels can cause devastating results such as stroke, high blood pressure, blindness, kidney disease, nerve damage and amputation. Diabetes is the fourth leading cause of death (often prematurely) in the United States. And heart disease is the leading cause of diabetes-related death, in part because diabetes predisposes people to high blood pressure and an abnormal lipid profile.

> **DID YOU KNOW?**
>
> **D**iabetes ranks as a major risk factor for developing coronary heart disease. Studies suggest that it raises the risk in men by 69% and in women by a whopping 174%.

Even though diabetics have heart disease death rates about two to four times higher than nondiabetics, most people who suffer from this disease are unaware of their increased cardiovascular risk. In a survey by the American Heart Association, diabetics identified loss of vision and amputation as the most serious complications of their disease. Only one-third of those surveyed named heart disease as a serious complication. Today, diabetes is considered a coronary risk equivalent.

There are three main types of diabetes. *Type 1 diabetes,* previously called insulin-dependent or juvenile-onset diabetes, occurs in childhood or early adulthood—often in children who have a diabetic parent or sibling. While the genetic component is strong, type 1 diabetes can also result from other diseases of the pancreas and may be set off by an environmental trigger such as a virus, toxin or food. People with type 1 have a severe shortage of insulin; their pancreas produces little or none at all. Since the absence of insulin means glucose cannot be used for energy, the

41

body burns fat for its energy, causing ketones (substances formed by the breakdown of fat) to build up in the bloodstream. Before the development of injectable insulin, children with diabetes usually died young. Now they can live relatively normal lives.

Type 2 diabetes, previously called non-insulin-dependent or adult-onset diabetes, accounts for up to 95% of all cases of diabetes. It usually strikes people in their forties or older, although it is increasingly showing up in overweight, sedentary teenagers and even young children. Genetics can play a role in the development of type 2 diabetes. (It has been found that certain populations, including African Americans, Hispanic/Latino Americans, Asian Americans, Pacific Islanders and Native Americans, have a higher incidence.) However, the main factor in the development of type 2 diabetes is excess weight.

Type 2 diabetics produce some insulin, but their bodies have developed a resistance to it; as time passes, these individuals require more insulin than the pancreas can produce, and the buildup of glucose in the bloodstream damages blood vessels and organs. Some quick-weight-loss diet books, in an attempt to justify their pop science, have claimed that

---

COMMON SYMPTOMS OF DIABETES

Type 1 and type 2 diabetes have many symptoms in common. One difference is that the symptoms of type 1 tend to come on suddenly, while those of type 2 appear quite gradually.

Frequent urination	Slow healing of cuts or bruises
Increased hunger and thirst	
	Tingling or numbness in the hands or feet
Weight loss	
Headaches; blurred vision	Recurring skin, gum or bladder infections
Weakness and fatigue	
	Irritability
Infections, especially yeast infections	

SPEAKING FROM EXPERIENCE

There's some terrifying information out there about the weight and health of our kids. The fact is that there have never been so many overweight and obese American children and adolescents. According to the Centers for Disease Control and Prevention, 16% of children aged 6 to 19 years are overweight or obese—a number that has tripled since 1980. Another 15% of children are considered at risk of becoming overweight.

One result of this excess weight is that record numbers of children (particularly Hispanic Americans and African Americans) have type 2 diabetes. Until a few years ago, this condition was called adult onset diabetes. Now, because so many children have it, it's called simply type 2 diabetes. **—J.P.**

insulin resistance leads to overweight. Increasing scientific evidence, however, suggests that the reverse is true. *Overweight leads to insulin resistance.* This points to a major link between overweight and the onset of type 2 diabetes.

To be clear, over 85% of type 2 diabetics are overweight. Burgeoning obesity is the central reason that more Americans are contracting type 2 at a younger age. But this situation can be reversed. You can lower your risk of getting full-blown diabetes by at least 80% if you lose as little as 5% of your body weight and exercise as little as 30 minutes a day.

A third type of diabetes is *gestational diabetes,* which affects 3% to 10% of pregnant women in the United States. In this condition, hormones from the placenta block the normal action of insulin in the body, creating insulin resistance. Because certain complications arising from gestational diabetes can be quite serious, every pregnant woman is tested for it.

DIABETES:
KNOW YOUR NUMBER, KNOW YOUR RISK

It's important to know your estimated risk for diabetes, particularly if you have a family history. Experts recommend that all adults over the age of 45, particularly those with a BMI greater than 25, be tested for diabetes every three years.

LIFESTYLE ALTERS HEART ATTACK RISK

About 65% of diabetics die of heart attack or stroke. The higher-than-normal risk of cardiovascular disease in diabetics is largely attributed to two factors: high blood pressure and an abnormal lipid profile. But researchers have now shown that regular exercise (150 minutes per week) and weight loss (6%) can delay or prevent type 2 diabetes by 58%. Moreover, exercise and weight loss may improve a person's ability to prevent clots and thus reduce cardiovascular risk.

The routine diagnostic test for diabetes is the fasting blood glucose test, which can be administered as part of your lipid panel. (Fasting means not eating for at least eight hours prior to blood sampling.) Researchers at the National Institute of Diabetes and Digestive and Kidney Diseases suggest that morning, rather than afternoon, is the optimal time for administering a blood glucose test because of the so-called "dawn phenomenon"—the fact that blood glucose levels of diabetics are highest in the morning hours.

Results of the fasting blood glucose test are represented as milligrams of glucose in one deciliter of blood. The American Diabetes Association suggests that the following scale be used for an estimation of risk:

GLUCOSE	RISK CLASSIFICATION
Below 100	Normal
100 to 125*	Prediabetes
126 or higher**	Confirmed diabetes
Your number: _____	Your risk: _____

*The relatively new risk category called prediabetes indicates glucose values greater than desirable or normal but below the level that is diagnostic of diabetes. Doctors are trying to learn how to predict which people with this condition will end up with diabetes. If you fall into this risk category, work with your doctor on a weight loss and exercise program to reduce your risk.

**A fasting blood glucose of 126 or higher indicates diabetes. Previously, a value of 140 was the standard. In some instances, doctors will elect to obtain an oral glucose tolerance test, in which case a glucose value of 200 or more indicates a diagnosis of diabetes.

According to diabetes expert Dr. Byron Hoogwerf, blood glucose levels can vary from hour to hour. Consequently, if the fasting blood glucose level is even slightly elevated (100 to 125), he recommends a follow-up blood test called hemoglobin A1c, or simply HbA1c.

In a nutshell, HbA1c testing measures the amount of glucose attached to red blood cells. The higher your blood glucose, the more sugar your red blood cells will accumulate over time. Because red blood cells typically live 90 to 120 days, this test reveals your "average" blood sugar during that time. For people without diabetes, target HbA1c numbers range from 4% to 6%. Diabetics and patients with coronary and other vascular disease should strive for a value below 7%.

Today, HbA1c testing can be done in a doctor's office using a blood sample from a finger stick. Diabetics should probably have an HbAlc test every six months; insulin-dependent diabetics should aim for three-month intervals. Your doctor can best determine the frequency that is most appropriate for you. Comparing the test results with your current blood glucose level offers a more accurate picture of diabetes control. The following chart provides an example of how the two measurements may relate to one another, as well as the level of control.

GAUGING YOUR LEVEL OF DIABETES CONTROL

Average Blood Glucose	Diabetes Type 1 or 2	HbA1c
mg/dl	Level of Control	%
360	POOR CONTROL	14
240		10
	MARGINAL CONTROL	
210		9
	GOOD CONTROL	
150		7
90	GOAL	5

7. Metabolic Syndrome

METABOLIC SYNDROME IS A COMBINATION OF MULTIPLE CARDIAC risk factors believed to be a product of insulin resistance. As discussed in the section on diabetes, our bodies convert the food we eat into glucose, which insulin transports to cells where fuel is needed. The cells, however, are protected by receptors that act as "gates," controlling which nutrients are allowed in. Normally, insulin is the key that opens these gates and allows glucose to enter the cells.

Unfortunately, these receptors can become resistant to insulin's action, probably as a result of weight gain and physical inactivity. If this occurs, the pancreas pumps out more insulin in an attempt to force glucose into the cells. This scenario, if repeated over time, is thought to trigger a series of metabolic abnormalities culminating in metabolic syndrome. The condition directly damages the coronary arteries, contributing to the buildup of plaque and promoting blood clots.

Metabolic syndrome affects more than 50 million Americans. It shows up as excess fibrinogen as well as elevated levels of plasminogen activator inhibitor1 (PAI1), a substance that slows clot breakdown, and a dangerous combination of cardiac risk factors including high triglycerides, low HDL, abdominal obesity and elevations in blood pressure, blood sugar and uric acid. It is widely believed that this cluster of metabolic abnormalities speeds the development of coronary heart disease, particularly in women and diabetics.

People with metabolic syndrome typically have a moderate level of total cholesterol, often under 200, so the syndrome may be overlooked in a medical exam. For example, data on a 51-year-old male in the Framingham Heart Study produced the following lipid profile:

Total cholesterol	195
LDL cholesterol	108
HDL cholesterol	32
Triglycerides	264

Because his total cholesterol was under 200 and his LDL level was "near optimal," it might be assumed that this man had a low cardiac risk. In fact, the man had coronary heart disease that was likely attributable to metabolic syndrome. Says Dr. William Castelli, "In Framingham, we found that when triglycerides are high and HDL is low, the predictive risk of heart attack doubles . . . even when total cholesterol is in line. We also found that when you fatten up in the abdomen, you start to move your triglycerides and HDL toward metabolic syndrome. And when you add in high blood pressure and diabetes, the effect is disastrous."

Metabolic Syndrome: Know Your Profile, Know Your Risk

In 2005, the American Heart Association/National Heart, Lung and Blood Institute published the following risk profile for metabolic syndrome:

Is your HDL number below 40 (men) or below 50 (women)?	Yes _____	No _____
Is your triglyceride number over 150?	Yes _____	No _____
Is your waist size 35 inches or above (women) or 40 inches or above (men)?	Yes _____	No _____
Is your blood pressure consistently 130/85 or greater?	Yes _____	No _____
Are you a prediabetic or diabetic (a fasting glucose of 100 or greater)?	Yes _____	No _____

If you answered "yes" to two of the five questions above, you probably have metabolic syndrome. If you answered "yes" to three or more, you definitely have metabolic syndrome. Recognize that the answer to the HDL, triglycerides, blood pressure and fasting glucose questions should be "yes" if you're taking drug treatment to correct them.

High triglyceride and low HDL levels, obesity, diabetes, high blood pressure—all are fairly common health problems and each increases cardiac risk. But in combination as part of metabolic syndrome, they can be deadly. A widely cited study followed more than 6,000 heart patients for 8 to 10 years after bypass surgery. It found that among people who had three or four of the characteristics of metabolic syndrome, the risk for death in the 10 years after surgery increased by 1.5 to 3 times compared with people with none of the conditions. The risk rose even more for women—a 5-to-12-fold increase.

Those who follow politics were stunned when journalist Tim Russert, host of *Meet the Press,* died suddenly from a heart attack. Russert had hypertension, abdominal obesity, elevated triglycerides and low HDL cholesterol—classic characteristics of metabolic syndrome.

8. Aerobic Capacity

PEOPLE WHO DEMONSTRATE PHYSICAL FITNESS—STRENGTH, stamina and flexibility—are most often in better overall health than those who can't heft a child or touch their toes. But that doesn't mean they're in good cardiovascular health. Much more important is their aerobic capacity, which is both a critical cardiac marker and a predictor of longevity.

Aerobic, which means "with oxygen," describes activities that cause the heart and lungs to process oxygen at a steady rate over a period of time. Brisk walking, jogging and swimming develop stamina and endurance, the ability to keep on going without placing undue strain on the cardiovascular system. Regular aerobic exercise develops aerobic fitness, the ability to work the muscles hard—but not so hard that the heart and lungs can't keep up with the oxygen demand.

In order to understand the benefits of aerobic fitness, we need to back up and examine what enables us to work and play. Through a series of chemical reactions, the food we eat is converted into energy reserves. Much more energy is formed if plenty of oxygen is available to body tissues—and that depends on the volume of blood the heart pumps per minute and the amount of oxygen the tissues extract from the circulating blood. These two variables determine the level of aerobic fitness. But since there is little difference from one person to another in the amount of oxygen extracted by the tissues, we know that aerobic fitness is largely reflective of the pumping effectiveness of the heart.

Quantifying Aerobic Fitness

People who run or jog, go out for a brisk walk or participate in a spinning class know very quickly if they have aerobic fitness. If you can run steadily for 30 minutes, for instance, you can probably call yourself aerobically fit. But if you have to stop to catch your breath 10 minutes into your walk, it's a safe bet that you haven't achieved aerobic fitness.

This type of casual determination is not sufficient, however, for evaluating your aerobic fitness as a cardiac marker, because it fails to measure oxygen consumption. The gold standard in this case is a progressive treadmill test that involves breathing through a mouthpiece or face mask. It factors your breathing and heart rates with your final speed and the grade of the incline, or the minutes achieved in the test. The results are expressed in *metabolic equivalents (of task),* or METs, a numerical rating of the body's ability to produce energy needed to perform certain activities.

One MET equals the amount of oxygen required for sitting at rest or lying down. The more effort it takes for a given activity, the greater the number of METs expended. Walking at a pace of two miles per hour, for instance, expends about 2 to 3 METs, the same as playing billiards or bowling. Boosting your walking speed to four miles per hour calls for about 5 METs, about the same as gardening or playing volleyball. And jogging at the speed of five miles per hour requires about 8 METs, about the same as playing basketball or competitive singles tennis.

The highest MET level you can achieve during an exercise stress test is referred to as your maximal MET level. Average men and women have an 8 to 12 MET capacity. This means that at maximal exercise, they can consume 8 to 12 times the amount of oxygen that they take in at rest. Older or unfit persons or heart patients generally average 5 to 8 METs. In contrast, marathoners and other highly trained endurance athletes have been measured at 15 to 20 METs or more.

Increasing your maximal MET level is crucial for cardiac health and longevity, as demonstrated in a series of landmark studies by Dr. Steven Blair and colleagues at the Cooper Institute. In one study, more than 13,000 healthy men and women were given a medical examination and a treadmill stress test. At the time, none of the subjects exhibited any evidence of heart disease or cancer. During a follow-up period averaging more than eight years, nearly 300 of the participants had died. The study concluded that, in general, the higher the subjects' initial level of fitness, the lower the death rate from heart disease or cancer (see below). This was true even after statistical adjustments were made for age and coronary risk factors.

Interestingly, there appeared to be no further decrease in mortality associated with fitness levels higher than 9 to 10 METs. Moreover, the greatest reduction in death risk for men occurred as they progressed from the lowest level of aerobic fitness (6 or less METs) to the next lowest level (7 METs). These findings show that even a slight improvement in aerobic capacity among the most unfit substantially reduces heart disease mortality.

In a subsequent study, Dr. Blair followed nearly 10,000 men who were given two treadmill tests about five years apart. Approximately five years after the second test, deaths from all causes were examined. The highest death rate occurred in men who were rated "unfit" at both examinations; the lowest death rate was in men who were rated "highly fit" both times. However, men who improved from "unfit" to "fit" between the first and second examinations had an intermediate death rate, supporting the hypothesis that improved aerobic fitness leads to decreased mortality.

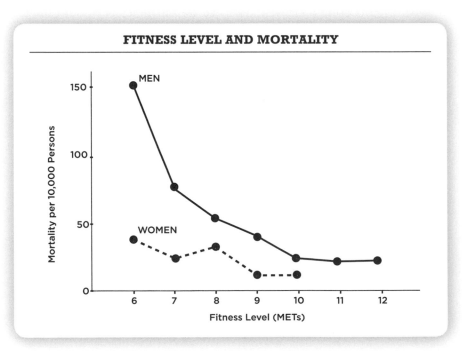

FITNESS LEVEL AND MORTALITY

> ## SPEAKING FROM EXPERIENCE
>
> It's not that hard to find beneficial physical activities of moderate intensity, which generally correspond to 3 to 6 METs. There are recreational activities—brisk walking (three to four miles per hour), biking, dancing fast, golf (pulling a cart or carrying clubs). There are also activities that are useful and productive—washing or waxing your car, washing windows, raking leaves and cutting the grass with a power mower. Numerous clinical trials have shown that a lifestyle approach to physical activity among previously sedentary people has similar effects on fitness, body fatness and coronary risk factors as a traditional structured exercise program.   **—B.F.**

More recently, researchers reported that exercise capacity more accurately predicts five-year mortality than does left ventricular ejection fraction, a key indicator of cardiac function, in heart attack survivors. Another study showed that aerobic fitness was a strong predictor of mortality in black and white men. Numerous studies also indicate that each 1-MET increase in exercise capacity confers an 8% to 17% reduction in mortality. Collectively, these findings indicate that assessment of exercise capacity (METs) can provide independent and additive information about cardiovascular risk, regardless of age, race, gender or health status.

Dr. Victor F. Froelicher, a world-renowned cardiologist at Stanford University Medical Center, explains it this way: "Aerobic capacity seems to be an independent predictor of mortality. A low exercise capacity of less than 4 METs indicates a higher mortality group, regardless of the underlying extent of coronary heart disease or cardiac impairment. On the other hand, an aerobic fitness level greater than 10 METs designates a group with excellent survival, regardless of their cardiac history."

AEROBIC CAPACITY: KNOW YOUR NUMBERS, KNOW YOUR RISK

Knowing your aerobic fitness level in METs is important in determining whether or not this cardiac marker is a risk for you. But being exercise-tested with a face mask can be an inconvenience, and the test itself requires complicated equipment, technical expertise and frequent calibration. So how can you estimate your fitness level in more practical ways?

One method is a simpler treadmill stress test that allows doctors to predict or estimate peak METs from the speed and grade or time achieved. The graph below illustrates one of the most common treadmill protocols, invented by Dr. Robert Bruce. The first stage of the conventional Bruce protocol starts at 1.7 miles per hour and 10% grade. Then, every three minutes, the speed and grade are increased until the subject exhibits abnormal signs or symptoms, suggesting that the test be stopped, or until the point of exhaustion for the subject. Needless to say, such tests should never be attempted without medical clearance, continuous electrocardiographic monitoring and the immediate availability of a physician.

A 50-year-old man who is able to achieve 9 minutes, or Stage 3, corresponding to 3.4 mph and 14% grade, has an estimated fitness level of 10 METs. This individual would be classified as "low risk." In contrast, the man who poops out after only 1½ minutes at Stage 1 would be classified as "high risk," suggesting that his mortality rate is greater than average.

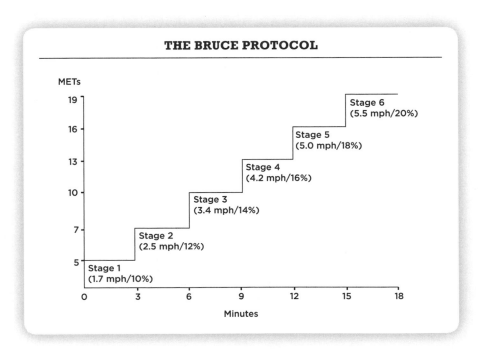

THE BRUCE PROTOCOL

METs

- 19 — Stage 6 (5.5 mph/20%)
- 16 — Stage 5 (5.0 mph/18%)
- 13 — Stage 4 (4.2 mph/16%)
- 10 — Stage 3 (3.4 mph/14%)
- 7 — Stage 2 (2.5 mph/12%)
- 5 — Stage 1 (1.7 mph/10%)

Minutes: 0 3 6 9 12 15 18

Although standard treadmill testing remains popular as a medical evaluation, it is quite costly (about $300 to $500 per test), time-consuming and not without risk.

Another method of estimating MET capacity is the use of a patient questionnaire like the Duke Activity Status Index shown below. For our purposes, the Duke questionnaire is a simple way to determine whether or not aerobic fitness is a marker that puts you at increased cardiovascular risk; if so, you may want to consult with your doctor about the appropriateness of a treadmill stress test. The key to the accuracy of this questionnaire lies in answering each of the questions as honestly as possible.

DUKE ACTIVITY STATUS INDEX

CAN YOU:	POINTS
1. Take care of yourself, i.e., eat, dress, bathe and use the toilet?	2.75
2. Walk indoors, as around your house?	1.75
3. Walk a block or two on level ground?	2.75
4. Climb a flight of stairs or walk up a hill?	5.50
5. Run a short distance?	8.00
6. Do light work around the house like dusting or washing dishes?	2.70
7. Do moderate work around the house like vacuuming, sweeping floors or carrying groceries?	3.50
8. Do heavy work around the house like scrubbing floors or lifting or moving heavy furniture?	8.00
9. Do yard work like raking leaves, weeding or pushing a power mower?	4.50
10. Have sexual relations?	5.25
11. Participate in moderate recreational activities like golf, bowling, dancing, doubles tennis or throwing a baseball or football?	6.00
12. Participate in strenuous sports like swimming, singles tennis, football, basketball or skiing?	7.50
Total points:	_____

Add up the points for each question to which you answered "yes." Your aerobic fitness, expressed as METs, can be approximated by using the following formula:

$$\text{METs} = (0.43 \times \text{total points} + 9.6) \text{ divided by } 3.5$$

As an example, if your total comes to 28.7 points, your equation would be: $0.43 \times 28.7 = 12.34 + 9.6 = 21.94$ divided by $3.5 = 6.26$ METs.

Now check your own MET level against the scale below:

AEROBIC FITNESS	MORTALITY RISK
4 or less	High
5 to 7	Average
8 or more	Low
Your METs: _____	Your risk: _____

Put simply, aerobically fit people generally live longer than their unfit counterparts. And it's not that hard to achieve. An exercise program can increase a sedentary person's maximal MET level by 10% to 30% in just three months. And most people who engage in only moderately intense exercise for at least 30 minutes a day can attain a cardioprotective fitness level of 8 to 10 METs or more.

9. Smoking

RESPONSIBLE FOR APPROXIMATELY 440,000 DEATHS ANNUALLY, smoking is the single most preventable cause of death in the United States. According to the American Lung Association, if a person starts smoking before age 20, each cigarette costs him or her at least 20 seconds of life. For the lifelong smoker, this means throwing away 10 to 14 years on average.

Most people assume that the greatest health risk from smoking is cancer. But while it's true that smoking leads to more than 150,000 cancer deaths each year, the impact of smoking on the risk of heart disease is much greater. Smoking contributes to about 40% of all cardiac deaths.

Smokers are twice as likely as nonsmokers to have a heart attack and are five times more likely to die from sudden cardiac death (SCD). In one study, the mortality from coronary heart disease in those smoking 25 or more cigarettes per day was nearly triple that of nonsmokers. It's the same for stroke. Results from the Harvard Physicians' Health Study of more than 22,000 doctors show that the risk of stroke among smokers is twice that of nonsmokers.

When combined with other risk factors such as high cholesterol or hypertension, the effect of smoking is compounded and lethal. Indeed, autopsy studies illustrate that coronary heart disease is far more severe and extensive in smokers than in nonsmokers. This increase is due to the inhalation of toxic compounds. A lighted cigarette gives off several hundred compounds, some in gaseous form and some in particles. The gases, which constitute 60% of cigarette smoke, include carbon monoxide, cyanide, ammonia, nitric acid, acetone and acrolein. The particulate compounds, inhaled as tar, produce ammonia, benzopyrene and at least 10 other known carcinogens, as well as the toxic chemical nicotine.

Studies point to carbon monoxide and nicotine as the chief culprits in producing coronary heart disease. Keep in mind that a single cigarette contains 640 times the amount of carbon monoxide that OSHA would allow in any industrial plant in the country, according to studies at UCLA by Drs. George Sieffert and Wesley Moore. Consider the following:

- As carbon monoxide (CO) moves through the bloodstream, artery walls become injured (pitted and cratered) and irritated. This causes inflammation, which increases cardiac risk.

- CO can irritate arteries to the point where they spasm and constrict, causing blood flow to be interrupted. This condition can also trigger malignant heart rhythms, causing sudden cardiac death. Cigarette smokers have two to four times the risk of SCD as nonsmokers.

- CO increases the heart rate, blood pressure and viscosity of blood, causing the platelets to become "sticky" and more reactive. Fibrinogen levels also transiently increase. The propensity to clot seriously increases the risk of heart attack.

55

■ Since smoking tends to reduce HDL cholesterol by up to 20% in regular smokers, it not only elevates risk but decreases protection as well.

The nicotine in cigarette smoke increases cardiac workload by increasing the heart rate by up to 15 to 25 beats a minute and raising blood pressure by 10 to 20 points. To maintain the increased workload, the heart needs more oxygen. In the blood of smokers, however, what's delivered is more nicotine and carbon monoxide. The consequence is an enormous strain on the cardiac muscle that can lead to a heart attack.

But there's hope for those who can give it up. Research shows that within two to three years of quitting, former smokers can markedly reduce their risk of heart attack and stroke. According to a recent landmark study, cessation at age 60, 50, 40 or 30 years gained, respectively, about 3, 6, 9 or 10 years of life expectancy.

SMOKING:
KNOW YOUR NUMBER, KNOW YOUR RISK

The risk of cardiac and other health problems increases with the number of cigarettes smoked and the length of time a person has been a smoker. But the reverse is also true. Risk can diminish with smoking reduction or cessation. The following scale approximates the cardiac risk from smoking:

CATEGORY	RISK
Non-tobacco user*	Optimal
Former tobacco user (at least four months tobacco-free)*	Lower
Cigar and/or pipe smoker or 1 to 10 cigarettes daily	Moderate
11 to 39 cigarettes daily	Higher
40 or more cigarettes daily	Extremely high
	Your risk:

*Nonsmoking is the only "recommended" category. All other categories place the individual at progressive levels of increased risk: the more cigarettes smoked, the greater the risk.

Choose Your Poison

Cigarettes pose the greatest smoking hazard, but other forms of tobacco are also injurious. Cigar and pipe smokers have a higher risk of heart disease than nonsmokers. This is probably due to the fact that they actually *do* inhale, even though many think they don't.

Smokeless tobacco is now used by millions of Americans, the largest percentage being young men who tend to think they're avoiding the health risks of cigarette smoking. The fact is that snuff and chewing tobacco contain nicotine, usually in more concentrated levels than in cigarette smoke. The body absorbs nicotine through the nasal passages and the lining of the mouth, rather than the lungs, but the result is the same: a kick in the heart rate and blood pressure, producing strain on the cardiac muscle. Smokeless tobacco, cigars and pipes also have deadly consequences, including lung, larynx, esophageal and oral cancer.

Secondhand smoke, or passive smoking, is another significant cardiac factor. A just-published study showed a dramatic drop (41%) in heart attack hospitalizations in the three years after the ban of workplace smoking in Pueblo, Colorado, took effect. There was no such drop in two neighboring areas, and researchers believe this is a clear sign that the ban was responsible. An earlier study at the University of California Medical School in San Francisco found that nonsmoking wives of cigarette smokers are three times more likely to suffer heart attacks than women whose husbands never smoked. Recent estimates suggest that approximately 35,000 nonsmokers die from heart disease each year as a result of exposure to environmental tobacco smoke.

10. Personality

IN RECENT YEARS, A NEW CARDIAC MARKER HAS ATTRACTED THE attention of both scientists and health professionals. Traditional cardiac markers such as smoking, high cholesterol and high blood pressure were found to account for about 80% of the heart attacks that occur in the United States, and these days research is being focused on a link between psychosocial variables—personality and behavior—and a rise in stress hormones that increase artery inflammation and blood pressure. Chronic stress, Type A personality (especially some of its components), anger/hostility, depression and social isolation not only have a direct negative influence on cardiac health, but also appear to increase the impact of the other, more traditional markers.

Chronic Stress

If there is a common element to modern life, it is that we are a hurried, harried and "stressed-out" society. Most people simply do not have enough time for their overcommitted, overscheduled and workaholic lives. Chronic stress hits everyone, from the mother trying to balance her personal and work life, to the elderly couple dealing with extensive medical bills, to the 55-year-old worker who has been "downsized," to the investor watching the stock market freefall, to the high schooler trying to get into an Ivy League college.

Unbridled stress has a significant influence on cardiac health. Its adverse effects include:

- Surges in heart rate and blood pressure
- Increases in cholesterol
- Promotion of artery wall inflammation
- Constriction of coronary arteries, which can result in heart attacks
- Heart rhythm irregularities, which can trigger sudden cardiac death
- Increases in blood clotting

In addition, people under stress tend to smoke, eat high-fat food and lead sedentary lives. If their weight goes up, which is likely, so do their triglycerides, BMI and waist circumference, as well as their chances of getting diabetes.

An eight-year study of day-of-the-week variations in heart attack incidence showed the incredible impact of stress. Significant peaks were found between 7 and 10 o'clock on Monday mornings, when the occurrence of heart attacks was 21% higher than during the rest of the week. The low was on Saturdays.

Acute emotional distress has also been implicated in the occurrence of heart attacks among people with coronary heart disease. Among individuals who return to work after a first heart attack, those with high chronic job strain had a twofold increase in the risk of recurrent coronary events over a six-year follow-up. Similar findings were noted in a comparison of the county coroner's records after the massive Los Angeles earthquake of 1994. On the day of the earthquake, there was a sharp increase in the number of sudden deaths from cardiac causes that were related to cardiovascular disease, from a daily average of 5 in the preceding week to 24 on the day of the earthquake.

PANIC ATTACKS

A study of 58,000 people with panic disorder found that it was associated with a 38% increase in the risk of heart attack.

Type A Personality

Type A personality, a behavior pattern associated with coronary heart disease and heart attack, was first identified in the 1960s by San Francisco doctors Meyer Friedman and Ray Rosenman, who saw it as an external manifestation of internal stress. Characteristically, Type A individuals are hard-driving competitors who feel that they have to do everything themselves. They are involved in an incessant struggle to accomplish more and more in less and less time against the perceived opposition of other people or things. They are combative, relentless "doers," impatiently steamrolling over any obstacles that may appear to stand in their way.

Type A people, who make up about 50% of the population, are often society's heroes and leaders—people who "get things done." The Western Collaborative Group Study found that the risk of heart attack was two times greater for a Type A than for a more relaxed Type B. However, numerous other studies have failed to confirm this association. Many experts now believe that particular components of Type A behavior—notably anger and hostility—are more closely linked to coronary artery disease than to Type A personality per se.

TYPE A:
KNOW YOUR PERSONALITY, KNOW YOUR RISK

A number of simple, effective tests have been developed to assess propensity for Type A behavior. A good example is the following self-scoring test, adapted from Dr. Andrew Goliszek's book *60 Second Stress Management*. This 30-question test asks you to describe yourself and your feelings on a rising scale (1 = never; 5 = always). The higher the total score, the greater the Type A tendency. While not clinically exact, this test will give a global representation of whether or not you exhibit Type A behavior.

TYPE A BEHAVIOR TEST

Read each statement below and grade yourself on how you would respond to each situation using the following:

1 = NEVER	2 = SELDOM	3 = SOMETIMES	4 = USUALLY	5 = ALWAYS

1. I become angry whenever I have to stand in line for more than 15 minutes. _____

2. I handle more than one problem at a time. _____

3. It's hard finding the time to relax and let myself go during the day. _____

4. I become irritated or annoyed when someone speaks too slowly. _____

5. I try hard to win at sports or games. _____

6. When I lose at sports or games, I get angry with myself and/or others. _____

7. I have trouble doing special things for myself. _____

8. I work much better under pressure or when I have to meet a deadline. _____

9. I find myself looking at my watch when I'm sitting around and not active. _____

10. I bring work home with me. _____

11. I feel energized and exhilarated after being in a pressure situation. _____

12. I feel like I need to take charge in order to get things moving. _____

13. I find myself eating quickly regardless of whether I have time or not. _____

14. I do things quickly regardless of whether I have time or not. _____

15. I interrupt what people are saying when I think they are wrong. _____

16. I'm inflexible and rigid when it comes to changes at work or at home. _____

17. I become jittery and need to move whenever I'm trying to relax. _____

18. I find myself eating faster than the people I'm eating with. _____

19. At work, I do more than one task at a time in order to feel productive. _____

20. I take less vacation time than I'm entitled to. _____

21. I find myself being very picky and looking at small details. _____

22. I become annoyed at people who don't work as hard as I do. _____

23. I find that there aren't enough things to do during the day. _____

24. I spend a good deal of my time thinking about my work. _____

25. I get bored very easily. _____

26. I'm active on weekends either working or doing projects. _____

27. I get into arguments with people who don't think my way. _____

28. I have trouble "rolling with the punches" whenever problems arise. _____

29. I interrupt someone's conversation in order to speed things up. _____

30. I take everything I do seriously. _____

Total: _____

SCORE	PERSONALITY TYPE
100 to 150	Type A
76 to 99	Type A/B
30 to 75	Type B

SPEAKING FROM EXPERIENCE

Looking back to the time before my bypass surgery in 1977, I can see that I demonstrated many of the classic characteristics of Type A personality:

■ **Feeling a great sense of urgency.** Time always seemed to slip away—I just never seemed to have enough of it. When the end of day came, I seldom had completed the 30 or 40 items that were on my daily "to do" list. (I actually used to cheat. I'd make a list in the morning that always included one or two things I'd already done. Then I could cross them out right away!) Type A's are always in a hurry, making a fetish of being punctual, and they're greatly annoyed if somebody keeps them waiting. I even used to set my watch ahead in order to induce more self-pressure to be on time. Several years ago, I read an article by Dr. Argir Kirkov Hadzhichristov, a Bulgarian doctor who studied people who live to be 100 or more. None of them wears a watch!

■ **Doing two or more things at once.** I would talk on the phone while signing letters, watch television while reading a book, and let my brain follow a completely different train of thought when I was chatting with someone.

■ **Acting as if I were constantly on deadline.** Type A's do everything fast. They even eat rapidly and will never linger at the dinner table. They dislike routine jobs at home because they think their time is too valuable. I used to show my impatience by interrupting people to answer questions before they were asked (a behavior I've worked hard to overcome). Type A's do not delegate well at all; if the job is not being done precisely as they would do it, they step in and take over.

Most health professionals do not believe that Type A behavior can be totally changed in a society that teaches it's better to wear out shoes than sheets, the early bird gets the worm and a man's reach should exceed his grasp. As long as our society views Type A behavior as a desirable personality trait, it will be encouraged. The basic problem, as Ralph Waldo Emerson wrote, is that "solitude is impractical and society is fatal."

Nonetheless, a decrease in the toxic elements of Type A behavior *is* attainable and well worth the effort in terms of cardiovascular health. In a study conducted at Stanford University, 600 cardiac patients received

- **Not being able to sit still.** I was constantly tapping and drumming my hands and feet. My speech was way too rapid, my words and gestures clipped, my smiles tense and tight. Type A's walk quickly and drive too fast. They just have to keep moving, preferably at top speed.
- **Measuring success in terms of numbers**—dollars, sales calls, size. The Type A's first thought upon seeing a Michelangelo painting will be: How much is it worth?
- **Turning hobbies into competitive events.** When my children were young, I built model cars for fun and relaxation. But then I entered a competition and won. Soon I was building more and more cars and competing every weekend! Type A's play to win, even with children. Some sons of Type A's reach adulthood without ever having beaten their fathers in a single game of one-on-one basketball. Winning is success; losing is disaster. As one psychologist warned, "Never enter a fun-run with Type A's. They will kill for a T-shirt or a blue ribbon."
- **Feeling guilty about relaxing and doing nothing.** Type A's take a briefcase on vacation or climb into a hammock with a sheaf of projects. And when at the beach or on a mountain peak, their overwhelming concern about starting back by a certain time will overshadow the beauty surrounding them.
- **Feeling insecure.** Type A's have a constant fear that sooner or later the time will come when they won't be able to cope in a given situation and will lose status in the eyes of people whose opinions matter to them. Fear of failure keeps them struggling to achieve more without ever savoring their accomplishments. **—J.P.**

intensive behavioral training to change Type A behavior—how to slow down, be more patient and have a more positive outlook—along with advice on diet and exercise. Only 12.9% of this group suffered a second heart attack. A second group of similar size received diet and exercise information only, with no instruction on modifying Type A behavior. More than 21% of this group experienced a second heart attack. A third group of 90 patients received no instruction at all; 32% had a second heart attack. Says Dr. Carl Thoresen, "This study clearly tells us that changing these destructive Type A habits can affect the chances of a second heart attack."

TYPE D BEHAVIOR

Historically, we've been concerned about the classic Type A personality, but now doctors are looking at the category called Type D, as in "distressed." Type D personalities demonstrate negative feelings about virtually everything. In other words, the glass is always half empty, never half full.

We've known that negative emotions, particularly depression, significantly increase the risk of developing heart disease while lowering long-term survival of cardiac patients. But studies now suggest that pessimistic people, "negative thinkers" who worry over trivial, everyday events, are more likely to have a heart attack than more positive thinkers. In contrast, people who are positive and optimistic have been reported to have less disease progression and faster recovery times after coronary bypass surgery.

Anger and Hostility

Are you the kind of person who becomes visibly upset when you're cut off in traffic by another car? Do you interrupt others mid-sentence or feel a flash of irritation when you're interrupted? Do you become enraged when someone yells into a cell phone right next to you or exceeds the maximum number of items permitted in the supermarket express line?

If so, accept the fact that these behaviors may be hazardous to your health. Duke University scientists have shown that hostile people—those with high levels of cynicism, anger and aggression—are at a much higher risk of developing heart disease and other chronic illnesses. Other researchers believe that dominant personality may also be problematic. "Having a dominant personality or a high level of irritability are two personality traits that make one prone to heart disease," says Dr. Aaron Wolfe Siegman. "We found that people with a dominant personality had a 47% higher risk of heart disease, and those easily irritated had a 27% increase in heart disease, compared with their less domineering, more easygoing counterparts. There is something about anger that thickens the walls of the heart and coronary arteries." These findings held true even after accounting for other risk factors including cholesterol, diabetes, obesity and smoking.

Feeling angry from time to time is normal. Things happen in life that make us mad. Some people express anger readily, shouting loudly and gesturing wildly at the slow driver in the fast freeway lane. Others fume silently over perceived slights. When anger is incurred by a specific event (as opposed to things in general) and is appropriate (a modest level for a moderate amount of time), then it usually is not a health risk. But if anger surfaces too frequently, too intensely and lasts too long each time it makes its presence felt, and if chronic hostility begins to take on the look of a personality trait, a commensurate rise in health risk is triggered, particularly for cardiovascular disease. Getting so angry that your "blood boils," it seems, may stress your heart and over time cause your arteries to clog, too.

Anger triggers a variety of physiological responses. When you're angry, your muscles tense, your breathing becomes shallow and rapid, your heart races and your blood pressure rises. In addition, stress chemicals such as epinephrine are released into the bloodstream. All these responses are normal. But if anger is chronic, it can penalize your heart, particularly if you already have coronary artery disease.

Heart attack risk is almost three times greater in people with high levels of anger than in those who control it. A study directed by Dr. Peter

WOMEN AND ANGER

Generally, men tend to get angry, blow up, get it over with and move on. Women often avoid anger or pretend it's not there, and this "anger diversion" actually creates more stress.

According to Dr. Deborah Cox, women divert anger by containing it, biting their tongue to keep from saying what they feel. "Women also internalize anger by absorbing guilt and blame meant for others with whom they're angry," says Dr. Cox. "If we feel unable to talk directly about anger to the person with whom we're angry, the next most likely target is ourselves." Many women become so afraid of their own anger that they lose their ability to know when they're angry.

And finally, some women externalize their anger by abusing and insulting others. While this may seem like a way to "get anger out," spilling it irresponsibly onto others—particularly children—is never a productive response.

Angerer of the University of Munich in Germany followed 150 people with diseased arteries and found that over a two-year period the subjects who reported high levels of expressed anger, particularly those with low levels of social support, were significantly more likely to have their coronary heart disease worsen. In addition, Dr. Murray Mittleman and associates at Beth Israel Deaconess Medical Center in Boston reported that the risk of a heart attack increased in the two hours following an episode of anger, suggesting that anger was a trigger that doubled and even tripled the risk of heart attack.

How does chronic anger penalize the heart? No one is certain, but it is thought that high levels of stress hormones injure the coronary artery walls and over time provide deposit sites for artery-clogging cholesterol. These hormones can also stimulate arterial inflammation, blood clotting and high blood pressure, and evoke potentially lethal heart rhythms.

ANGER AND HOSTILITY: KNOW YOUR PERSONALITY, KNOW YOUR RISK

The following test, from the Arnot Ogden Medical Center, will help you to assess your general tendency to "fly off the handle." You will score a value of "1" if the statement is never true for you, "2" if it's rarely or sometimes true, "3" if it's often true and "4" if it's always true. Circle the appropriate number and add up your scores to find your total.

NEVER	RARELY	OFTEN	ALWAYS
1	2	3	4
It doesn't take much to get me mad.			
1	2	3	4
People tell me I should calm down.			
1	2	3	4
I blow up at terrible drivers.			
1	2	3	4
If I am upset, I'll take it out on the dog or the cat.			

1	2	3	4

People call me hotheaded.

1	2	3	4

I'm furious about the way I get treated at restaurants or stores.

1	2	3	4

When others' mistakes slow me down, I'm upset all day.

1	2	3	4

If the situation is bad enough, I'll throw things.

1	2	3	4

I swear loudly to blow off steam.

1	2	3	4

I feel like hitting someone who makes me very angry.

1	2	3	4

I've been told I have a bad temper.

1	2	3	4

If you embarrass me in front of someone, I'll be furious.

1	2	3	4

I'm a very ambitious person, so sometimes I get impatient
and angry with other people.

1	2	3	4

I've been known to break things when I'm frustrated.

If you scored 18 or below on this test, you have a high temper threshold and are able to stay calm in situations that would frustrate many others. This is a big help in managing your stress levels. If you scored 19 to 27, you get angry about as often as most other people. If you scored 28 to 35, there's a good possibility that you're under too much stress, or it may be that getting angry has become a habit; take this score seriously and begin to make changes now, before it adversely affects your health.

If you scored over 35 on the test and continue with the same behaviors and attitudes, you risk serious stress-related disease. It may be helpful to speak to a counselor about ways to deal with your anger.

Depression

Doctors have associated heart attacks and clinical depression for some time, usually in that sequence. After all, who wouldn't be depressed after a heart attack? But new research is showing that depression may actually be a *cause* of the attack.

- Depression has been reported to precede a heart attack in up to 50% of cases.

- Depression has also been associated with an increased number of cardiovascular events after an initial heart attack or following coronary bypass surgery. In two landmark studies, patients who were depressed were three to five times more likely to die during the first year after suffering a heart attack than were nondepressed patients.

- A study of about 4,500 elderly people free of coronary disease found that the risk of heart disease and death increased by 40% and 60%, respectively, for those who became depressed when compared with those who did not become depressed.

- Scientists at the Johns Hopkins Medical Centers found that, all else being equal, people who have some depression symptoms are twice as likely to suffer heart attacks as those with no symptoms, and people diagnosed with major depression were 4.5 times as likely.

- After a person suffers angina or a heart attack, depression is a better predictor of prognosis than many other known risk factors for heart disease.

- According to a recent report, depression produces a greater decrement in health than many chronic diseases, including anginal chest pain. However, the presence of depression and any medical condition incrementally worsens that condition. The bottom line? Depression is very disabling.

One reason for the link between depression and cardiac risk is that depression contributes to poor lifestyle choices. Depressed people are more apt to eat poorly, be sedentary, drink, smoke and use drugs. Depressed heart patients are also less likely to see their physician or take prescribed medications. "It may also be that stress hormones play a role," says clinical psychologist Dr. Judith Schwartzman. "Depression can be thought of as an extreme and prolonged response to stress. Many of the physiological changes that happen when you are in fight-or-flight mode, such as an increase in cortisol, also happen when you are depressed." Heart disease and depression may have common origins. "You get mood changes with heart disease," says Dr. Schwartzman. "And people also often experience something called vital exhaustion, which essentially means they're worn out, shortly before heart disease surfaces. But is it a symptom of early heart disease or of depression? It could be either."

On the positive side, people with depression symptoms who have had one heart attack can greatly reduce their chance of a second heart attack by managing stress. "We found that people who walked regularly as a stress dissipation technique after an initial heart attack benefited from the exercise and the social contact and support," says Dr. François Lesperance of the Montreal Heart Institute. "Lack of walking is a symptom of more severe depression. The coronary survivor's true best friend is a dog. Then he'd have to be out walking about an hour a day."

Nearly a decade ago, investigators in the Standard Medical Intervention and Long-Term Exercise (SMILE) Study reported on 156

HIGH ANXIETY

Intense psychological stress resulting from high anxiety levels can cause alterations of the heart's rhythm and trigger sudden cardiac death. Data show that men who have high anxiety levels are up to six times more likely to experience sudden cardiac death than are men of calmer disposition. That's twice the increased risk of sudden cardiac death from smoking.

Anxiety is an inappropriate manifestation of one of our most ancient instincts—to flee danger when it confronts us. Just how it increases cardiac risk remains unclear, but researchers hypothesize that anxiety triggers a host of physiological responses, including increased heart rate and blood pressure. What makes anxiety a medical condition is its presence in the absence of any real danger.

patients with major depression who were randomly assigned to three groups: those who received exercise training, those who received drug treatment and those who received both. Most of the patients demonstrated a reduction in depressive symptoms, with no significant group differences at the end of four months of treatment. Patients who continued to exercise on their own tended to maintain their improvement.

DEPRESSION:
KNOW YOUR PERSONALITY, KNOW YOUR RISK

How do you know if depression is a problem for you? The following screening test, adapted from the Harvard Department of Psychiatry National Depression Screening Day Scale, commonly called the HANDS™ questionnaire, is designed to help identify individuals who are likely to be suffering from a depressive disorder that may require treatment.

DEPRESSION SCREENING TEST

1. I feel sad most of the time.	Yes _____	No _____
2. I don't enjoy the things I used to.	Yes _____	No _____
3. I sleep too little or too much.	Yes _____	No _____
4. I don't feel like eating or I eat too much.	Yes _____	No _____
5. I can't make decisions.	Yes _____	No _____
6. I have difficulty concentrating.	Yes _____	No _____
7. I feel hopeless.	Yes _____	No _____
8. I feel worthless.	Yes _____	No _____
9. I get tired for no reason.	Yes _____	No _____
10. I think about killing myself.	Yes _____	No _____

Scoring: If you answered "yes" to four or more of these questions, *and you have felt this way every day for two weeks or more,* you may be suffering from clinical depression and should consult a health care professional for a complete evaluation. If you answered "yes" to question 10, seek help immediately, regardless of your answer to any of the other questions.

DEPRESSION AND GENDER

According to a study published in the *International Journal of Psychiatry in Medicine,* women tend to report symptoms of depression in the following order: self-disappointment, irritability, hopelessness, dissatisfaction, sleep difficulties. Men tend to report symptoms in this order: dissatisfaction, difficulties completing work, fatigue, irritability, hopelessness, self-disappointment.

Social Isolation

Numerous studies show higher cardiovascular death rates among people who are socially isolated. One of the first studies to identify the importance of social networks in buffering the deleterious effects of heart disease involved a small town in eastern Pennsylvania called Roseto. Health researchers were startled to find a strikingly lower death rate there than in neighboring towns. From 1955 to 1961, Roseto had 157 cardiovascular deaths per 100,000 population, while three neighboring towns averaged over 600 cardiovascular deaths. After careful analysis, researchers concluded that social support and close family ties were the primary reasons for Roseto's lower rate. They also predicted that, over time, social ties would diminish and cardiovascular death rates would rise, a prediction that proved true over the next 20 years.

Since the Roseto report, a number of scientific investigations have confirmed this effect. For example, a six-month mortality rate of 16% was noted among patients who lived alone after their heart attack versus 9% for those living with others.

Another study of more than 1,300 cardiac patients, conducted at Duke University by Dr. Redford Williams and colleagues, showed that married patients with heart disease fared far better than their unmarried counterparts. But the people with the highest death rate were unmarried patients who had no close family or friends. These patients had a five-year survival rate of just 50%, compared with 83% for those who had a spouse, a confidant, or both.

It remains unclear how social isolation harms health. Perhaps lonely people are less likely to get rapid medical assistance. Another possibility is that those without social ties may not seek medical attention, take prescribed medications or be encouraged to follow their doctors' advice. Or it may be that social isolation produces an injurious mental and physical effect. Much research is still to be done. Then again, there may be a lot more to Barbra Streisand's contention that "people who need people are the luckiest people in the world."

PSYCHOLOGICAL RISK FACTORS: POTENTIAL LINKS TO CARDIOVASCULAR DISEASE

Psychological risk factors may not, by themselves, have direct effects on the atherosclerotic disease process. Nevertheless, these risk factors may worsen or exacerbate the development of heart disease by two pathways: 1) encouraging unhealthy behaviors such as cigarette smoking, sedentary living, eating foods that are high in calories and/or fat, and increased alcohol intake; and 2) eliciting physiologic responses that may lead to various clinical consequences, including insufficient blood flow to the heart, threatening heart rhythms, more vulnerable plaque, and the potential for blood clotting.

Unfortunately, the influence of psychosocial risk factors on cardiovascular morbidity and mortality remains underrecognized compared with conventional risk factors. Recognizing this relationship offers an important target for cardiovascular education, counseling, and behavioral interventions, even after controlling for major risk factors. This focus should serve to maximize the potential for cardiovascular risk reduction by addressing at least a portion of the 10% to 25% incidence of heart disease that is unexplained. Although the incidence of disease due to psychosocial risk factors is small compared with established cardiovascular risk factors, it is an important public health problem because of the enormous number of people affected by heart disease and because of the exaggerated responses to these stressors over time.

Your Cardiac Marker Profile

The first step is to take all the information you've gained about yourself in relation to the 10 controllable heart-health markers and create your own risk profile. Individually and in concert, these markers wield considerable influence over your cardiac destiny.

Recommended marker values (identified by asterisks) reflect the optimal levels, representing the lowest cardiac risk. It's important to understand that these values are not hard-and-fast. We cannot say that people with a total cholesterol of 240 will definitely have a heart attack any more than we can label people with a cholesterol of 199 as "home free." But cardiac risk *is* greater for the individual with the higher cholesterol number. And that's why your cardiac marker profile is so significant—it can help you evaluate your own risks.

1. CHOLESTEROL AND OTHER LIPIDS/LIPOPROTEINS

TOTAL CHOLESTEROL	RISK
Below 200 mg/dl*	Desirable
200 to 239 mg/dl	Borderline high
240 mg/dl and above	High
Your number:	Your risk:

LDL CHOLESTEROL	RISK
Below 100 mg/dl*	Optimal
100 to 129 mg/dl*	Near optimal
130 to 159 mg/dl	Borderline high
160 to 189 mg/dl	High
190 mg/dl and above	Very High
Your number:	Your risk:

HDL CHOLESTEROL	RISK
60 mg/dl and above*	Low
40 to 59 mg/dl	Moderate
Below 40 mg/dl	High
Your number:	Your risk:

TRIGLYCERIDES	RISK
Below 150 mg/dl*	Desirable
150 to 199 mg/dl	Borderline high
200 to 499 mg/dl	High
500 mg/dl and above	Very high
Your number:	Your risk:

2. CORONARY INFLAMMATION

C-REACTIVE PROTEIN	RISK
Below 0.70 mg/dl*	Lowest
0.70 to 1.1 mg/dl	Low
1.2 to 1.9 mg/dl	Average
2.0 to 3.8 mg/dl	Higher
3.9 to 15.0 mg/dl	Highest
Your number:	Your risk:

PLAC	RISK
Below 160*	Very low
160 to 199 ng/ml	Low
200 to 235 ng/ml	Moderate
Above 235 ng/ml	High
Your number:	Your risk:

3. BLOOD CLOTTING

FIBRINOGEN	RISK
Below 200 mg/dl*	Desirable
200 to 400 mg/dl	Borderline high
Above 400 mg/dl	High
Your number:	Your risk:

4. WEIGHT

BODY MASS INDEX	RISK
19 to 24.9	Desirable
25 to 29.9	Borderline high
30 to 39.9	High
40 or more	Very high
Your number:	Your risk:

WAIST CIRCUMFERENCE	RISK
Men Less than 40 inches*	Lower
40 inches or more	Higher
Women Less than 35 inches*	Lower
35 inches or more	Higher
Your number: _____	Your risk: _____

5. BLOOD PRESSURE

SYSTOLIC	DIASTOLIC	RISK
Below 120 mm Hg*	Below 80 mm Hg*	Normal
120 to 139 mm Hg*	80 to 89 mm Hg*	Prehypertensive
140 to 159 mm Hg	90 to 99 mm Hg	Stage 1 hypertension
160 mm Hg and above	100 mm Hg and above	Stage 2 hypertension
Your number: _____	Your risk: _____	

6. DIABETES

FASTING GLUCOSE	RISK
Below 100 mg/dl*	Desirable
100 to 125 mg/dl	Borderline high
126 mg/dl and above	Confirmed diabetes
Your number: _____	Your risk: _____

7. METABOLIC SYNDROME

FACTORS

Is your HDL number below 40 (men) or below 50 (women)?	Yes _____	No _____

FACTORS

Is your triglyceride number over 150?	Yes _____	No _____
Is your waist size 35 inches and above (women) or 40 inches and above (men)?	Yes _____	No _____
Is your blood pressure consistently 130/85 or higher?	Yes _____	No _____
Are you a diabetic or prediabetic (a fasting glucose of 100 or higher)?	Yes _____	No _____

"YES" ANSWERS	RISK
None*	Desirable
1 to 2	Borderline high
3 to 5	Confirmed metabolic syndrome
Your number: _____	Your risk: _____

8. AEROBIC CAPACITY

MET LEVEL	RISK
(Treadmill testing or calculated from the Duke Activity Status Index)	
4 METs or less	High
5 to 7 METs	Average
8 METs or higher*	Low
Your number: _____	Your risk: _____

9. SMOKING

CATEGORY	RISK
Non-tobacco user*	Optimal
Former tobacco user* (at least 4 months tobacco-free)	Lower
Cigar and/or pipe smoker or 1 to 10 cigarettes daily	Moderate
11 to 39 cigarettes daily	Higher
40 or more cigarettes daily	Extremely high
Your number: _____	Your risk: _____

10. PERSONALITY

TYPE A PROFILE TEST SCORE	PERSONALITY TYPE
100 to 150	Type A
76 to 99*	Type A/B
30 to 75	Type B
Your number: _____	Your personality: _____

There is presently insufficient data to categorically link heart disease with a specific personality type. Not all Type A's have heart attacks; not all Type B's are free of heart disease.

However, the consensus is that people with Type A personality (especially certain components, e.g., anger/hostility) are at increased risk and should be considered as such for the purposes of this assessment.

ANGER PROFILE TEST SCORE	LEVEL OF ANGER
18 or less*	Desirable
19 to 27	Average
28 to 35	High
36 and above	Severe
Your number:	Your anger level:

As with Type A personality, there is insufficient data to link numeric results from the anger profile test to incidence of heart disease. However, some experts believe that high and severe levels of anger demonstrate increased cardiovascular risk, and that is how you should evaluate your score for the purposes of this assessment.

DEPRESSION TEST SCORE (HANDS QUESTIONNAIRE)	RISK
Below 4*	Average
4 or higher	Elevated
Your number:	Your risk:

NOTE: Another assessment, using several of these markers, for calculating the risk of developing heart disease over the next 10 years can be obtained using estimates of the Framingham Risk Score. It is available on the NHLBI website (www.nhlbi.nih.gov) and has been validated in white and black men and women without known heart disease.

YOUR ASSESSMENT SUMMARY

CRITICAL MARKERS	Is this a risk for you?	
	YES	NO
Total cholesterol		
LDL cholesterol		
HDL cholesterol		
Triglycerides		
C-reactive protein		
PLAC		
Fibrinogen		
Body mass index (BMI)		
Waist circumference		
Blood pressure		
Diabetes		
Metabolic syndrome		
Aerobic capacity		
Smoking		
Type A personality		
Anger		
Depression		

Time for Action

IRST OFF, DON'T PANIC. If your profile exceeds the recommended values in any category—that is, if you've identified a risk—keep in mind that you can make things better simply by taking action. Remember, each step you take is a step in the right direction. According to the Harvard Nurses' Health Study, published in the *New England Journal of Medicine*, as many as four out of five heart attacks could be prevented if people followed a heart-healthy lifestyle.

But how to do that? To start with, the most important thing you can do is make the commitment. On the following pages you'll find the first 13 Heart Savers, designed to help you mitigate your risks. Read them carefully. Take them to heart. Decide to control your destiny.

Lower Your Cholesterol Numbers

If your total cholesterol is 200 or above, it's too high and you need to take action to bring it down. Many experts now recommend a value below 160, especially if you've had a heart attack, bypass surgery or angioplasty procedure. A healthy diet is the first line of defense, complemented by drug therapy if appropriate. Center your diet on foods that can lower cholesterol, such as fish high in omega-3 fatty acids and whole grains and vegetables rich in soluble fiber. Limit foods rich in saturated fat (red meat, for example, and whole-milk dairy products) and trans fat (as in hydrogenated margarine). At one time, the American Heart Association (AHA) recommended a diet of no more than 30% of calories from fat, but today the emphasis is on reducing saturated and trans fats. The AHA now says you can get up to 35% of your total calories from fat (unless overweight is an issue), but less than 7% of these calories should come from saturated fat and less than 1% from trans fats. Cholesterol should be limited to less than 300 milligrams per day.

Some experts still advise a diet lower in total fat for cardiac health. Dr. Dean Ornish, among others, suggests a less than 10%-fat diet—

certainly effective in bringing down cholesterol but very difficult to follow. Dr. Gerhard Schuler of Heidelberg University in Germany recommends more moderate fat levels. "A 20%-fat diet lowers cholesterol," he says, "and is much easier to achieve in the real world."

If diet and exercise do not improve your cholesterol after six months, it may be time to consider drug therapy. Some of the most widely used cholesterol-lowering medications include statin drugs, bile acid sequestrants and nicotinic acid. (See pages 312–320 for more information.) One study of more than 6,000 subjects was cut short a year before its intended end date because those receiving a statin drug had a 40% lower incidence of heart attacks. According to Dr. William C. Roberts, "Statin drugs are to atherosclerosis what penicillin was to infectious diseases." Talk with your doctor about the pros and cons of cholesterol-lowering drugs.

Reduce Your LDL Level

Get your LDL level as low as you can, ideally below 100.

For individuals with known heart disease, further reduction of LDL cholesterol to below 70 is reasonable. Again, the first line of defense is dietary change. Step 4 of our protocol offers numerous tips for modifying your diet, but to begin with, here are some simple yet effective ways to get your LDL level under control:

- Moderate caloric intake and increase physical activity to lose weight. Weight loss (5% to 10% of body weight) and regular exercise training (1,000 to 2,000 calories per week) have each been shown to reduce LDL cholesterol by 5% to 15%.

- Cut down on foods rich in saturated fat, trans fat and dietary cholesterol (all animal foods).

- Increase foods rich in complex carbohydrates (such as fruits and vegetables), soluble fiber (oat bran, oatmeal and beans), bioflavonoids (strawberries and eggplant), antioxidants (foods high in vitamins C and E and beta-carotene), vitamin D (fat-free milk) and sterol or sterol esters (Smart Balance, Take Control, Benecol and other cholesterol-lowering margarines and yogurts).

- Substitute soy protein for animal protein. Studies suggest that this could lower LDL and total cholesterol by 8% and 9%, respectively.
- Increase consumption of omega-3 fatty acids in the form of fish, especially oily fish, two or more times each week.

In addition, you may want to talk to your doctor about drug therapy, particularly statins. Many doctors are now recommending that heart patients and others at high risk immediately start drug therapy along with dietary changes. Depending on the drug and dosage, statins typically reduce LDL cholesterol by 27% to 60%. Studies confirm that statins also reduce the risks of heart attack, stroke, bypass surgery or balloon angioplasty by 20% to 30% with minimal side effects.

Increase Your HDL Level

Exercise, moderate alcohol consumption, losing weight and drug therapy all can increase your HDL (much more on those later), but here's a preview of what you should know:

- Exercise, exercise, exercise! A regular program of exercise is effective in boosting HDL concentration. Researchers at Stanford University reported that approximately 1,000 calories of additional energy expenditure—equivalent to walking or running 8 to 10 miles weekly—may represent the "threshold" exercise dosage required for increasing HDL cholesterol. So, first see your doctor about an exercise program, then get started.
- Moderate alcohol consumption has been shown to boost HDL. The key is "moderate," since the risks of heavy drinking (increased triglycerides, hypertension, cancer, stroke, liver disease, accidents) outweigh the potential cardiac benefits. Limit alcohol consumption to two drinks per day for men and one per day for women, ideally with meals. The Brigham and Women's Harvard Study found that the form of alcohol you drink doesn't matter; wine, beer and hard liquor have equally beneficial effects on raising HDL cholesterol.
- Lose weight if you're overweight. Choose monounsaturated oils (such as olive oil) over polyunsaturated oils (such as corn oil) and saturated fats.

- Quit smoking!
- Drug therapy can be effective. Niacin, many statin drugs and gemfibrozil (Lopid) have been shown to modestly elevate HDL. The best counsel if your HDL is low is to talk to your doctor about an appropriate course of action.

Bring Down Your Triglycerides

There are many ways to lower your triglyceride level: moderate your caloric intake; cut down on foods rich in sugar, saturated fat and trans fat; increase your consumption of fish and healthful oils; eat foods rich in fiber; restrict alcohol; exercise regularly; don't smoke; and utilize drug therapy if necessary. The message is familiar, but here are some additional facts to consider:

- Most studies report reduced triglycerides (approximately 20%) after a single aerobic exercise session. These beneficial reductions usually occur 24 hours after exercise and can last up to 72 hours postexercise. Even a modest weight loss (e.g., 5% to 10% of body weight) can reduce triglycerides by as much as 30%.
- In this case, some fats are good—notably the omega-3 fatty acids found in salmon, sardines and tuna.
- Drug therapy has proven effective. If your triglycerides are above 500, you're likely to have a high rate of cardiovascular complications and are at risk of developing acute pancreatitis, a serious inflammatory condition. Confer with your doctor about medication. Niacin, fibric acid derivatives such as gemfibrozil (Lopid) and fenofibrate (Tricor) and statin drugs can help.
- If your triglycerides are above 200, non-HDL cholesterol should be less than 130, if possible.

Manage Your CRP Level

If your levels of C-reactive protein (CRP) are high, you have to first cover the basics. Eat a low-fat diet, control your cholesterol and other lipids, stop smoking, lose weight if needed, control your blood pressure and any diabetes, manage stress and, very important, exercise regularly. A study from Finland showed that moderate-intensity exercise can reduce levels of CRP. Men in the exercise group showed a 16% reduction in CRP, compared with a 2% reduction in the sedentary control group. Several investigations, including data from the Aerobics Center Longitudinal Study, have now shown that fitness levels in men and women are inversely related to CRP levels and the prevalence of elevated CRP values.

Beyond these considerations, aspirin therapy has been found to be very effective as an anti-inflammatory agent, and several studies now suggest that statin drugs may lower CRP levels. For example, the Cholesterol and Recurrent Events Trial showed that pravastatin (Pravachol) lowered CRP and reduced cardiac events independent of its cholesterol-lowering effects. These trial findings lend support to the notion that statin drugs may confer cardioprotective benefits that go well beyond their cholesterol-lowering ability. See your doctor about treatment options.

If the inflammatory process is in fact a causative factor in heart disease, the treatment of America's number one killer could change dramatically. In the future, it's possible that patients might be treated with antibiotics to prevent infections that cause inflammation and that CRP levels might be routinely measured to assess coronary risk. It should be emphasized, however, that other medical conditions, unrelated to cardiovascular disease, can cause acute elevations in CRP.

Lower Your PLAC Level

New results from numerous major clinical trials show that when measured approximately 30 days after an acute coronary event such as angina or heart attack, elevated levels of lipoprotein-associated phospholipase A_2 (PLAC) are a novel risk marker for death or recurrent cardiovascular events. The data acquired by this marker, obtained via a simple nonfasting blood sample (called a PLAC test), provides independent and additive information to that obtained from traditional risk factors such as LDL cholesterol and C-reactive protein.

If your PLAC test reveals an elevated level, your doctor may prescribe lifestyle changes such as an aerobic exercise program and/or a low-calorie, low-fat diet, with or without prescription medications. Statins alone or the combination of a statin and niacin have been shown to reduce PLAC by approximately 30% and 50%, respectively. Darapladib is the first agent in a new class of drugs under clinical development that inhibit PLAC. In one randomized clinical trial of nearly 1,000 coronary patients, darapladib reduced PLAC by more than 50% when compared with a look-alike placebo pill. Trials to establish if this outcome reduces mortality or stabilizes high-risk coronary plaque are currently under way.

Control Your Fibrinogen Level

At this time, there are no established medical treatments for lowering fibrinogen, but if your classification is borderline or high, it makes sense to take normal risk-reducing steps (such as changes in diet and exercise). You should also discuss antiplatelet agents/anticoagulant therapy with your doctor. Aspirin and/or clopidogrel (Plavix) lessen the chance of clots forming and blocking narrowed arteries.

Keep Your Weight Down

While excess weight can cause cardiac risk to soar, maintaining an ideal body weight can reduce heart disease risk by an amazing 35% to 55%. If that's not inspiration enough, note that even a 10% loss of body weight can provide major health benefits in overweight and obese individuals.

A huge chunk of this book is devoted to helping you devise a plan of eating for a lifetime. But before you get started, it's important to understand that it is not "weight" that you want to lose, but extra "body fat." Theoretically at least, losing body fat is pretty simple. You must burn more calories than you take in—3,500 calories per pound of body fat, to be exact. In other words, if you can cut 500 calories a day, you'll lose a pound a week. You can do that by reducing your caloric intake, increasing calories burned in exercise, or both.

Here's a preview of what you should know before making the decision to start a diet:

■ **Don't crash-diet.** Fads like the "high-protein" diets might help you lose a few pounds in the short run, but they may not be safe for your heart. Many are exceptionally high in fat, including the dangerous artery-clogging saturated fat that can greatly accelerate your risk of heart disease. In addition, crash diets do not work in the long run; such diets may ultimately cause you to regain lost weight and even put on more pounds.

■ **Don't rely on "fat-burning" products** that promise to melt pounds without exercise or dietary change, even if endorsed by celebrities. These people get paid very well for their testimonials. If it's too good to believe, it probably means it doesn't work.

■ **Develop an active lifestyle.** For weight reduction, the American College of Sports Medicine recommends 200 to 300 minutes of moderate-to-vigorous exercise per week, or approximately 45 minutes per day. Other major organizations now suggest 60 to 90 minutes of moderate-intensity activity per day to prevent weight gain or weight regain in formerly obese individuals. This amount of exercise can be

SPEAKING FROM EXPERIENCE

It seems that there's a new weight-loss diet or product introduced every day—rubber suits, metabolic powders, diet books, even machines that exercise for you! With so many such products, you'd think America would be a nation of skinny folks. Instead, we're fatter than ever. The truth is that fad diets and fast-weight-loss programs seldom lead to long-term success in weight control. And they often can be a health hazard. I think most people know in their heart of hearts that controlling weight for a lifetime requires more than dieting. Weight control takes a change in behavior, a commitment to being physically active, a new way of eating and dealing with stress effectively. These are lifetime goals, not just something to do for a week or two. **—J.P.**

accumulated in shorter bouts of physical activity (10 to 15 minutes) throughout the day. Adding strength training to exercise programs can further increase metabolism.

- **Watch ballooning portion size.** A recent study showed that, compared with the mid-1950s, portion sizes and calories for many foods have tripled! Says Dr. Brian Wansink of Cornell University, "We are seeing portion distortion, especially in restaurants. . . . Studies show that 67% of Americans eat everything on their plates, no matter what the size. Supersizing has gotten to the point where many can't remember what's a normal serving size."

- **Plan sit-down meals.** Don't rush.

- **Drink five to eight glasses of water daily.** Avoid high-calorie drinks such as soft drinks, sugared juices and certain alcoholic beverages. Using the Framingham Heart Study database, researchers recently reported that drinking more than one soft drink daily was associated with a higher risk of developing obesity and other risk factors for heart disease. Interestingly, it didn't matter if the soda consumption was regular or diet!

- **Keep a food journal.** People eat less when they account for it in writing.

- **Take your time.** One to two pounds of body-fat loss per week doesn't sound like much, but it adds up to success.

- **Don't eat while you're watching television.** Studies show that people who are distracted while they're eating tend to consume more calories.

- **Limit eating out.** Increasing research suggests that haste makes waists. Recognize that restaurant meals tend to be higher in fat and calories than foods prepared at home. A recent study showed that children consume nearly twice as many calories at restaurants as they do during meals at home.

- **Get more sleep.** Numerous studies now show that people who get less than seven hours of sleep a night are more likely to be overweight or obese. Those who average less than four hours per night are at the greatest risk for weight problems. Why? "Night owls" are generally engaged in sedentary activities (television, computer interactions) while simultaneously eating and/or drinking. Researchers also believe that this may be attributed, at least in part, to hormone imbalances. For example, people who are sleep-deprived have insulin and blood sugar levels that are similar to those found in diabetics. Others have reported that people who do not get enough sleep seem to have high levels of ghrelin and low levels of leptin, both of which can cause hunger and trigger eating.

Monitor Your Blood Pressure

Fewer than 5% of patients with hypertension have a definable cause. Genetics plays a part, since hypertension can be inherited, but lifestyle is much more important. Sometimes high blood pressure develops or is made worse by certain over-the-counter medications like decongestants, diet pills and nonsteroidal anti-inflammatory drugs such as ibuprofen. Overweight and obesity are critical indicators. So is excessive salt intake, because too much salt can cause the body to retain too much fluid, increasing blood volume and raising pressure because the heart is working harder. The caffeine in coffee can also cause an increase in blood pressure.

On the other hand, healthy eating promotes control. Several years ago, researchers demonstrated that the DASH eating plan, including a diet rich in fruits, vegetables and low-fat dairy products with reduced levels of saturated and total fat, could decrease systolic blood pressure by 8 to 14 points. The investigators emphasized that the reduction in blood pressure was similar to that commonly reported with single drug therapy!

Chronic emotional stress is another factor that can cause blood pressure to rise. When you're under stress, your arterioles narrow, causing a temporary increase in blood pressure. When stress is occasional, such an increase usually does not present a health problem. But when stressful events take place too frequently, stress hormones continue to constrict arterioles and send blood pressure upward. Studies by Dr. Robert S. Eliot, author of *Is It Worth Dying For Anyway?*, show that about 20% of Americans can be classified as "hot reactors" who respond to chronic stress with skyrocketing blood pressure. Over time, the result can be higher blood pressure.

Excessive alcohol consumption is also a factor. A 12-year study of 325 Japanese men, all of whom had normal blood pressure at the start, found that those who drank the most had nearly twice the risk of high blood pressure as nondrinkers. Light drinkers had the lowest risk, demonstrating once again the power of moderation.

If lifestyle modifications do not sufficiently reduce blood pressure, you may want to consult with your doctor about drug therapy. Some medications help relax and dilate vessels to facilitate blood flow. Others can lower heart rate or help eliminate excessive fluid and salt. Commonly recommended drugs include diuretics, beta-blockers, calcium channel-blockers, ACE inhibitors and vasodilators. The choice of medication depends on the individual and other medical conditions that may be present. Another important consideration is which drug(s) lower blood pressure effectively with the fewest side effects. If drug therapy is appropriate, be sure to take your medication regularly.

Deal with Diabetes

It is critical to your cardiac health to prevent diabetes or, if you have it, to manage it well. Nearly a decade ago, researchers showed that people at high risk can cut their odds of developing type 2 diabetes by 58% simply by losing weight and walking at least 30 minutes a day. More recent studies suggest that drug therapy may also prevent the development of diabetes in individuals with prediabetes. According to a just-published report, impaired glucose tolerance is 81% less likely to turn into full-blown diabetes if patients take the prescription drug pioglitazone (Actos). But here's the most exciting news: Researchers at William Beaumont Hospital in Royal Oak, Michigan, have now reported the clinical resolution of type 2 diabetes, without bariatric surgery, with a diet-induced BMI reduction of approximately 18%! These provocative data should be encouraging to both patients and physicians pursuing a possible "cure" as opposed to "control" of type 2 diabetes.

Be Smart About Metabolic Syndrome

When metabolic syndrome strikes, there are key steps that you can take to reduce insulin resistance and improve the metabolic abnormalities associated with this condition.

- **Eat the right foods.** According to Dr. Gerald M. Reaven, the "ideal" diet to combat metabolic syndrome supplies 45% of calories from carbohydrates, 15% from protein and 40% from fat. The last should primarily include foods rich in mono- and polyunsaturated fats, found in fish, nuts, seeds and canola, corn, olive, safflower, soybean and sunflower oils, as opposed to saturated fats. A high-fiber diet is also extremely helpful in fighting metabolic syndrome, adds Dr. Dennis Sprecher of the Cleveland Clinic.

Recently, Dr. Eric Westman of the Lifestyle Medicine Clinic at Duke University and Dr. Neil Stone of Northwestern University presented data supporting the argument that certain key dietary elements have to be reduced or eliminated as the best approach to resolving metabolic syndrome. Patients who intentionally reduce or eliminate sugar, starch (baked goods, pasta, rice, potatoes, chips) and saturated fats (fried foods, bacon, cheese) showed considerable improvement in all blood tests, often indicating resolution of metabolic syndrome.

- **Lose weight.** Shedding pounds lessens insulin resistance. In the ongoing Framingham Heart Study, weight losses of just four or five pounds produced beneficial results in people with metabolic syndrome. Other studies have shown that insulin resistance falls an average of 20% for each 10 pounds of weight loss in overweight individuals.

- **Move!** Regular exercisers use insulin more efficiently than their sedentary counterparts. For the vast majority of middle-aged and older adults, a goal of 30 minutes or more of moderate exercise each day can be achieved just by walking at a pace of 2.5 to 4.5 miles per hour. Why? Because moderate-to-vigorous physical activity diminishes the magnitude of all five risk factors associated with metabolic syndrome.

- **Don't smoke.** Not smoking decreases insulin resistance.

- **Consider medications.** If lifestyle changes aren't enough, triglyceride-lowering medications, which may reduce the likelihood

91

of abnormal blood clotting and boost HDL levels, should also be considered. These include nicotinic acid, gemfibrozil (Lopid) and fenofibrate (Tricor), which have the added benefit of lowering LDL cholesterol. The latter drugs can, in rare cases, cause muscle soreness and damage to the liver, which should be periodically checked. Because many people with metabolic syndrome also have high blood pressure, selected antihypertensive medications, including those that may simultaneously increase insulin sensitivity, might also be helpful. Talk with your doctor about which medications might be best for you.

Give Up Smoking

12

In terms of cardiac risk, smoking is a black-and-white issue. If you smoke, you are much more likely to develop coronary heart disease and have a heart attack than if you do not smoke. But smoking is an addiction, and it takes more than cognitive understanding about the hazards of smoking to cause a change in habits. There are, however, some practical actions you can take.

- **Get help.** Your doctor, the American Heart Association, the American Cancer Society and the American Lung Association can point you to groups and programs and treatments that work.
- **Start a regular exercise program.** In addition to dissipating stress and burning up nervous energy (triggers for smoking), physical activity causes the release of endorphins, which promote feelings of well-being.
- **Go crunchy.** Many smokers find that crunchy, low-fat whole foods such as apples, carrots and celery help to dissipate the craving to smoke by keeping the hands and mouth occupied.
- **Drink water.** Staying hydrated cuts down on the craving for nicotine.
- **Avoid those cigarette moments.** If your craving is worst after dinner, take a walk instead.
- **Consider medications.** Two prescription medications—bupropion and varenicline—are available as smoking cessation aids. Other helpful therapies include nicotine-containing gum, inhalers, nasal spray, lozenges and patches.

ACCENTUATE THE POSITIVE

There are hundreds upon hundreds of successful smoking cessation programs throughout this country. Such programs generally produce quit rates of 15% to 25% in the general population of smokers. Even higher quit rates have been reported for people with smoking-related diseases, with up to 70% of patients quitting one year after a heart attack when provided with an intensive nurse-managed program.

Consider the whole new generation of medical aids. Think positive. Seventy percent of all smokers would like to quit, but each year less than 5% are able to do so without assistance. What successful quitters have in common is the decision to live without cigarettes. This decision is fundamental if you are to view the process as an opportunity for self-improvement rather than as a painful ordeal marked by nothing but deprivation.

Cope with Stress

It's a given that chronic stress is part of the fabric of contemporary American society. The modern era of high-speed living, with its increased demands from family and job commitments, contributes to a hectic lifestyle. Most people are simply out of time and deeply feel the stress of overcommitted, overscheduled and workaholic lives. We're multitasking, working on weekends, grocery shopping or doing laundry at nine P.M., commuting longer distances (while using a cell phone so that no time is wasted!). In addition, we're bombarded by "bad" news: terrorism, crime, staggering investment losses, an uncertain economy. So many factores seem to be beyond our control, contributing to a ceaseless stress that saps our strength and threatens our health.

At the same time, support organizations of the past are not always available to us today. Organized religion and the educational system have their own challenges. The extended family, once a bulwark against the world, has broken up and moved all over the country, leaving many of us feeling alone and helpless.

Unfortunately, the daily events that cause stress cannot be avoided. There will always be traffic jams, jangling telephones, e-mails to answer, overdrawn checking accounts, sick children and an up-and-down stock market. The key to success is learning how to *respond* to chronic stress rather than react to it. You do have the ability to take action to manage your stress more effectively. It all starts with a decision to take charge. Mental and physical activities such as regular exercise, keeping a journal, deep breathing and creating a realistic perspective will give you the tools to handle your stress and take control of your life.

THE EASTERLIN PARADOX

It has long been accepted that an increase in personal economic growth leads to an increase in happiness. "Not so," says University of Southern California economist Richard Easterlin. "If that were true, then it should follow that Americans should be happier than a generation ago as today we are much wealthier. But surveys over the last four decades show that people are *less* happy today than in 1970, even though we are vastly richer."

The disconnect between economic growth and happiness is called the Easterlin Paradox. It attributes the phenomenon of happiness levels not keeping pace with economic gains to the fact that people's desires and expectations change along with their material fortunes. Where an American in 1970 might have once dreamed about owning a house, he or she might now dream about owning two. "People are wedded to the idea that more money will bring them more happiness," says Easterlin, "so they are constantly stressed trying to achieve more economic success. But they are failing to factor in the fact that when they get more money, they are going to want an even bigger house. So they want even more money. In the end, they never have enough money to achieve happiness. But the increase in chronic stress penalizes family life and health, often making them less happy."

Manage Daily Stress

Making Sense of Stress

WHEN YOU'VE WRITTEN AND LECTURED extensively for more than three decades on the positive effects of diet and exercise on cardiac health, it's hard to admit that you've been neglecting something equally important. But that's the position we find ourselves in. Recent research and experience have convinced both of us that stress management is crucial to cardiac well-being. Even more important, they've convinced us that you can't expect people—including cardiac patients—to stick to an exercise and diet plan if they're under chronic stress. They can't. And they won't.

Stress can have a terrible impact on the heart. It causes increases in cholesterol and blood pressure. It promotes arterial inflammation. It constricts arteries and promotes abnormal heart rhythms, which in extreme cases can result in sudden cardiac death. It increases blood clotting.

But its *indirect* impact is just as devastating.

Stress drives people to make poor lifestyle decisions. Strung-out people smoke. They're "too tired" to work out. They eat high-fat foods and sit around the house, both of which promote weight gain with increased triglycerides, body mass index and waist circumference as well as diabetes. Stress causes people to become supercompetitive and driven, to feel a heightened sense of time urgency, to be angry, hostile and depressed.

SLEEPLESS NIGHTS, FOGGY DAYS

Americans are sleep-deprived workaholics. According to the National Sleep Foundation, only about a third of us are sleeping the recommended seven to eight hours a night, and 40% say they have trouble staying awake on the job. Instead of working to live, we are living to work—a practice that is having a profound impact on escalating stress levels.

Simply put, stress places people at much higher risk for heart disease. It also helps to explain why people who know what to do for a healthy heart (and that means most of us) don't do it. We know we're supposed to eat a lean, balanced diet. Exercise regularly. Not smoke. But we eat fatty food, sit on our duffs and stoke our bad habits *because of chronic stress*. This is why Step 2—right after risk assessment—concerns stress management. When you've got that figured out, and only then, you'll be in a position to manage exercise and diet successfully.

What Is Stress?

STRESS IS ANY CIRCUMSTANCE THAT IMPOSES SPECIAL PHYSICAL OR psychological demands on us or throws off our equilibrium. Or, as defined by Dr. Wayne Lesko of Marymount University, stress is "anything that causes us to change."

"Not all stress is bad. Some stress is good," says Dr. Esther Sternberg of the National Institutes of Health. Positive stress, or *eustress,* is often reflected in a confident attitude and superior performance. Athletes, for example, use it to "get up" for a big game, but all of us feel its effect; when we're under pressure, we experience heightened energy and motivation levels that enable us to function at our optimum. A certain amount of stress also makes life interesting. With too little stimulation, we tend to become bored and frustrated.

On the other hand, too much stress pushes us into overdrive. It's not unlike the strings on a violin. When they're too loose, the sound they make is poor; too tight, and the strings break. "Stress can be the spice of life," says Dr. Mark Ketterer, a neuropsychiatrist at Henry Ford Hospital in Detroit, "or it can be the kiss of death." It's the latter possibility we're worried about.

Dr. Hans Selye's research in the 1930s was the first to link negative stress, or *distress,* to a common biological response that could result in illness. For example, a downsized worker experiences acute stress at the sight of a pink slip. Yet so does a 15-year-old at cheerleading tryouts. The situations differ greatly, but the physical responses to acute stress—tightness in the neck, a pounding heart, a knot in the stomach, dry mouth, shallow

HOLIDAY STRESS

Are people more stressed—and more at risk—during the winter holidays than during other times of the year? Yes. There's even a name for the condition, which is characterized by rapid heartbeat, lightheadedness and palpitations: "holiday heart syndrome."

Eating and drinking too much, shopping and preparing for holiday festivities, partying with relatives and friends—all are tough on health. "Everything becomes exaggerated this time of year," says cardiologist Dr. Stephen Winters. "It's like cramming for a test, where people are trying to be sociable, to do a lot of entertaining, to do in a couple of weeks what they might want to do all year long. This results in a kind of performance pressure that can lead to increased stress."

Doctors suggest better planning as a way to minimize stress. "Ask yourself basic questions when you plan your day," suggests Dr. Winters. "Do you really want to go to the mall on a busy Sunday afternoon? Do you need to make two trips through the buffet line at an afternoon party?" If the answer is no, don't do it.

breathing—are surprisingly similar. Dr. Selye found that humans are equipped to deal with acute stress if it's only occasional and not prolonged. But chronic stress can lead to illness—from headaches to heart attacks.

Unfortunately, modern society tends to produce constant distress. From morning to night (and sometimes throughout the night), many people experience a continuum of stressful events. Some are serious— death, divorce, bankruptcy. But others are more trivial—being delayed in a bank line or even doing something "fun" like shopping for the "perfect" Christmas gift. Research suggests that the cumulative effect of life's trivial hassles—the parking tickets and traffic jams—is often harder on health than a life-threatening family medical crisis. "The human body," says Dr. Pamela Peeke, "was never meant to deal with prolonged chronic stress. We weren't meant to drag around bad memories, anxieties and frustrations. When we do, long-term stress takes its toll. We end up with health problems."

The presence of distress in American society can actually be quantified, as shown in the scientific findings that follow.

- The Centers for Disease Control and Prevention estimates that up to 75% of all disease and illness is stress-related.
- Eighty-nine percent of adults state that they chronically experience high stress levels.
- According to the American Academy of Family Physicians, the use of St. John's wort and other herbal remedies for altering mood are one of the fastest-growing segments of alternative medicine.
- Alcoholism is linked to stress. There are almost 18 million alcoholics in the United States.
- People under chronic stress are more likely to abuse drugs in an effort to reduce that stress, according to a report in the *Journal of Psychopharmacology.*
- One in four people suffers from sleep deprivation as a direct result of stress.
- The American Academy of Child and Adolescent Psychiatry identifies an overload of stress leading to depression as a key element in tripling the suicide rate of people aged 15 to 24 over the past 30 years.
- More than 25% of adults have high blood pressure due to or aggravated by stress.
- An estimated 75% to 90% of visits to physicians are stress-related.
- Job stress costs American businesses about $350 billion annually in absenteeism, compensation claims, mental health claims, health insurance and direct medical expenses, and reduced productivity.
- According to the American Medical Association, more than half of the national medical bill can be attributed to an unhealthy, stressful lifestyle.
- A recent study published in the *Journal of the American Medical Association* found that job strain, a combination of high psychological demands and low attitude/decision-making, increases the risk of a first heart attack.
- About 60% of women say that job stress is their number one problem.

Is increased stress an inevitable hazard of modern life? Perhaps, when you think about 60-hour workweeks, looming deadlines, long commutes, chirping cell phones, late-night e-mails, lost weekends and an uncertain economy. But in many ways life was more stressful 200 years ago, when children routinely died before reaching adulthood. The challenge we face is to master not the threats themselves, but our all-too-human response to them.

An additional problem for many women working outside the home is that they are also primarily responsible for running the home. They "punch out" of their outside job, only to "punch in" at a second one as homemaker. Even in this day of more sensitive males, studies show that women still perform the vast majority of household tasks. This is further complicated by female child-rearing responsibilities, an aspect of society that has remained unchanged. Men and women alike still see the mother as having the primary role in child-rearing. It is estimated that nearly 63% of women employed outside the home have children under six years of age. Even with good child care (not always easy to find), working women often feel guilty about leaving their children with someone else. This problem is even greater for single mothers. Many women, attempting to build two "perfect" worlds with limited time and energy, run themselves ragged and into Type A lifestyles.

> ### KILLER DEBT
>
> An Ohio State University study suggests a connection between health and the strain of debt. Dr. Paul J. Lavraks, director of the study, says, "We found that people who are stressed about debt, particularly from credit cards, tend to be in worse physical condition than those without money worries. We've known that such folks tend to be more likely to smoke and be overweight. What was a surprise was that we found heart attack to be the single most prominent health problem stemming from credit-card debt."

Physical Responses to Stress

Stress itself is not a health hazard; it's our response to it that's potentially dangerous. The physiological changes due to stress were first described by Harvard University's Dr. Walter B. Cannon, who labeled them the "fight or flight" syndrome. To understand this response, picture yourself in the following situation. It's 20,000 B.C., and you're asleep in a cave in the middle of the night. Suddenly you're awakened by the low growl of a saber-toothed tiger. Then, well before you're fully awake, your

STRESS AND FORGETFULNESS

Researchers have found that elevated levels of the stress hormone cortisol can impair verbal declarative memory, or the ability to remember words, details and phone numbers. Every day for four days, volunteers in one study were given a dose of cortisol mimicking a mildly stressful event, a higher dose mimicking a major stress, or a placebo. About 93% of those given the higher dose of the stress hormone had more difficulty in recalling information in a paragraph read to them than did those given low doses or a placebo.

brain transmits a biochemical message to your body in the form of stress hormones—cortisol, adrenaline and norepinephrine—to put it on notice that quick action will soon be taking place.

Stored fats and sugars immediately pour into your bloodstream to provide fuel for energy. Your breathing quickens to meet anticipated oxygen needs. Your heart rate and blood pressure increase in preparation for carrying extra oxygen. Activity in your digestive system slows down to make extra blood available to your muscles and extremities. Blood-clotting mechanisms become activated in anticipation of injury. In short, all senses are primed, all muscles are tensed, all systems are go. You're ready to either take a stand and fight the tiger or take flight to save your skin.

This is a very appropriate response to external physical danger if your goal is to survive the next 20 minutes. It is not, however, a healthy response to the emotional stress that all of us face in modern society. While contemporary life has changed greatly from prehistoric times, our physiological makeup has not. The stress caused by a broken traffic light produces virtually the same bodily response as a confrontation with a saber-toothed tiger—a response that is no longer appropriate to the stimulus.

The hormone cortisol gets the body all worked up, heart racing and muscles tensed, but in modern society there are few ways for the stress to be released. "Fight or flight" is no help with a jangling telephone, a crashed computer or a vaguely threatening note from the IRS. In the modern world, we do not respond to a nagging boss with a spear; we grin and bear it. In the modern world, stress is not a situation that is soon over. It is continual and chronic. And it is detrimental to your heart. Every heartbeat at elevated blood pressure takes its toll on the coronary arteries.

The excess fats and sugars released for energy are not metabolized right away, so they stay in the bloodstream, contributing to arterial deposits and diabetes. And, as already noted, ongoing stress can cause arterial inflammation, which can lead to a heart attack.

Stress can also foster overweight and obesity. People under stress often have lower levels of serotonin (a brain chemical that boosts mood) and higher levels of cortisol, a combination that promotes overeating of high-fat, high-calorie foods. There is another problem as well. "We found that women in particular who have high levels of cortisol after a stressful event tend to eat more sweets," says Dr. Elissa Epel of the University of California at San Francisco. "Emotional eaters have trouble keeping the weight off." Since one facet of the stress response is to use the body's fat reserves as energy, people under chronic stress are prone to storing fat in the abdomen, where it can quickly be utilized by the liver. Called "deep-belly" fat, the accumulation of fat around the middle—a potbelly—increases the risk of metabolic syndrome and heart disease.

The same primeval response that served ancient man so well is detrimental to the health of modern man—nothing less than a prescription for an overdose of stress chemicals. What once meant survival has become suicidal.

Emotional Responses to Stress

The first emotional response of a person under severe stress—imagine a mother seeing her toddler dart into traffic—is *acute alarm*. This is an emergency system that prepares the body to fight or take flight.

Too often today we feel acute alarm over less severe stressors—this time imagine a traffic light on the fritz. Indeed, acute alarm is the result of any real or perceived situation that threatens us with loss of control and incites anger and aggression. The body is prepared to fight, but how can you punch a traffic light? Instead, the intended blows are internalized. Each time this happens, powerful stress hormones are secreted and the body literally ends up stewing in its own juices.

The second emotional response to stress is *long-term vigilance*, a mental state in which we project the future and adapt to that projection.

This is what separates humans from other creatures, yet many people look into the future with fear, watching and waiting for something disastrous to happen. Vigilance, a response to lack of control, can occur on a temporary basis, as in the case of accountants imagining that they won't be able to meet a tax deadline. Or it can occur as a way of life, as with air traffic controllers. Chronic vigilance can lead to a passive outlook, an "it's out of my hands" mentality that is responsible for self-doubt, a sense of failure, depression and feelings of entrapment.

The emotional response to stress dictates how we see the world and how we think it sees us. Programmed as predators, we wind up preying on ourselves. At best, the result is chronic tension. At worst, we suffer damage to the cardiovascular system that can lead to serious physical and psychological disorders and, not infrequently, to premature death.

The Stress of Life

ACCORDING TO NUMEROUS POLLS, TIME IS THE SCARCEST AND MOST coveted commodity in our modern culture. As Swedish economist Staffan Linder explains in his book *The Harried Leisure Class,* the time we need to produce and consume has by necessity reduced the amount of "free" time, which has become too valuable for us to do "nothing."

But who even has free time? Extended work hours, multitasking, longer commutes, both parents working, single-parent households, increased organized activities for children—these are just some of the factors that have produced a serious shortage of time and, for many, an increase in stress. Americans report a constant struggle to balance career, marriage and family, and an ongoing battle against fatigue. A harried and "out of control" feeling has become an ongoing challenge for many people.

Add to that the undeniable fact that life is constantly changing. People move, change jobs, get married or divorced, buy and sell houses, have children and watch them grow up. There is birth; there is death. Whether trivial or significant, happy or sad, planned or unplanned, all change stresses the body by causing it to adapt. It is the process of adaptation that the body finds stressful. Change, adaptation, stress—these elements always go together.

The body adapts to most changes fairly well. However, when change occurs too often or too rapidly, the overload has implications for your health. The relationship between the frequency of major changes in life and the predictive risk of illness has been shown in a number of study findings:

- The death rate for widows and widowers is highest during the first six months following the death of a spouse.

- The death rate from cardiovascular disease is two to three times higher for divorced women than for married women.

- Even Mondays are stressful. Most people know this intuitively, but research by Dr. Simon Rabkin lends medical credence. Over almost 30 years, Dr. Rabkin followed 3,983 men with no previous history of cancer or heart disease. Cancer deaths were distributed evenly throughout the week, but this was not true of sudden cardiac death: Monday saw twice as high an incidence as any other day of the week.

- Just thinking about work can elevate people's stress hormones. A study conducted by University College, London, measured levels of the stress hormone cortisol in participants' saliva. Samples were taken every two hours from waking until sleep. The highest levels were found early on Monday mornings when participants were preparing to return to work.

The definitive work on stress and the predictability of illness was authored by Dr. Thomas H. Holmes at the University of Washington. He found that hospitalized patients, regardless of their illness, had one major thing in common—the occurrence of a number of life changes just prior to their hospitalization. Carrying his findings forward, Dr. Holmes developed the Social Readjustment Rating Scale, which ranks specific life events in relation to predictable illness. Some events are significant, such as divorce; some are smaller, such as being cited for a minor traffic violation. This scale also shows that stress is cumulative; just a few significant events, or a number of smaller events, can overload the adaptive system. In addition, it illustrates that events need not be negative to be stressful. Vacations, Christmas and marriage are positive but still stressful events.

Use the Holmes scale on the following pages to estimate how life events may be influencing your health. Obviously, the scale cannot predict illness with certainty, but it is a good tool for raising your awareness about the potential external sources of stress in your life.

LIFE EVENTS

If one of the following events occurred in your life within the last year, give yourself the mean value in points in the *past* column. If you can reasonably expect it to happen in the year to come, give yourself the value in the *future* column.

MEAN VALUE	PAST	FUTURE	LIFE EVENT
100	____	____	1. Death of spouse
73	____	____	2. Divorce
65	____	____	3. Marital separation (or separation from any major intimate relationship)
63	____	____	4. Detention in jail or other institution
63	____	____	5. Death of a close family member
53	____	____	6. Major personal injury or illness
50	____	____	7. Marriage
47	____	____	8. Being fired from work
45	____	____	9. Marital reconciliation
45	____	____	10. Retirement from work
44	____	____	11. Major change in the health or behavior of family member
40	____	____	12. Pregnancy
39	____	____	13. Sexual difficulties
39	____	____	14. Gaining a new family member (birth, adoption, remarriage, oldster moving in)
39	____	____	15. Major readjustment (merger, reorganization, bankruptcy)
38	____	____	16. Major change in financial state (a lot worse or lot better off than usual)
37	____	____	17. Death of a close friend
36	____	____	18. Changing to a different line of work

MEAN VALUE	PAST	FUTURE	LIFE EVENT
35	_____	_____	19. Increase in the number of arguments with spouse
31	_____	_____	20. Mortgage or loan for major purpose
30	_____	_____	21. Foreclosure on mortgage or loan
29	_____	_____	22. Major change in responsibilities at work (promotion, demotion, lateral transfer)
29	_____	_____	23. Son or daughter leaving home (marriage, college)
29	_____	_____	24. In-law troubles
28	_____	_____	25. Outstanding personal achievement
26	_____	_____	26. Starting or ceasing formal schooling
26	_____	_____	27. Spouse starting or ceasing work outside home
25	_____	_____	28. Major change in living conditions (building a new home, remodeling, deterioration of home or neighborhood)
24	_____	_____	29. Revision of personal habits (dress, manners, associations)
23	_____	_____	30. Troubles with boss
20	_____	_____	31. Major change in working hours or conditions
20	_____	_____	32. Change in residence
20	_____	_____	33. Change to a new school
19	_____	_____	34. Major change in usual type or amount of recreation
19	_____	_____	35. Major change in church activities
18	_____	_____	36. Major change in social activities (clubs, movies, visiting, etc.)

MEAN VALUE	PAST	FUTURE	LIFE EVENT
17	_____	_____	37. Purchase of major item (auto, computer, etc.)
16	_____	_____	38. Major change in sleeping habits (amount or time of day)
15	_____	_____	39. Major change in number of family get-togethers
15	_____	_____	40. Major change in eating habits (amount, hours or surroundings)
13	_____	_____	41. Vacation
12	_____	_____	42. Christmas or major holiday
11	_____	_____	43. Citation for minor violations of the law

Chance of a physical illness in the next 12 months if your score for the past year is:

300 or higher:	80%
150 to 299:	50%
Below 150:	30%

A Changing View

STRESS IS USUALLY THOUGHT OF AS A MODERN PROBLEM, BUT ITS impact on health has been recognized for hundreds of years. Medical observations from the 18th century describe people "paled with fear," or "reddened with rage," or "weeping with joy or sorrow." Such observations also noted that people under extreme stress could go mad or pine away. In 1813 James Johnson, a London physician, was the first to note the relationship between the "wear and tear" of life and premature old age. But documentation of the impact of stress on cardiac health goes back even further. Dr. William Harvey, the first physician ever to present a theory of blood circulation, wrote in 1628, "Every affection of the mind

STRESS AND GENDER

Since acute stress produces the same physiological responses in both men and women, scientists have long assumed that the behavioral responses of both sexes are similar. New studies, however, show that this is not the case when stress results in depression.

■ "When life's burdens lead to depression, men and women respond quite differently," says Dr. Susan Nolen-Hoeksema, a professor of psychology at Yale University. "Men drink. And women think." That's not to say that men never ruminate and women never drink, but in a study of 1,300 adults aged 25 to 75, Dr. Nolen-Hoeksema found that when upset, women tend to sit and stew while men are more likely to use alcohol to take the edge off.

■ Research at UCLA Medical School indicates that women typically employ a "tend and befriend" response. When stress mounts, women are more prone to protect and nurture their children ("tend") and turn to other females for support ("befriend"), perhaps because evolution has valued behavior that leads to a higher rate of offspring survival and the passing on of desirable traits.

■ When men or women are subject to stress, a powerful hormone called oxytocin is produced by the pituitary gland. Secreted at high levels during childbirth (to aid in labor), oxytocin exerts a calming influence. Estrogen, a female sex hormone, seems to amplify this effect, while androgens, male sex hormones, tend to diminish it.

This difference in response to stress could in part explain why American women, on average, live 7.5 years longer than men. "The fact is that women have their own ways of responding to stress," says lead researcher Dr. Shelly Taylor. "We didn't realize this in the past because the vast majority of subjects in the 'fight or flight' studies were males. Women made up only 17% of participants in those studies." While much more research must be done, many health professionals are leaning toward the acceptance of this theory.

that is attended with either pain or pleasure, hope or fear, is the cause of an agitation whose influence extends to the heart."

Despite this history, not until very recently did physicians rank the treatment of stress as a high priority. Perhaps that is because it has been hard to measure. The same event can produce totally different reactions in two people. For one, the event is upsetting and stressful; for the other, it is viewed simply as a new challenge. In addition, traditional medicine has resisted the notion that a mental condition alone could have a measurable effect on arteries and organs. As Dr. Esther Sternberg explains, "Until recently, scientists and physicians dismissed the idea that stress could make you sick. They had the same motto as the state of Missouri: 'Show Me.' Now researchers are able to do just that."

Evidence reveals that chronic stress wreaks havoc on the body. While stress is seldom listed as the official cause of death, its negative role is now undisputed. Researchers estimate that mental stress has either caused or aggravated the symptoms of 50% to 90% of all hospital patients in the United States.

Indeed, stress may be the single greatest contributor to illness in the industrialized world.

How Stress Works Against Your Heart

WE'VE ALREADY TOUCHED ON THE NEGATIVE EFFECTS THAT STRESS can have on cardiovascular health. Now it's time to get specific. Chronic stress is a very tough foe to combat, and we want you to be motivated.

Stress elevates blood pressure. The "fight or flight" response causes a temporary increase in blood pressure. When stress is occasional, such an increase does not usually present a health problem, but frequent elevation of blood pressure can lead to the permanent establishment of a new and higher level. According to Dr. Robert S. Eliot, a noted stress expert, about 20% of Americans are "hot reactors" whose response to even mild stress is a skyrocketing blood pressure. Each time stress is encountered—often many times a day—their blood pressure rises. Over time, their blood pressure settles permanently at the higher level, elevating heart attack risk significantly.

This seems to be particularly true when there is a genetic predisposition to high blood pressure. Researchers at the University of North

Carolina studied men aged 18 to 22 who had at least one parent with a history of high blood pressure and a high response to stress themselves. Ten years later, this group had three times the risk of hypertension, compared with people who had a low response to stress. But following this finding, members of this group who underwent 10 weeks of stress management therapy were able to significantly lower their blood pressure. Says Dr. Wolfgang Linden of the University of British Columbia, "Results in many stress management studies were similar to those that you would find in many hypertensive drug studies, and without side effects."

Blood pressure response to stress may also be gender-specific. Women's blood pressure seems to rise less than men's in reaction to stress. But women feel stress more often, according to Dr. Ronald Kessler of Harvard University. His study of 166 married couples found that women take a holistic view of everyday life. "A man may worry if someone in his family is sick," he says. "His wife takes on the burdens of the whole neighborhood. Men take care of one thing at a time. Women put the pieces together."

Stress causes arterial inflammation. Powerful hormones travel through the bloodstream every time the body reacts to acute stress. These hormones have the ability to injure coronary artery walls, creating places where cholesterol can collect, plaque can develop and inflammation can occur. The more chronic the stress, the greater the chance for injury and inflammation.

Stress injuries may be a key determinant of whether or not blockages form on artery walls. In a study conducted by Dr. Jay Kaplan, one group of monkeys was fed a low-fat diet but subjected to constant social stress. Another group was fed the same diet but lived stress-free. The

> ## DOMESTIC STRESS
>
> **A** five-year study on women and stress found that family stress increases a woman's chance of a heart attack more than stress on the job. While high work stress doubled the risk of a first heart attack, women with the worst family stress were four times more likely to have a first heart attack.
>
> In addition, a Swedish survey of 292 women who had suffered heart attacks revealed that those with the most marital stress averaged a three times greater risk of a second heart attack during the following five years.

WARNING SIGNS

Chronic stress, anxiety and pressure are common by-products of the modern American lifestyle. But when does stress become so pervasive that it can injure your health? It makes sense to be aware of the physical, emotional and behavioral signs of overstress:

- Ringing in the ears
- Increased muscular tension; neck and back aches
- Numbness or tingling
- Chest pains; shortness of breath
- Stomach and intestinal problems
- Irregular menstrual periods
- Skin eruptions and cold sores
- Loss of self-esteem; a feeling of worthlessness
- Difficulty making decisions
- A feeling that there "just aren't enough hours in the day" to get things done; trouble meeting deadlines
- A sense of paranoia; increased sensitivity to criticism
- Feelings of fatigue and boredom, unhappiness and sadness
- A hard time concentrating or being productive or creative
- A short temper; a tendency to criticize and be argumentative
- Problems with moodiness or depression
- Poor memory
- Rigid behavior
- Poor lifestyle habits: overeating, abusing alcohol and/or drugs, being "too tired" to exercise, smoking
- Oversleeping or not getting enough sleep

Often a person under great stress can exhibit many of these warning signs simultaneously. The cruel irony is that the reaction to stress may itself produce more stress in an ever-escalating spiral. Be sure to talk with your doctor or health professional if you experience more than the occasional sign of being overstressed.

stressed monkeys developed arterial injuries and extensive plaque, whereas the unstressed animals did not, even though both groups ate the same diet and had similar cholesterol levels.

Stress can elevate cholesterol. People with ongoing stress often have higher cholesterol counts. This is illustrated by a study involving a group of certified public accountants whose cholesterol was measured in April, when the group was facing tax deadlines, and again during their August vacations. The result: April cholesterol levels were much higher than those in August, even though there had been no change in the accountants' diets. Studies of auto racers produced similar results. Cholesterol levels were significantly higher on the day of a race than on the day after. And one study found that levels of LDL cholesterol rose about 5% in a group of middle-aged airline pilots during a time of high occupational stress.

Some researchers believe this effect is caused by a reduction of the liver's capacity to prepare for cholesterol excretion. One of the physical responses to stress is the shunting of blood to the arms (to fight) and legs (to take flight) and away from internal organs. Reducing blood supply to the liver causes a slowing down of function, impairing the organ's ability to rid the body of cholesterol. This may explain why some people under chronic stress have difficulty reducing cholesterol. It's not that they produce more cholesterol than others do; it's that they have a problem eliminating it.

Studies suggest that coping skills can improve protective HDL cholesterol. Says Dr. Carolyn Aldwin, "Stress can raise total cholesterol and LDL cholesterol. In a study of 716 men, we expected that those who coped well with stress would have lower levels of LDL cholesterol. But what we found was that coping skills contributed to a higher level of protective HDL."

Stress promotes blood clotting. This response makes good sense as part of the "fight or flight" pattern. After all, if you face a physical threat that could result in a wound, the ability to produce and sustain coagulation provides protection. But that same ability, based on an increase in the stickiness of blood platelets, also creates a higher risk for heart attacks.

Stress can trigger sudden cardiac death. Coronary arteries are often pictured as passive, rigid tubes, like PVC pipe. They are not. Lined with muscle tissue, arteries dilate and constrict rhythmically. Powerful stress hormones can cause muscle tissue to contract abruptly, producing a spasm that cuts off blood to the heart. Stress can also trigger heart rhythm irregularities. In either case, sudden cardiac death can result.

Of more than 5,000 male heart attack fatalities examined at Brigham and Women's Hospital in Boston, 30% were found not to have substantial coronary plaque at the time of death. Their deaths were attributed primarily to lethal heart rhythm irregularities or coronary spasm brought on by an episode of acute stress. Other research reveals many examples of stress-induced sudden cardiac death:

- Ten days after the assassination of President John F. Kennedy, the 27-year-old army captain responsible for the ceremonial troops at the funeral died of a cardiovascular complication.
- After 31 years of trying to bowl a 300 game, a 40-year-old man in Detroit collapsed and died of a massive heart attack about 15 minutes after finally achieving his goal.
- A 56-year-old man collapsed and died of a heart attack while celebrating his first hole-in-one.
- A man watching his favorite baseball team lose on TV got so overwrought that he suffered a fatal cardiac event.
- During the 2006 soccer World Cup in Germany, on days of matches involving the German team, there were three times as many cardiovascular events as on days they did not play.

Stress contributes to obesity. The powerful stress hormone cortisol is an appetite stimulant that historically increased food intake to supply extra energy in dealing with enemies like the saber-toothed tiger. But the stresses we face today aren't the kind you fight or run from. Instead, we usually just sit there and get upset and anxious. Meanwhile, our brain assumes we've gotten really physical with such high levels of cortisol circulating, so it gives us a big appetite for the special fuels of the stress response—fats and carbohydrates. And this means lots of extra calories. Stress hormones also cause the body to hold on to fat cells as an energy reserve, thereby hindering weight-control efforts.

Stress can also foster overweight by promoting poor lifestyle choices such as overeating and exercise avoidance. "There is increasing evidence that stress may affect weight through changes in behavior that influence health," says Dr. Jane Wardle, writing in *Psychosomatic Medicine.* "For many people, that means unrestrained, emotional eating." Anger, depression, loneliness, anxiety—any of these negative emotions can be caused or aggravated by chronic stress and can motivate a person to eat. In this case, food isn't eaten because of hunger; instead, it has become a reward or a consolation, good for whatever ails. Stressed people are unconcerned about the quality of what they eat. They choose "high-comfort" foods because of nervous energy, not even tasting them and often losing track of calories.

Experts say that people who reach for food in response to stress do so as a means of self-medication. "It's nature's way of getting you to feel better," says Dr. Judith Wurtman, a research scientist at the Massachusetts Institute of Technology. "When the right foods are eaten, they act like an edible tranquilizer." In particular, foods that are rich in carbohydrates increase levels of serotonin in the brain, and serotonin minimizes symptoms of stress. "Contrived diets that are low in carbohydrates—such as the high-protein, low-carbohydrate diets—cause a depletion of brain serotonin," adds Dr. Wurtman, "contributing to increased tension, insomnia and anxiety. Add current levels of persistent uncertainty characteristic of our society, and you have a recipe for high stress." Unfortunately, comfort foods do not provide instant relief. The effects of serotonin on the brain can take about 30 minutes to be felt. If you keep eating until you feel better, that half-hour later can also mean two or three doughnuts eaten.

In addition, overweight people can feel additional stress because they hate being overweight. Unfortunately, this is a society that tends to equate physical characteristics with character, intelligence and self-worth, and overweight people often suffer the consequences. Many have low self-esteem, actually despising their bodies. They see their lives and their appearance as being out of control. Tension and unhappiness—the stress of the situation—drive them to overeat often to the point of bingeing. Feelings of guilt, accompanied by even lower self-esteem, soon result and the cycle begins anew.

Lack of exercise compounds the problem. Stress causes mental fatigue, a chronic feeling of tiredness that keeps many overweight people from participating in physical activities that would help to dissipate stress and renew energy levels. As a result, these people choose to be sedentary. They restrict activities that would burn fat, help to control their weight and give them a sense of being in charge of their lives. When stress produces a cycle of overeating and underexercising, extra weight becomes a predictable result.

Time for Action

I F YOU ASK A ROOMFUL OF PEOPLE, "How many of you would like to reduce the stress in your lives?" a lot of hands will go up. If you then ask, "How many people would like to win the lottery?" more hands will go up. The truth is that the chances for one are as good as for the other. Stress is part and parcel of modern life, particularly in the United States, where a fast-paced, out-of-time lifestyle and a Type A–fostering culture combine to induce high levels of frustration, anxiety and anger. There will always be traffic jams and overdrawn checking accounts. And there will always be stress. But we do not have to succumb to it.

The secret is not to avoid stress, but to manage it; not to react to stress, but to respond to it. Effective stress management means figuring out the level of stress below which you can function safely and then controlling the way in which you react to stress above that level. Woody Allen once remarked that death is nature's way of telling us to slow down, but we definitely shouldn't wait that long before making the decision to slow down, assess stress in terms of causes and reactions, and figure out how to manage it.

The first step is to make a decision to take control, to decide to manage your stress rather than have it manage you. As author Arlen Price has said, "Where the heart is willing, it will find a thousand ways to succeed. Where it is unwilling, it will find a thousand excuses."

Next, identify what causes you to feel stressed. Is it coming from your job, your home, or both? Are too many things happening in your life? Are you always out of time? Are you setting unrealistic goals for yourself? Do you have Type A personality traits?

And finally, do something positive about combating stress. The Heart Savers in this section are all designed to help you do that. Remember, though, it takes some flexibility to devise a stress-busting strategy. No single approach works for everybody. Jogging and meditation are great for some people, but dull, boring and stressful for others. You have to find what works for you. But even using a handful of tips on a regular basis will allow you to better cope with stress when the going gets tough.

Take Time Out to Relax

According to Dr. Herbert Benson of Harvard University, the key to handling stress lies in learning how to produce a relaxation response to offset the stress response. Anything you can do to relax your mind and body on a regular basis will enhance your chances of managing stress in your life. Set aside time for yourself in the midst of your busy schedule. You deserve it! Then look for an activity that will help you switch off and relax. Go for a walk, read a book, listen to music, soak in a warm bath, practice yoga. Never use lack of time as an excuse to keep you from practicing relaxation techniques. *Make* the time, even when your schedule is hectic. Do it for yourself, because no one else will do it for you. Says syndicated columnist Marilyn Preston, "When the going gets tough, the tough must get still, using whatever calming technique you choose to find that deeply restful state."

Reserve Judgment

The Chinese character for crisis means "danger," but it can also be translated as "opportunity." This contrast in definition is basic to an understanding of stress and stress management: *It's not the event that is stressful, but the perception of the event.* Each of us sees the same event differently, as in the movie *Rashomon*, and this difference dictates whether or not the event produces stress. In other words, one person's stress can be another person's pleasure.

A famous anecdote illustrates this point. An elderly wealthy woman who lived in an elegant New York hotel was awakened at one o'clock in the morning by piano music from the adjoining suite. Boiling mad to be hearing "noise" at that hour, she called up the night manager and was told that the offender was none other than the world-renowned concert pianist Arthur Rubinstein; apparently disappointed in his performance that evening at Carnegie Hall, he was replaying the entire three-hour concert. Hearing this, the woman promptly forgot her complaint, pulled up a chair next to the wall and happily listened to Mr. Rubinstein play.

Had a change of events reduced the stress she originally felt? No, nothing had changed but her own response. She had taken a highly charged, stressful event and turned it into one of deep, satisfying pleasure. As author Carlos Castaneda has suggested, "Things don't change. You change your way of looking, that is all."

Focus on Concerns, Not Worries

16

A *concern* is a problem that can be addressed or a situation that can be changed. For example, being habitually late for work or car pool is a legitimate concern. It's a problem, but it can be addressed with an action such as setting the alarm clock for 15 minutes earlier or laying out clothes the night before. In this way, the concern is dealt with realistically, the problem is solved and the situation is de-stressed.

A *worry*, on the other hand, is immune to direct action. A good example is a woman who has been working to lose weight. She's been eating fewer calories, exercising regularly and making steady progress, until one day, in a moment of weakness, she eats a dozen Oreo cookies. Her mind turns this relatively minor slipup into a major event and time-travels to unlock unpleasant images of the past or bring up future "foul-ups." By dwelling on the incident, she feels guilty and her self-esteem suffers.

A better idea would be for this woman to zero in on the present and make it her *concern* to get back on track for weight control. Why worry about the event? It's over. It can't be undone. Worrying will not affect the outcome, but planning to eat fewer calories and exercise a few more minutes over the next couple of days will put things in perspective.

Expect the Unexpected

17

Build a cushion into your day for the unexpected. Instead of cramming your schedule, fill it to 80%, leaving 20% for traffic jams, family illness and other surprises.

Keep a Journal

Researchers have long recognized the health benefits that come from writing about significant personal experiences in an emotional way. Journaling is especially valuable in coping with the aftershocks of extremely stressful events such as divorce or the death of a spouse or close relative. Dr. James Pennebaker, a psychologist at the University of Texas, studied rape victims and others who experienced upsetting and traumatic events. He found that people who wrote about those experiences reduced their stress and consequently had fewer health problems than those who did not.

The same holds true for relieving daily stress—as long as you focus on feelings, not facts. You may want to start with where you were or what you were doing. But move quickly to a description of your reaction to the event and how it is affecting you. That will let you consider how those feelings square with your personal rules, values and beliefs.

The best way to get started is simply to write every day, at the same time and in a place set aside as a sanctuary. Use a notebook or computer. Some experts argue that the physical act of writing with a pen on paper is therapeutic, but we believe there are no rules. There is no right way or wrong way. Just let it rip. Even if words don't come easily to you, keep at it. The more you write, the quicker it will become second nature to you.

Practice Positive Self-Talk

Each of us is continually involved in self-talk, a running internal conversation that interprets events and actions. Most people are generally aware of some self-talk, yet a great deal of it occurs beyond conscious awareness. If you tune in to it, however, you become more aware of what you're telling yourself. After you've done that, you can begin practicing *positive* self-talk, a technique that will help you quiet your mind and gain a healthier perspective on life.

Unfortunately, much of our self-talk consists of negative, harmful put-downs. If corrected by a boss or parent, we might say to ourselves,

119

"Can't I do anything right? I'm always fouling things up!" These messages—not the event—trigger the stress. Indeed, whenever we tell ourselves "This is terrible," "How could they do this to me?" or "The workload is killing me," we set ourselves up for a nasty set of emotions. The procedure takes place in a step-by-step sequence of events:

A		B		C
SITUATION	→	BELIEF	→	EMOTION
(the event)		(self-talk)		(the result)

Suppose you're scheduled for an important job interview. You jump in your car and turn the key, but nothing happens. The interview is scheduled for nine A.M., and there's no way you can make it. This is the situation (A). The belief you have about the meaning of the event, your interpretation, takes the form of self-talk (B). In this instance, the talk is negative: "Mr. Brown will be disappointed in me. He'll think I'm rude and I don't care about the job. Why does this always happen to me? I'll never have such a great opportunity again." The result is, of course, skyrocketing stress (C).

But what if the self-talk is positive? "Mr. Brown will be unhappy with me because I'm late, but the battery is dead. Getting upset won't help. I'll call him to say I have to come by taxi. I won't be there on time, but I'm sure he'll understand. He's probably been caught in the same situation himself. And besides, he *wants* to talk to me. He knows I'll be a great addition to his company." This self-talk produces a very different perspective of the event and keeps it from generating overstress.

The A-B-C model illustrates how thinking influences feeling and explains why two different people can respond to the same situation with far different emotional reactions. The model also suggests that emotions can be changed by altering self-talk. This is known as *cognitive restructuring.* It calls for being aware of our negative self-talk, challenging those self-defeating comments and replacing them with positive statements that decrease or prevent a negative emotional response.

The first step toward positive self-talk is listening. Spend some time focusing on your inner monologue. Don't judge, don't apologize; just listen and learn. Then, the next time you notice a negative thought, try countering it with something positive. The trick is to stay in the moment, the zone of noncritical thinking, and not let yourself be dragged down by worries about what you did in the past or might do in the future.

Clarify Your Goals and Values

People who are under the greatest stress, say many psychologists, are those who drift through life without direction. They have no standard against which to measure their lives, which means that the act of living itself carries no reason and little joy. As Viktor Frankl, author of *Man's Search for Meaning*, wrote: "There is ample evidence that in many cases, depression, aggression and addiction are caused by feelings of emptiness and meaninglessness. Today, many people have enough to live on, but nothing to live for. They have the means, but no meaning."

Stress-resistant people, on the other hand, have goals that concern quality of life as well as material success. They concentrate on what is

WRITE YOUR OWN EPITAPH

One exercise we use in seminars may help you put your values and goals into perspective. Write your own epitaph, based on how you're presently living. Then ask yourself if that's how you'd like to be remembered. If you're a hardworking, perpetually stressed-out person who isn't home very much because of your job's travel requirements, you may end up writing "Here lies the best marketing consultant on the west coast." If you would rather have written "Here lies a great parent and a wonderful spouse," you may realize that your true values, priorities and goals are inconsistent with how you actually live. By putting balance in your life and reducing your stress, you will find more tranquillity—and often more productivity at work!

121

worth *being,* not just what is worth having. Sure, having goals of any sort can put us under some pressure, but when our goals are ones that make life meaningful, they work for us by allowing us to work toward them.

Dr. Robert S. Eliot used an exercise to clarify and crystallize priorities. He called it the "Six Months to Live" test. Suppose you had just six months to live and had to decide how to spend your time. You make three lists to identify 1) the things you have to do, 2) the things you want to do, and 3) the things you neither have nor want to do. Dr. Eliot recommended throwing the third list away, since the items on it are what's preventing you from doing what you really want to do. The first list should be taken care of, but once it's out of the way, the rest of the time should be spent on the second list—those things that give life meaning for you. It's important to select goals that are truly important and that reflect personal values, interests and talents.

Tranquilize with Exercise

Frequent exercisers have more positive moods and less anxiety than those who exercise little or not at all. In one study, researchers found that after 30 minutes on a treadmill, people scored 25% lower on anxiety tests and exhibited favorable changes in brain activity. "The relationship is clear across the board," says psychologist Thomas Stephen. "The more you exercise, the better your mood is and the less likely you are to be anxious or depressed."

No one is certain why this is so. One reason may be that the physical act of exercise allows the body to "throw off" tension. Anyone who runs, walks or swims regularly knows that post-exercise feeling— the body feels tired, even drained, but good and less stressed out.

Another possibility is that exercise reduces stress hormones, which is particularly important for those who suffer from chronic stress. Since these people are always geared up in a "fight or flight" mode, they generally have high levels of stress chemicals circulating in the bloodstream. When no physical response is necessary, the stress hormones bombard the coronary arteries, causing injury, inflammation and, in rare instances, sudden cardiac death. Exercise appears to burn up excess stress hormones. Obviously, the next time stress appears, the stress chemicals will reappear. With regular exercise, however, the body learns to metabolize these hormones more effectively, potentially reducing the likelihood of coronary injury.

A third possibility is that exercise stimulates the brain's production of endorphins, chemicals that produce a positive feeling and a happy, self-satisfied attitude and thus enhance one's sense of calm and well-being. Simply put, people who exercise regularly feel better about life. The result is an enhanced ability to cope with stress.

Other scientific studies support the notion that exercise can have a positive effect on emotions and moods:

- A University of Southern California study found the effect of a 15-minute walk to be comparable to that of a strong tranquilizer in reducing tension.

- A Duke University study showed that Type A behavior, characterized by aggressiveness and impatience, can be modified by aerobic exercise. In this study, 50 men and women aged 25 to 61 were tested to determine whether they were A or B types, then put on an exercise program (45 minutes, three times a week). After 10 weeks, the Type A's were found to be substantially calmer and more relaxed than they were at the start of the study.

- A study in England found that regular exercise boosts people's moods and may even fight clinical depression by elevating the body's levels of phenylethylamine, a natural chemical linked to energy, mood and attention. Men in the study who exercised had levels 14% to 57% higher than those who never exercised at all. Researchers speculate that phenylethylamine may play a role in the purported "runner's high."

- A review of research by the American Psychological Association on the effect of exercise on depression found that just five weeks of mild to moderate aerobic exercise and/or a weight training routine could boost mood. The research suggested that regular exercise can also benefit those who suffer from panic disorder.

The bottom line is that exercise makes you feel self-reliant, powerful, in control and generally better about yourself—all of which can reduce stress. Having the discipline to commit to regular exercise means you are in control. As clinical psychologist Dr. Kenneth R. Pelletier has observed, "When people begin to pay attention to their health, they seem to have a much better ability to look at things that used to bug them and simply be more detached. If you're taking time out of your life to exercise, you're taking a psychological stance that in itself is going to have you reacting differently to your job, your office, your sense of achievement, your career."

Breathe Deeply

When you're feeling stressed, your blood pressure increases and your muscles tense. There's little you can do about that, but you can control your breathing. And because breathing is one of the internal communications systems that tell your organs how to function, controlling your breathing can promote a relaxation response. Deep breathing can be used as a calming technique in response to a stressful situation, or it can be practiced regularly as a stress-preventive, done once or twice a day to break tension's hold. But in order to use the technique successfully, you must know how to breathe. Most people, particularly during stressful situations, tend to breathe incorrectly by expanding the rib cage. Chest breathing results in short, shallow breaths. It is constricting and actually *heightens* stress.

On the other hand, deep breathing, also called abdominal or diaphragmatic breathing, creates a state of calm. The technique is easy

LEARN HAPPINESS

Although the Declaration of Independence provides for the pursuit of happiness, there are no guarantees that the pursuit will be successful. Researchers such as Dr. Sonja Lyubomitsky at the University of California contend that happiness can be learned. "It's a product of both nature and nurture," says Dr. Lyubomitsky. "About 50% of happiness comes from the genetic variables—some people are born programmed to be happy. Another 10% of happiness comes from individual circumstances. And a whopping 40% is a result of behavior modification."

to practice and can be done standing, sitting or lying down. Find a comfortable position and take deep breaths through your nose with your mouth closed. As you inhale, push out your stomach. This lowers the diaphragm. Hold the breath for a few seconds, then expel it slowly and easily through your mouth with your lips pursed, as if you were whistling or kissing. Make your exhalation twice as long as your inhalation. Both intake and expulsion should be rhythmical. If you've never practiced deep breathing, a good way to learn it is to lie on your back, relax and place two or three books on your stomach. When you breathe in and push out your stomach, the books will rise. When you exhale, their weight should press in. Once you get the hang of it, you can practice deep breathing in any position, even sitting in a comfortable chair with your feet up.

By regulating your breathing, making it slow and regular, you're actually modulating your feelings. Do it for just a few minutes and tension will lessen. The key to success, however, is daily practice. If you want to be good at using deep breathing in an emergency, you have to be good at using it in ordinary circumstances.

Get Enough Sleep

A nationwide survey by the National Sleep Foundation found that 44% of Americans reported trouble falling asleep, 48% said they wake up in the night too often and 50% said they wake up feeling unrefreshed. Chronic sleeplessness is linked to psychological distress, such as depression and anxiety. Research at Pennsylvania State University suggests that blood levels of cortisol and other stress hormones are significantly higher in insomniacs than in healthy sleepers. But it's a catch-22. Getting seven to eight hours of sleep on a regular basis is critical to managing chronic stress, yet this kind of stress often keeps us awake.

So what can you do to get a good night's sleep?

■ **Avoid stimulants.** Don't drink any caffeine after two P.M. Avoid nicotine. And don't drink alcohol any later than three to five hours before bedtime.

- **Lose excess weight.** Overweight people are more prone to snoring and other nighttime breathing problems that can interfere with sleep.

- **Try not to nap during the day.** While napping for 15 to 20 minutes can increase alertness and productivity, a nap that lasts an hour or more can cause you to lapse into a deep sleep and wake up feeling worse than when you first fell asleep.

- **Exercise regularly.** Studies have shown that 30 to 40 minutes of daily exercise can help some people fall asleep more easily. But remember, the best time for exercise is in the morning or afternoon, not in the evening.

- **If you can't fall asleep, get out of bed,** no matter what time it is. Don't go back to bed until you feel sleepy.

- **Avoid eating heavy meals.** If you have to eat a meal an hour or so before bedtime, make it a light one.

- **Relax your mind** with meditation, deep breathing or prayer. Try not to watch TV or listen to the radio. Don't read or do work in your bed.

- **Establish a routine.** Have a regular time for getting out of bed each morning, regardless of how many hours you've slept. Try to go to bed and get up at the same time every day, even on Saturday and Sunday.

- **Establish a peaceful setting.** Minimize the amount of light and noise in your bedroom, and keep the temperature moderate.

- **Take a hot bath.** Researchers found that insomniacs who took a 30-minute warm bath about an hour before bedtime slept better than they had before.

- **Talk to your doctor.** Some over-the-counter or prescription medicines can interfere with sleep. Find out if anything you're taking could be having an effect on your ability to sleep.

Develop Resiliency

Because differences in the perception of stress explain why some people can weather devastating experiences with serenity and others cannot, researchers are looking carefully at resiliency—the ability to get through, get over and thrive after trauma, trials and tribulations. Instead of asking why bad things happen to good people, these scientists are now focusing on how good people can best overcome bad events or situations.

Stress-resistant, resilient people often share distinctive habits of the mind. They tend to focus on immediate issues rather than global ones. Work by Drs. Suzanne Kobasa and Salvatore Maddi shows that many such people are stress-resistant because of "hardy" personalities. In a study of the breakup of the Bell System, Drs. Kobasa and Maddi found that the executives who flourished under the change demonstrated three attitudinal characteristics:

- A sense of control—the belief that they can influence and shape events, and turn situations, even bad ones, to their advantage
- A commitment to life—the belief that their actions are worth doing at full tilt since they are useful to themselves, their families and to society, and the knowledge that no one aspect of life should become an obsession
- Love of a challenge—a willingness to accept and anticipate change as natural and exciting, not threatening

No one can be successful in everything. Failure is a product of the human condition. But failing does not have to be a weakness; it can provide for tremendous growth. It isn't the failure that's important; it's how you handle it. Imagine what would have happened if certain people had allowed themselves to think of themselves as failures:

- Albert Einstein's poor performance in all his high school classes except math prompted a teacher to predict failure for him and encourage him to leave school.
- Thomas Edison's father called him a dunce and his teachers described him as "addled," warning that he "would never amount to anything."
- Sir Winston Churchill, who twice failed the entrance exams to Sandhurst, was considered "dull" by his father.

If you're curious about how resilient you might be in the face of adversity, take the test on the next page, adapted from *The Survivor Personality* by Al Siebert, Ph.D.

HOW RESILIENT ARE YOU?

Circle the appropriate numbers below to rate how much each of the following applies to you (1 = very little; 5 = very much).

1 2 3 4 5   Curious; question how things work; experiment.

1 2 3 4 5   Constantly learn from own experience and experience of others.

1 2 3 4 5   Need and expect to have things work well for self and others. Take good care of self.

1 2 3 4 5   Play with new developments; find the humor, laugh at self, chuckle.

1 2 3 4 5   Adapt quickly; highly flexible.

1 2 3 4 5   Feel comfortable with paradoxical qualities.

1 2 3 4 5   Anticipate problems and avoid difficulties.

1 2 3 4 5   Increase self-esteem and self-confidence every year. Develop a conscious self-concept of professionalism.

1 2 3 4 5   Listen well; read others, including difficult people, with empathy.

1 2 3 4 5   Think up creative solutions to problems and challenges. Trust intuition and hunches.

1 2 3 4 5   Manage the emotional side of recovery. Grieve, honor and let go of the past.

1 2 3 4 5   Expect tough situations to work out well; keep on going. Help others, bring stability to times of uncertainty and turmoil.

1 2 3 4 5   Find the gift in accidents and bad experiences.

1 2 3 4 5   Convert misfortune into good fortune.

Add numbers for your score:

60 to 70: Highly resilient   30 to 39: Struggling
50 to 59: Better than most   Under 30: Seek help
40 to 49: Adequate

Can you learn resiliency and hardiness? Drs. Kobasa and Maddi say yes. First focus on signals from the body that something is wrong, then mentally review the situation that might be stressful. Next, mentally reconstruct the stressful situation to think about how it could have gone better or worse. This often illustrates that things did not go as badly as they might have. And finally, compensate for stress through self-improvement. When life seems out of control, taking on a new challenge can result in regaining self-esteem and a sense of accomplishment.

The source of the stress—loss of a job, divorce, health problems—may be impossible to avoid. But by taking on a new task, a person is assured that he or she can still function.

Meditate

Studies at UCLA and Harvard University show the physiological effects of meditation. When you're asleep, your oxygen consumption is decreased by 8%. With meditation, however, it's down by 12%, an indication that your body is equally if not even more deeply relaxed. These studies also illustrate that meditation can decrease blood pressure significantly.

One centuries-old technique, called repetition, involves the repeating of a single word for a concentrated but brief period of time. Designed to clear the mind and anchor it in the present, it produces an immediate calming effect on the nervous system. Start by selecting a quiet spot. Loosen your clothing and remove your shoes. Assume a comfortable sitting or reclining position, close your eyes and prepare to focus on something—an object, a word or your breathing. Empty your mind of everything else. Take a deep breath and slowly repeat a single word. In *The Relaxation Response,* Dr. Herbert Benson recommends using words or sounds that end in *m* or *n,* such as "calm" or "ocean," but any appropriate word will do. Slowly repeat the word mentally, over and over again. Other thoughts will occasionally interfere, but just let them pass through your mind. After a while, repetition will have an almost hypnotic effect and create a state of deep rest and relaxation. In a few minutes, you'll feel renewed energy and optimism. Meditation requires only 10 to 30 minutes, but is most effective when done every day at the same time.

Author Deepak Chopra says, "Meditation is not a way of making your mind quiet. It's a way of entering into the quiet that's already there—buried under the 50,000 thoughts the average person thinks every day."

SPEAKING FROM EXPERIENCE

I know several heart patients who are big believers in the positive effects of meditation, but frankly it's hard for me to do. As a Type A personality, I have difficulty clearing my mind. Lists of things I should be doing just seem to pop in, and the next thing I know, I'm thinking about a project instead of meditating. So, for me, deep breathing, progressive muscle relaxation and exercise work best as ways to create a relaxation response. But for many, many others, meditation is an effective means of coping with stress.   **—J.P.**

---

26 Listen to Your Spiritual Side

Good family relationships, playing bridge with friends, belonging to the Elks or Rotary—all are associated with less stress. New studies are finding that having a religious faith and a sense of spirituality can also reduce stress. According to Dr. Fred Luskin of the Stanford University School of Medicine, "People who go to church, synagogue, mosque or Buddhist monastery once a week average 83 years of longevity. For those who do not go at all, longevity averages 75 years. You do the math!"

Historically the belief in a faith-health connection centered on God's healing power. Most of us have heard stories of people who, by sheer faith alone, have miraculously recovered from terminal illnesses or survived longer than thought possible by physicians. Their prayers, and the prayers of others in their behalf, caused divine intervention. And while that certainly may be true, it cannot be proven scientifically. It is a matter of faith.

More recently, however, medical studies are showing that spiritual beliefs and participation in organized religion have a measurable, beneficial health effect. More than 30 scientific studies have linked spiritual or religious commitment and more effective management of stress with better health or a longer life:

- A 29-year study of people aged 25 to 55 in Alameda, California, found that those who attended religious services once a week had 36% lower mortality than nonattendees.

- Those with a religious commitment had fewer symptoms and better health outcomes in seven out of eight cancer studies, four out of five blood pressure studies, four out of six heart disease studies and four out of five general health studies.

- One study showed that people with normal blood pressure who worship regularly are less likely to experience high blood pressure in the future.

- Over 200 studies by Dr. Jeffrey Levin of Duke University Medical Center found that a positive connection between religion and health cuts across age, sex, cultural and geographic boundaries.

According to Dr. Herbert Benson, praying elicits a relaxation response in the body similar to meditation or deep-breathing exercises. It decreases blood pressure, heart rate and breathing rate, and diffuses stress chemicals. "It is a legitimate stress-management technique," says Dr. Benson.

Religious faith also promotes a sense of hope and control, which provides a better ability to cope with stress and adverse events such as health problems. Research has shown that when people over 60 are hospitalized, over 50% report they use religious faith as their primary coping mechanism. Says Dr. Harold Koenig of Duke University, "Commitment to a system of beliefs enables people to better handle the stress of traumatic illness, suffering and loss. The opposite is also true. Loss of religious faith, feelings of doubt and anger are normal when dealing with serious illness. But when people get stuck there, it creates stress that interferes with the body's ability to recover."

Attending religious services provides the social support associated with stress reduction. Says Dr. Fred Luskin, "Social bonding is a well-documented key to health and longevity. Church, synagogue or mosque often provides an 'us' in an 'us vs. them' world. It is a family, a circle of friends. It provides community and support so helpful to allowing us to move safely through our lives. This protective effect results in less stress and better health."

Many religious people also practice "sin avoidance," staying clear of excessive drinking, smoking, taking drugs and engaging in risky sexual practices. In addition, religious faiths tend to encourage marriage, which in itself has been linked to longer life.

Visualize Life as You Want It

27 Jim Carrey visualized himself receiving $20 million before he ever made it in Hollywood. Life *is* as you picture it, and programming your brain with positive mental images can help reduce your stress. The MacArthur Foundation Study findings suggest that longevity and successful aging are more mental than genetic.

Take Up Tai Chi

28 Tai chi, sometimes called "meditation in motion," is a Chinese martial art that improves physical function and promotes mental and spiritual well-being by lowering blood pressure, enhancing self-confidence and reducing levels of the stress hormone cortisol.

The highly disciplined movements and forms of tai chi help to unite the body and mind, thereby bringing harmony and balance to life. Unlike karate and other "external" martial arts, tai chi has an "internal" focus emphasizing complete relaxation. It is characterized by soft, slow, flowing, precisely executed movements.

Tai chi is a particularly good way to dissipate stress for people who prefer a physical basis for promoting a relaxation response. Says Dr. William Kaplindis, "We recommend that people go home and listen to a relaxing tape or do meditation, but many people are not going to do that. They want to do something physical for relaxation, and tai chi is perfect for them."

Because it is low-impact, tai chi has multiple advantages for elderly people who want to improve balance and prevent osteoporosis. One study found that when compared with nonstudents, tai chi students (average age, 76) went an average 48% longer before experiencing a first fall.

"People generally learn tai chi in a class, where beginners can learn the forms," says Dr. Kaplindis. "But ideally, they will incorporate tai chi into their daily practice, even doing it on days when there is no class, in order to get the maximum benefit." To find a qualified tai chi instructor in your area, consult your local alternative health association.

29 Practice PMR

Progressive muscular relaxation (PMR) is one of the best ways to clear tension from the body. In this technique, you tense a group of muscles, hold them in their contracted state for a few seconds, then release and relax them. By concentrating on groups of muscles, you can imagine them relaxed, which in turn causes an actual relaxation to take place.

Begin by finding a quiet place where you can spend an uninterrupted half-hour. Lie on your back in a comfortable position with your arms at your sides and legs uncrossed. Loosen any restrictive clothing. Close your eyes and adjust your body position to be comfortable. Focus your attention on breathing. Notice the movement of air through your nostrils down into your lungs, filling them up, and then back out again. Breathing should be deep and easy, rhythmic and smooth. Bring attention to the muscles of your scalp and forehead; tune in to feelings of tension there. Tighten your scalp and forehead muscles. Squeeze and hold the tension, then release it, relaxing the area.

JAW STRESS RELIEVER

The Academy of General Dentistry suggests putting your tongue between your teeth or at the roof of your mouth toward the back during times of stress. This will keep your upper and lower teeth apart, thereby preventing your jaw from tightening and your teeth from grinding.

133

Repeat this cycle with all parts of your body, starting with your head and moving systematically through your arms, shoulders, abdomen, buttocks and legs down to your feet. Be aware of each area, tighten the area, then relax. Go slowly. Let go more and more until your whole body is in a state of deep relaxation. Allow the tension to flow out with each breath. After you've gone through these steps, you will feel very calm, refreshed and rejuvenated.

30 Release Stress Now!

Don't wait until the end of the day to tackle stress.

Whenever you're feeling uptight, frustrated, overwhelmed or mentally drained, ask yourself, "What can I do *right now* to relax and manage my stress burden?" Some good choices include changing your posture, listening to soft music, being kind to or doing something for someone, taking a short walk, soaking in a warm bath, having a drink of water, taking a relaxation break, making a change in your routine and taking a few moments to breathe deeply.

31 Laugh

According to Dr. William F. Fry Jr. of the Stanford School of Medicine, a good laugh—like a good workout—produces an overall sense of well-being. Laughter flexes the muscles of the chest and abdomen, including the diaphragm, and causes deep breathing to take place. By exercising the shoulders, neck and face, it releases tension in the muscles. And humor itself can help create a different perspective on life and its challenges. As cardiologist Dr. Steve Yarnall says, "Laughter is the shortest distance between two people."

Until recently, many health professionals discounted laughter's therapeutic effect. Now things are changing, in large part because of the groundbreaking work done by Norman Cousins, once editor of *Saturday Review* and subsequently a professor at the UCLA School of Medicine. In his book *Anatomy of an Illness,* he recounts how laughter helped to cure an unexplained sudden illness for which he had been hospitalized.

After a period of time with no progress, he abandoned conventional thinking, stopped taking medication and ordered in reel upon reel of old Marx Brothers films. According to Mr. Cousins, his heavy, sustained laughter was the key to his recovery.

On average, adults laugh 15 times a day. If we can up that number, we can reduce the stress that underlies so many diseases. You can do that by cultivating friends and acquaintances who smile and joke, putting playfulness into your relationships and leaving work concerns at the office. Just remember the words of comedian Milton Berle: "Laughter is an instant vacation."

Practice Yoga

Yoga comes from a Sanskrit word that means "yoking," in this case joining or balancing the mind, body and breath through the practice and mastering of three principles. First are the specific physical postures called asanas; held for an extended period of time, they are designed to relax and tone the muscles. Second are the pranayama, or breathing exercises, that slow breathing and increase the body's vital energy. And third is resting completely between postures.

Practiced for a thousand years, yoga's stretching, strengthening and meditative exercises encourage complete focusing on movement and the body parts involved. Yoga trains the mind and body to work together to create a healing environment.

There are few scientific studies regarding the health benefits of yoga, but participants report feeling better, more relaxed and centered, with fewer headaches, less back pain and less severe menstrual cramps. Yoga dissipates stress by increasing flexibility and reducing muscle tension and tightness, which the body interprets as a generalized reduction in tension and mental stress. It also teaches you to be more in touch with your breathing and to breathe more easily throughout the day to relieve tension. And finally, it can free your thoughts. Yoga teaches that your thoughts have the ability to affect your overall contentment and health. During the deep relaxation pose, every part of the body is systematically relaxed, serving as a kind of meditation to relieve stress.

135

Experts suggest that the best way to learn yoga is to take a class with a trained leader. Audiotapes and videotapes are available for practicing yoga at home, but most people make better progress with personal instruction. Classes are offered at private studios, health clubs and community recreation centers in many areas. Your instructor will be able to advise you on different moves and techniques to practice at home.

Be Assertive

33

For many people, feelings of stress arise from not knowing how to say no. These people feel put upon yet powerless to change the circumstances. Learning how to be more assertive, to make your own needs known to others in a forceful, honest and polite manner, can significantly reduce the level of stress.

If you don't express your feelings and needs when it's your right to do so, or if you discount your feelings as being unimportant or less worthy than someone else's feelings, emotions get bottled up and you feel miserable. On the other hand, aggression to the point of insults or criticisms fosters neither effective communication nor positive relationships.

Being assertive means stating your feelings and requesting appropriate change. If a meeting is scheduled for a time convenient for others but not for you, an assertive statement of feelings can avert later feelings of stress: "I'd really like to be at the meeting, but this isn't a good time for me." Follow up with a request for appropriate change: "I know we've tried to find a time good for everyone, but let's give it one more try."

Assertiveness is not rudeness. It's simply taking your own needs and desires into consideration, but often the mind has to overcome the heart in order to get there. Your mind knows you have a right to put yourself first sometimes, but your heart feels the familiar childhood programming that "nice people always put others first." Assertive thinking and action will place you in control.

Take a Vacation

Skipping vacations can have a devastating impact on cardiovascular health. Studies show that people who don't take an annual vacation are 21% more likely to die over the next nine years and 32% more likely to die of coronary heart disease than those who take time off each year. "This is either because vacations reduce heart problems or because people with heart problems don't take vacations," says Dr. Brooks Gump of the State University of New York at Oswego. "Either way, the more often you skip your vacation, the higher your risk of death. People need to start thinking of vacation as preventive medicine."

While no one is certain of the mechanism involved, evidence shows that the very qualities that lead us to bypass vacation also tend to promote heart disease. As Dr. Gene Ondrusek of the Scripps Center for Executive Health has observed, "Executives will say, 'Gosh, it's been years since I've had a vacation,' and it's almost said with pride, as evidence of their commitment and ambition. There's a driven quality there. There is also a cynical hostility, a paranoia: 'If I leave, someone working in the background is going to take my position.' Or they don't trust that whoever is filling in for them will do a good job. Unfortunately, cynical hostility is linked to chronic stress and is known to promote heart disease." Equally unfortunate is the survey finding that

SPEAKING FROM EXPERIENCE

As long as it relaxes you, any type of vacation can promote stress management. Obviously, touring 20 cities in Europe in 18 days is more stressful than lying on a beach in Maui for a week. But the real point of going on vacation is just to leave your normal life at home. If you bring your briefcase, cell phone and laptop, are you taking a break . . . or just setting up a new office location? One executive told me that on her last vacation she answered more than a hundred e-mails a day! That, I think, is at odds with using vacation time to produce a relaxation response. **—J.P.**

many workers believe it will reflect positively on them if they don't take their allotted vacation time.

Some researchers believe that the scenic beauty encountered on many vacations can promote health; it focuses attention, helping people plan better and deflect distractions while lowering irritability. Others say that relaxation can be found in the escapism of reading on vacation (history or "trashy" novels, but not business books). And to Dr. Herbert Benson the benefit lies in the fact that vacations "break the train of everyday thought that often drives you up a wall, such as finances, family and deadlines."

"We don't know if it's just the absence of stress on vacations or some positive, restorative quality when you get away," says Dr. Gump. "But whatever it is, it works. Regular vacations help people handle stress and reduce the risk of heart disease."

Stretch

35 *HEART SAVER*

In addition to decreasing the risk of injury, helping to relieve low-back pain and improving agility, regular stretching exercises promote a relaxation response. Stretching acts as an internal massage for the body.

There are many good books and videos to get you started. Health clubs and community recreation centers often offer instruction. Whether on your own or in a class, here are a few guidelines:

- **A regular program is most effective.** Plan to stretch at least two to three times per week and more often if you're under chronic stress. Stick to a schedule.
- **Muscles stretch best when they're warm.** Stretch after a cardiovascular routine, such as brisk walking, or after a hot bath or shower. If your muscles are "cold," jog in place before stretching.
- **Don't bounce when you stretch.** View your stretching routine as a time for relaxation. Go slowly and gently.
- **Avoid pain.** Stretch to the point of tension but not pain.
- **Perform stretches in a slow, controlled manner.** Remember to breathe. Relax and exhale as you go into a stretch, then breathe normally and slowly.

- ■ **Never stretch injured or strained muscles.**
- ■ **Take your time.** Hold each stretch for 10 to 30 seconds, to the point of mild discomfort or where you "feel the stretch." Pause and then repeat the stretch at least three more times.

36 Volunteer

People under chronic stress often make themselves the center of the universe. Almost everything in life—events, relationships, workloads—is seen in terms of how it impacts them. As a result, they are constantly vigilant and prone to anxiety.

Changing from an inward to an outward perspective can break this cycle. A great way to do this is by becoming a volunteer. Coach a youth soccer team. Read to elderly shut-ins. Man the information desk at the hospital. Get involved in a political campaign. Find an area of interest and give something of yourself to it. You'll forget your problems, widen your perspective and establish meaningful relationships. As cardiologist Dr. Fred Pashkow likes to tell his patients, "Volunteering helps to establish a realistic perspective and bring balance to your lives. Helping others simply makes it harder to dwell on your own troubles. And anytime you can put your own troubles aside, even temporarily, you reduce your stress."

37 Get a Massage

Whether the method is Swedish, pressure-point, sports massage, shiatsu, acupressure, reflexology, deep-tissue or craniosacral, massage therapy is designed to improve health and well-being through the hands-on manipulation of muscles and other soft tissues of the body. It may also reduce heart rate, lower blood pressure, increase blood circulation, relax the muscles and improve range of motion. Many people use therapeutic massage as part of their regular health-care maintenance. As defined in the *Journal of the American Massage Therapy Association*, "Massage is to the human body what a tune-up is to a car."

But there are many other positive results. Massage also:

- Fosters peace of mind and a sense of well-being.
- Promotes a relaxed state of mental alertness.
- Reduces levels of anxiety and helps to relieve mental stress.
- Improves the ability to monitor stress signals and respond appropriately.
- Enhances the capacity for calm thinking and creativity.
- Satisfies the need for caring/nurturing touch.
- Increases awareness of the mind-body connection.

The cost is typically $50 to $120 for a one-hour session. Be sure that your practitioner is licensed.

Don't Be a Stranger

The MacArthur Foundation's landmark study on successful aging identifies meaningful social relationships as being of equal importance to diet and exercise in a healthy life. Associate with people who share common interests, make you laugh and help you feel good about yourself. Stay in touch with friends and family. Talk things over. When tensions build up, discuss the problem with a close friend or with the people involved.

Positive social connections keep you from feeling that you're going through life alone. You have help and support.

Be Realistic

Set practical goals and expect to meet them. Don't overload yourself with more work or commitments than you can handle. Let go of perfectionism; your home doesn't always have to be spotless, and you don't always have to be the last one to leave the office. And don't expect perfection from others, either.

Try to meet daily challenges in a logical manner. Even personal problems, if approached intelligently and systematically, have reasonable solutions. Focusing on one small part at a time will make each challenge seem less overwhelming.

Get a Pet

This is not as offbeat as it may sound. Scientific evidence suggests that those who keep pets are likely to benefit from improvements in physical and emotional well-being. Indeed, pets seem to be particularly therapeutic for people with or at risk of heart disease. Several years ago, researchers studied patients in a coronary-care unit at a major hospital. All had experienced a heart attack or had severe chest pain. In the one-year follow-up, 28% of those who did not own pets had died, as compared with only 6% of pet owners. Critics said these findings might simply reflect an association; in other words, those who felt better had taken on the responsibility of caring for a pet. Yet even when other factors like physical health and severity of heart disease were accounted for, pet ownership remained an independent predictor of survival.

People with pets seem to handle stress better and have lower blood pressure. In addition, many behavioral scientists contend that loneliness, isolation, depression and hostility—all powerful predictors of adverse health outcomes—may be partially alleviated by the companionship of pets. Some experts believe this may stem from active involvement in the daily care of pets and from the unconditional love and acceptance that the animals offer their owners.

And finally, dogs in particular have a positive effect on health because of a second factor: walking them is great exercise!

SPEAKING FROM EXPERIENCE

In my house, it's impossible to walk past our miniature dachshunds Luke and Cody without petting them or inviting them for a walk. When they're bad, they instinctively roll over on their backs so I can rub their stomachs, and immediately my anger turns to laughter. I'm convinced that I'm the one who benefits most from these pedestrian interactions. Surveys show that most people who keep pets describe them as family members. And, says Dr. Redford Williams of Duke University, contact with animals helps to restore our bond with nature.   —B.F.

Control Your Anger and Hostility

Anger and hostility greatly increase cardiac risk. But you can learn to gain control:

■ **Exercise regularly.** This can increase the natural painkillers called endorphins, which may help to reduce anxiety and frustration.

■ **Accept conflict as a normal part of life.** Conflict is part of every relationship.

■ **Find your triggers.** Keep a record of your "hot buttons" and what seems to trigger them. Then work to avoid them.

■ **Don't insist that everyone agree with you.** Learn to disagree without being disagreeable.

■ **Think before you speak.** Make sure your own attitude isn't the root cause of your anger. Don't assume people are out to get you or to insult you intentionally. Try to understand the other person's point of view.

■ **Take time out.** Deep breathing, counting to 10 or removing yourself from an adverse situation can let you calm down and regain control.

■ **Do more laughing.** Try to put some humor in the situation to defuse anger before it arises.

THE DANGERS OF ANGER

Angry young medical students are apt to become angry old doctors with heart attacks, according to a long-term study conducted by the Johns Hopkins University School of Medicine. The study found that medical students who became angry quickly when under stress were three times more likely than normal to develop premature heart disease and five times more likely than their calmer colleagues to have an earlier heart attack. Said Dr. Patricia Chang, lead author of the study, "Our findings suggest that people who have a very high level of anger, in contrast to people with little anger or none in settings of stress, are at risk for premature cardiovascular disease, even when controlling for other risk factors like family history, hypertension and diabetes."

- **Practice positive self-talk.** Angry, negative words often cause a stress response from the body. Keep a positive perspective.
- **Don't blame others.** Take full responsibility for how you feel or for what happens to you.
- **Be forgiving and patient.** Remember that most people are doing the best they can.

If you can't control your anger, you may want to consult a psychiatrist or psychologist trained in cognitive behavior therapy. This can help you change the way you look at and react to situations. Medications are also available to help stabilize mood. Talk with your physician.

Turn Off the TV

Thanks to television, America is perhaps the most informed nation on earth. The morning news, the evening and late-night reports—not to mention extended cable and Internet coverage—these are staples of modern life.

Unfortunately, what is presented on TV is often unbalanced, not necessarily in the "to the left or right" sense, but because TV news presents hyped-up versions of today's headlines that are invariably sensationalized and negative. Instead of producing clarity, it increases anxiety. Every day we are subjected to unforgettable images of violence and destruction; the more raw the footage (the shootings at Columbine or the destruction of the World Trade Center), the more we see it. "TV news is a fear factory," says Gavin de Becker, author of *Fear Less*. "It impersonates information when, in fact, most of the time it is delivering sensation."

When natural disasters—floods, earthquakes, tornadoes, hurricanes—cause terrible headlines, we feel sad for the people whose lives are affected by them. But these events don't register as viscerally as when humans commit violent acts. Stories about such acts can fray the nerves and produce overwhelming uncertainty. "People can be vicariously traumatized," says Dr. Edward Hallowell. "With the access we now have to bad news, you can be put into a worried state each night."

But you can always turn off your TV set and get more of your news from written reporting, which tends to provide a calmer, less-hyped account of current events. It also helps you concentrate on your immediate surroundings—family, work, friends and community. By being involved in "real life" events, you will feel less anxious and more in control.

Make Exercise a Habit

The Exercise Advantage

"**I**F EXERCISE COULD BE PACKAGED INTO A PILL," says Dr. Robert Butler, former director of the National Institute on Aging, "it would be the single most widely prescribed and beneficial medicine in the nation." With physical activity ranking so high on the list of smart things to do for your heart and health, you'd think most Americans would have gotten the message to exercise regularly. And if you judged us by our appearance—jogging shoes, biking pants, warm-up suits—you'd think the country was in the middle of a fitness boom.

Think again. Americans do not exercise. We just buy exercise stuff. According to government data, about 70% of the adult population admits to being inactive or not regularly active. "The interesting thing is that 97% of people place good health as their number one priority," says Joe Cirulli of the International Health, Racquet and Sportsclub Association, "but still a lot of people fail to make the vital connection between exercise and health."

Only about 30% of the U.S. adult population gets the recommended level of daily physical activity. The percentage is even less among African Americans, Hispanics and Latinos. Moreover, new members of health and fitness clubs typically use these facilities less than twice per month! Says Dr. Steven Schroeder of the University of California at San Francisco, "Physical inactivity, along with obesity, accounts for 365,000 premature deaths each year in the United States." Dr. Frank Booth of the University of Missouri echoes the thought: "The impact of inactivity-related diseases is so great that we've actually created a new category called sedentary death syndrome, or SeDS."

In truth, our grandparents didn't spend time jogging or working out at the gym, but there was a lot of physical activity built naturally into their lives. Then lifestyles changed radically with the advent of automation, labor-saving devices and all the electronic paraphernalia of the information

SITTING CAN BE HAZARDOUS TO YOUR HEALTH

Recent studies indicate that people who sit for long periods have a significantly greater risk of premature heart attack and diabetes.

age. "What occurred," explains Dr. Michael Jensen of the Mayo Clinic, "was the culmination of a century of invention and industrial development. Technology took most people out of fields and factories and plopped them behind desks. As work became more sedentary, so did workers." In the contemporary work environment, we are generally paid to think, to provide specific sedentary skills and to communicate or process information. Smart phones, BlackBerrys and laptop computers have become part of our vocational garb. The elimination of physical activity in the workplace is also compounded by the fact that so many suburbanites commute to their jobs. As Dr. Gregory Heath of the University of Tennessee College of Medicine has pointed out, "The average American rides about 22 miles a day in a car, bus or other form of motorized transportation."

Leisure-time activities have also shifted in the direction of non-physical pursuits. In past generations, families went to the park or out to the backyard after dinner to catch or kick a ball. Nowadays, popular sedentary pastimes include watching TV or DVDs, viewing sports, listening to MP3 players, using cell phones, playing video games, e-mailing, searching the Internet and gambling. Automobiles, elevators, remote controls and energy-saving devices such as dishwashers, microwave ovens, self-propelled lawn mowers, electric snow blowers, automatic garage door openers and online ordering/bill paying have helped to engineer physical activity out of daily life.

The Benefits of Exercise

MANY PEOPLE HAVE COME TO THINK OF EXERCISE PROGRAMS AS synonymous with vigorous physical activity like jogging or running, but numerous health benefits can be derived at more moderate exercise intensities, including better management of coronary risk factors. Critical for weight loss, exercise also extends longevity and increases self-esteem.

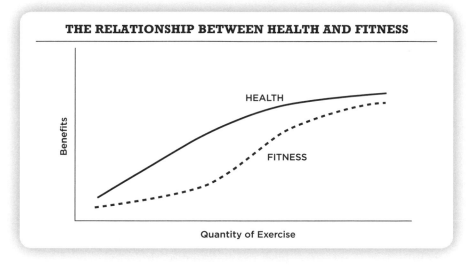

THE RELATIONSHIP BETWEEN HEALTH AND FITNESS

The graph above shows the theoretical relationship between health and fitness from increasing doses of exercise. It is apparent that health benefits can occur at lower levels or intensities of exercise—amounts that may not necessarily improve aerobic fitness. Such programs, however, are usually associated with an increased exercise duration, frequency, or both.

Exercise and the Heart

Exercise is particularly important because it both directly and indirectly influences all cardiac markers. Studies show that people who attain cardiovascular fitness through exercise reduce their risk of a heart attack by up to 50%—more than the best cholesterol-lowering drugs can accomplish. Conversely, physical inactivity is linked directly to an increase in cardiac risk. Says Dr. Steven Blair of the University of South Carolina, "From a public health perspective, the emphasis on getting sedentary adults to become moderately active is highly appropriate; the evidence shows that on a population-wide basis, this is where the majority of the health benefits are to be obtained."

Two landmark studies solidified the strong relationship between physical activity and protection from coronary heart disease. Dr. Ralph Paffenbarger and associates examined almost 17,000 Harvard alumni and found that the active men in the group had 35% fewer heart attacks and

149

lived about two and a half years longer than their sedentary counterparts; moreover, fit persons who suffered heart attacks were more likely to survive. And Dr. Steven Blair showed that even a minimal improvement in fitness, which may be achieved by a half-hour walk daily, could reduce cardiac mortality substantially.

Results of the long-running Nurses' Health Study have shown that three hours of brisk walking each week or half that time spent in more vigorous exercise (such as jogging or aerobic dance) reduces the risk of heart disease by 35% to 40%. This study is important because 1) it's the first large study to look at women and exercise, and 2) it found that intensity matters, but moderate intensity can be highly effective—it just takes more time. "Strolling won't do it, no matter how long you walk," says Dr. JoAnn Manson. "You have to stride out at three miles per hour or more, or 20 minutes or less per mile. But three hours of brisk walking and an hour and a half of vigorous exercise use the same amount of energy." Recent studies suggest that vigorous activity confers added cardiovascular benefits over more moderate exercise.

A program of regular exercise benefits the heart in the following areas:

Cardiac muscle. All muscle responds to physical activity by increasing in size and strength. When exercised, cardiac muscle gets stronger and more efficient. Says Dr. Steven Blair, "If you exercise, what you get is a bigger, better, stronger pump. Exercising regularly promotes improvement in the heart's ability to transport and use oxygen. The more fit the cardiovascular system, the more oxygen the heart can deliver to the body's muscles and the more easily muscles can extract oxygen from the blood."

The ability to perform with less effort can greatly reduce strain on the heart because a strong heart can pump the same volume of blood in fewer strokes. This is how it works: An "average" resting pulse is 72 beats per minute, or 103,680 beats a day; however, if the heart becomes more efficient through regular exercise, the resting pulse might be reduced to 58 beats per minute, or just 83,520 beats a day. Even if a vigorous daily one-hour workout requires an increase of 5,000 heartbeats a day (as compared with rest), this still represents a net saving of 15,160 heartbeats each day.

SPEAKING FROM EXPERIENCE

We put exercise before diet because it can positively influence what we call dietary compliance—the ability to make permanent dietary changes once and for all. Anyone can eat healthfully for a week. The real challenge is to do it for a lifetime. Just look at the huge number of Americans who go on and off diets every year.

Although starting and sticking with an exercise program is challenging, it's probably easier than making long-term dietary changes. Exercise and recreational activities are about doing something positive and enjoyable, whereas dieting is often seen as a negative experience. It's easier to establish a walking routine than it is to give up (or even cut back on) favorite foods.

But that isn't the only reason for this sequence. As the old axiom says, "Nothing breeds success like success." And success in establishing an exercise routine can provide a foundation for changing the way you eat. So, at this point in the protocol, I'd suggest putting questions of diet aside until you've learned to manage your stress and exercise regularly. Within a month or so, you can work up to walking 45 minutes, three to five times (or more) a week. Not only will this activity further help you to cope with chronic stress (which is often a trigger for mindless eating), but you'll have greater self-confidence and self-esteem. Once you feel better about yourself, you'll be ready to tackle your diet   **— I P**

Heart rate. Regular exercise can reduce the likelihood of extremely rapid heart rates resulting from physical or emotional stress. For instance, when the heart is called upon to beat faster because of a strenuous activity like shoveling snow, it may speed up to 180 beats a minute or more in an effort to supply blood to the muscles. This can strain the heart and cause plaque rupture, which may lead to a heart attack, potentially fatal heart rhythm irregularities, or both. It's the same for emotional stress. We've all experienced near-misses with a car and that "heart in your throat" feeling. In a conditioned heart, the slowdown mechanism helps to keep racing heartbeats in check. But a deconditioned heart may refuse to slow down and instead speed up dangerously.

HDL cholesterol. High HDL is protective of cardiac health, while lower levels raise risk. Researchers at Stanford University reported that walking two miles a day, three times a week, can raise HDL by up to 10%. Greater increases may occur with more extensive exercise or in persons with low baseline values. However, you don't have to run marathons to get the HDL boost. Dr. Kenneth Cooper suggests that running no less than two miles four times a week, and no more than three miles five times a week, can have a profound impact on HDL, comparable to running even higher mileages. The key message is that moderate-to-vigorous regular exercise can boost HDL levels and positively influence cardiac health.

Coronary arteries. The exact mechanism is not well understood, but exercise appears to reduce arterial inflammation. For example, recent studies in both men and women indicate that increased fitness levels are associated with lower C-reactive protein values. It may be that by helping to dissipate stress, exercise prevents hormones such as cortisol from injuring the artery wall. It may be because exercise helps to control high blood pressure, which is also a source of injury. And it may be that exercise improves the ability of the coronary arteries to dilate, increasing blood flow to the heart muscle.

Other studies now indicate that vigorous exercise promotes the proliferation of tiny coronary blood vessels and vascular regeneration. In addition, aerobic exercise conditioning can reduce the heart rate at rest and during any given level of exercise. The result appears to be increased cardiac electrical stability and a decreased likelihood of sudden cardiac death.

Blood clotting. Exercise is one of the best ways to lower your fibrinogen level and reduce blood viscosity and the risk of easy platelet aggregation. In addition, people who exercise regularly have the ability to dissolve blood clots more easily.

Blood pressure. A recent review of studies by the American College of Sports Medicine concluded that endurance exercise prevents the development of high blood pressure and lowers blood pressure in adults with and without hypertension. These effects of exercise are most pronounced in people with hypertension, averaging five to seven points. Moderate-intensity training, like walking, seemed to be just as effective as higher-intensity training, and possibly even more so.

Exercise also promotes weight loss, which in turn reduces blood pressure. But exercise may trigger an independent blood-pressure-lowering mechanism as well. Studies at Boston University have found that regular exercise can cause blood vessels to dilate over time, thereby reducing resistance to flow.

Stroke. Data from the Nurses' Health Study show that women who exercise regularly (five days a week) and moderately (30 to 60 minutes of brisk walking) have half the risk of stroke as their sedentary counterparts. More recently, this finding was echoed by researchers at the Cooper Clinic, who reported that, during an average follow-up of 10 years, men who were moderately or very fit had a lower risk of stroke mortality (approximately 65%) when compared with men who had a low level of fitness.

Exercise and Weight Loss

Can we say it often enough? Americans are habitually sedentary and getting fatter. This is echoed by the Surgeon General's Report, which cites reduction of physical activity as a major cause of overweight and obesity. According to the report, low levels of physical activity, resulting in fewer calories used than consumed, contribute to the high prevalence of obesity in the United States.

According to Dr. James Hill, an internationally recognized expert on obesity, our increased reliance on technology has resulted in a positive energy balance (taking in more calories than we expend), as illustrated in the diagram on page 154. Dr. Hill suggests that the most likely explanation for the current obesity epidemic among Americans is a continued decline in energy expenditure that has not been matched by an equivalent reduction in caloric intake.

This may surprise you, but many overweight people do not on average consume more calories than people of normal weight. Obviously, they consume sufficient calories to stay overweight, but they do not necessarily eat more than other people do. A study of San Francisco runners showed that the men consumed an average of 2,960 calories per day but weighed 20% less than inactive men their age who consumed only 2,360 calories per day; the women averaged 570 calories more per day but weighed 30% less than their inactive counterparts. Experts say that in about 70% of

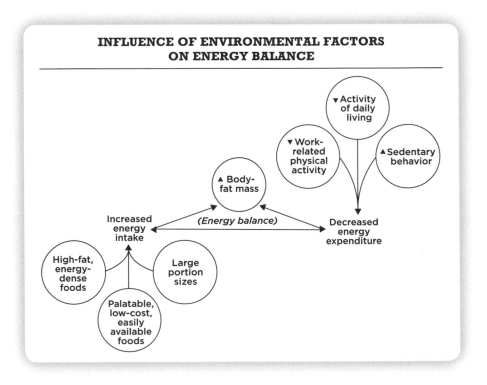

**INFLUENCE OF ENVIRONMENTAL FACTORS
ON ENERGY BALANCE**

instances, being overweight is related to inactivity; in only about 30% is it linked primarily to increased food intake.

Many studies have demonstrated the effectiveness of exercise in promoting reductions in body weight and fatness. One study examined overweight women in three separate groups, each instructed to "lose" 500 calories a day. Participants in the first group, using diet alone, reduced their caloric intake by 500 calories a day but did not increase physical activity. The second group reduced calories by 250 a day but increased exercise by the same amount. The third group used exercise exclusively, leaving their eating pattern unchanged but increasing physical activity to burn 500 calories a day. The results showed that the two groups that exercised lost significantly more body fat than the group that only dieted. Moreover, the diet-only group was the only one that experienced an "unhealthy" loss of lean body mass (muscle tissue).

Your level of physical activity affects your weight for all of the following reasons.

Exercise burns calories. Walking for 30 to 45 minutes a day burns 200 to 300 calories in a 150-pound person. The chart below shows how long it would take that person to burn 250 calories in a variety of activities:

ACTIVITY	CALORIES PER HOUR	MINUTES TO BURN 250 CALORIES
Walking (4 mph)	355	42
Tennis (moderate)	425	35
Swimming (crawl, 45 yards per minute)	530	28
Downhill skiing	585	26
Handball/squash	600	25
Tennis (vigorous)	600	25
Jogging (5.5 mph)	650	23
Biking (in excess of 13 mph or up a steep hill)	850	18

Burning calories is essential to reducing body fat. When you take in more calories than are used, the excess is stored as body fat. It takes 3,500 extra calories to create a pound of body fat, and an energy expenditure of 3,500 to use up this pound of fat. Daily exercise can produce an energy deficit that requires the burning of body fat, which over time will lead to weight loss. Pretty simple, wouldn't you say?

Exercise raises metabolism. If burning calories directly were the only benefit, exercise would not be a very efficient way to lose weight. A 150-pound person has to walk for more than nine hours at a pace of four miles per hour to lose a pound. But regular exercise also raises metabolism, the *rate* at which the body burns calories, even after the activity stops. This means that even during rest the body needs to burn more calories.

How and why exercise increases metabolism is not clear, in part because metabolism is hard to measure and tends to vary greatly among people of the same weight, age and sex. But studies show that those

DO IT FOR YOUR KIDS

Raised on fast food, television and computer games, kids today are more sedentary, overweight and out of shape than a generation ago. Today, more than twice as many children—and almost three times as many teens—are overweight as compared with 1980. Sixty percent of overweight children already have one coronary risk factor. If this trend continues, experts warn that the current generation of children may become the first in history to live shorter lives than their parents.

Parents can change this dangerous trend. "Kids don't do what you tell them to do," says Paul F. Rosengard, director of the Sports, Play and Action Recreation for Kids (SPARK) program at San Diego State University. "They do what you do." Parents who work out regularly and who find daily physical activities to do with their children—play catch, take a walk or kick a ball—are sending the clear message: *In this family, fitness and health matter.*

individuals who exercise vigorously experience a 7.5% to 28% increase in metabolic rate for up to four to eight hours after the activity is concluded. Dr. Jack Wilmore, formerly of Texas A&M University, has translated this as follows: "If exercising regularly changes your metabolism even slightly, so that you burn an extra 100 calories a day, that small change can add up to 10 pounds of weight loss a year."

Exercise builds and maintains muscle. The body works like a car. The engine is muscle, which burns the fuel, which is fat. The more muscle you have, the bigger your engine, and the easier it is to burn fat. Studies show that every added pound of lean muscle burns an additional 30 to 50 calories each day.

Body fat, on the other hand, needs fewer calories to maintain itself; indeed, overweight people need one-third to one-half fewer calories to maintain their weight than do people of normal weight. This is why, of two people who eat the same amount of food, the fat person gets fatter and the lean person stays thin. "Diets can't build muscle tissue," says Georgia Kostas, a registered dietitian in private practice. "But exercise will." Aerobic exercise (walking, jogging, aerobics classes) combined with resistance training (light weight lifting, push-ups) will build and preserve muscle tissue.

Exercise reduces stress. People under pressure tend to overeat, binge or live on a diet of fast food and snacks. A calm, relaxed, de-stressed person is less likely to "pig out" on brownies or ice cream. A study at Case Western Reserve University of the dietary habits of sedentary versus physically active people clearly shows that active people choose to eat more healthful foods and fewer foods high in fat.

Exercise may reduce food cravings. The misconception that exercise always increases appetite and caloric intake has now been discounted. Most research indicates either no change in caloric consumption with moderate exercise or slight decreases with vigorous exercise.

Exercise and Aging

Regular physical activity is a characteristic shared worldwide by people who live long with good health. As Shay McKelvey of the American Council on Exercise says, "A good 70% of what we think of as normal aging is really a result of inactivity." In fact, large population studies have now shown that exercisers regularly live two to three years longer than their inactive counterparts. According to Dr. Ralph Paffenbarger, "For every hour of your life you spend exercising, you increase your life span by two hours."

A study of 6,000 men conducted by the VA Hospital in Palo Alto, California, found that the death rate of obese men who were fit was about one-third that of their lean but unfit counterparts. This led Dr. Kenneth Cooper to quip, "You're better off fat and fit than skinny and sedentary. I'm not promoting obesity. I'm just illustrating how important it is to become physically fit. Lack of exercise is deadly."

Specific age-related benefits of exercise are seen in the following areas:

Bone strength. The aging process tends to leach minerals from bones, causing them to become so brittle and weak that

> **PHYSICAL ACTIVITY AND COGNITION**
>
> The prevalence of dementia rises exponentially after the age of 65 years, affecting as many as one in every two people older than 80. Observational studies suggest that regular physical activity reduces the risk of cognitive decline and dementia in later life.

even a moderate fall can produce a break or fracture. Osteoporosis is a particularly serious condition for older women. The first line of defense against this condition is to ensure an adequate intake of calcium. But exercise is also needed. Many studies show that bone, like muscle, tends to get thicker and stronger the more it is used. People who weight-train have thicker arm bones than joggers; joggers have thicker leg bones than swimmers. The critical point is that, without exercise, extra calcium in the diet may be useless in reducing the risk of osteoporosis. Taking this one step further, to keep bones strong and protect against osteoporosis, regular exercise is a necessary, even critical, need.

Oxygen uptake. Our ability to process oxygen, called maximal O_2 uptake, declines at a rate of about 1% a year after age 20, accelerating to 2% after age 55. Regular exercise can prevent or slow down this deterioration.

In a study conducted at San Diego State University by Dr. Fred Kasch, the oxygen-processing capabilities of participants in an adult fitness program were measured over 10 and 15 years. The study found that for those who exercised regularly, there was no difference in maximal oxygen uptake between ages 45 and 55. From the standpoint of cardiovascular performance, the two groups showed the same capabilities. In effect, exercise had retarded the aging process for the older group.

Muscle strength. Between the ages of 20 and 70, people lose about 30% of their lean body tissue (muscle). This process, called sarcopenia, is associated with marked declines in muscular strength. But a study by Dr. Herbert deVries at the University of Southern California found that this erosion was due largely to inactivity, not aging. People who continued to exercise in their senior years experienced little or no decrease in muscle strength.

ACTIVE ADULTS HAVE MEASURABLY "YOUNGER" CELLS

A sedentary lifestyle may accelerate the aging process. Startling new studies of twin volunteers indicate that the individuals who exercise regularly are biologically younger—by approximately 10 years—than their siblings who don't. This provides a powerful message to promote the potentially antiaging effect of regular exercise.

A Balanced Exercise Program

THERE HAS LONG BEEN AGREEMENT THAT REGULAR EXERCISE IS beneficial; still, questions arise about what types of exercise are most effective, how hard you need to work out and how often an exercise should be performed. Most experts recommend a balanced program that includes four components:

- **Daily physical activity** as part of life's routine.
- **Aerobic exercise** to promote cardiovascular endurance and fat-burning.
- **Weight training** for building strength and reducing demands on the heart.
- **Flexibility exercises (stretching)** to prevent injury and allow aerobic exercise and weight training to be more enjoyable.

Daily Physical Activity

In 1996, the surgeon general issued guidelines to encourage people to be physically active every day, or on most days, for a minimum of 30 minutes. Regular moderate-intensity activities—walking up stairs, doing errands on foot, walking the dog, parking at the far end of the lot, raking leaves and doing household chores—were suggested. Recently, these recommendations were echoed and updated in a joint statement by the American College of Sports Medicine and the American Heart Association, which alternatively listed vigorous exercise for a minimum of 20 minutes at least three days each week.

One big difference from past recommendations is that these activities do not have to be continuous. Numerous studies have shown that shorter periods of activity (minimum of 10-minute exercise bouts) can be accumulated throughout the day to achieve these goals. In other words, the deskbound executive who takes a lunch-hour jog three days a week may not be better off than the person who performs periodic moderate-intensity activity throughout the day on most days of the week.

Increased daily physical activity is *key* to cardiac health. Two landmark studies in the *Journal of the American Medical Association* showed that

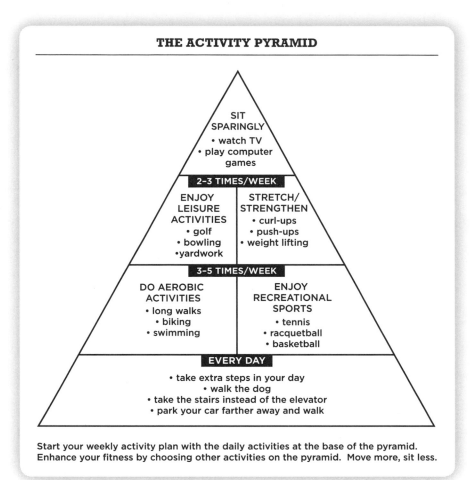

THE ACTIVITY PYRAMID

SIT
SPARINGLY
• watch TV
• play computer
games

2-3 TIMES/WEEK

ENJOY
LEISURE
ACTIVITIES
• golf
• bowling
•yardwork

STRETCH/
STRENGTHEN
• curl-ups
• push-ups
• weight lifting

3-5 TIMES/WEEK

DO AEROBIC
ACTIVITIES
• long walks
• biking
• swimming

ENJOY
RECREATIONAL
SPORTS
• tennis
• racquetball
• basketball

EVERY DAY

• take extra steps in your day
• walk the dog
• take the stairs instead of the elevator
• park your car farther away and walk

Start your weekly activity plan with the daily activities at the base of the pyramid.
Enhance your fitness by choosing other activities on the pyramid. Move more, sit less.

doing moderate-intensity lifestyle activities for at least 30 minutes daily is as effective in the long run at lowering body fat, improving blood pressure and boosting aerobic fitness in sedentary people as doing more traditional, structured exercise three to five days a week. Moreover, such activities are great for dissipating daily stress. This is not to suggest that daily physical activity should replace more traditional workouts, but rather that it is a wonderful complement to any health and fitness program.

The Activity Pyramid above may help you visualize what we mean. Starting at the base of the pyramid, you'll see that you should accumulate at least 30 minutes of moderate-intensity activity on most and preferably all days of the week. The next tier of the pyramid represents structured aerobic activities and/or recreational sports, which you should be doing three to five days each week. Complementary leisure-time activities, such as playing golf, bowling or working in the yard, as well as calisthenics and weight training, are recommended in the third tier, at the lesser frequency of two to three days a week.

Collectively, the activities listed in the first three tiers should reduce the amount of non-exercise time at the top of the pyramid, that is, time spent on sedentary activities such as watching television or playing computer games.

Aerobic Exercise

As illustrated in the Activity Pyramid on the facing page, vigorous, longer-lasting exercise—three or more sessions per week of aerobic activity—is required in order to attain cardiovascular fitness. Indeed, according to Dr. Paul Williams, an exercise expert at the Lawrence Berkeley Laboratory, an increase in your level of fitness has nearly twice the impact on reducing your risk of heart disease as does merely increasing your daily physical activity.

Aerobic exercise, involving continuous, rhythmic movement of the large muscle groups, conditions your heart, lungs and vascular system, and promotes your body's ability to burn fat by causing your heart and lungs to process oxygen at a steady rate over a sufficient period of time. Some of the best examples of aerobic exercise are listed below:

Brisk (power) walking	Jogging
Cycling (stationary and spinning)	Running in place
Skipping rope	Swimming
Aerobic dancing (high-impact, step)	Cross-country skiing (indoor)
Rowing (indoor)	Stair-stepping
Stair-climbing	Elliptical exercise

Many popular leisure-time activities can also be considered aerobic if they're done at a moderate-to-vigorous pace and maintained continuously for the proper duration. See the list that follows.

Basketball	Handball/squash/racquetball
Hiking	Skating (ice/roller/in-line)
Soccer	Rowing (outdoor)
Tennis (singles)	Aerobic dancing (medium-impact)
Jumping rope	Cycling (outdoor)
Cross-country skiing (outdoor)	

In order to be classified as aerobic, an activity must meet the F.I.T. criterion: *frequency, intensity* and *time*. How often, how hard, how long—these are the three critical elements.

F = Frequency. Most health professionals recommend an aerobic program of at least three to five days a week. This takes into account recent guidelines from the American College of Sports Medicine. Exercising every other day is very effective for cardiovascular conditioning. (People who need to lose weight may need to exercise daily.) However, anyone who exercises more than four days a week should be certain to alternate high-impact activities with non-jarring ones, such as brisk walking and swimming, to minimize strain and other injuries.

Recent studies suggest that the risk of cardiovascular complications is somewhat increased during vigorous exercise compared with that at other times. This appears to be particularly true among sedentary people with known heart disease who perform unaccustomed vigorous physical activity. Dr. Gerald Fletcher of the Mayo Clinic in Jacksonville, Florida, warns: "You can't 'catch up' with exercise by cramming a week's worth of exertion into one day."

I = Intensity. "Intensity plays a role in making people fitter and healthier," says Dr. Miriam Nelson, author of *Strong Women Stay Slim.* "How hard you exercise is important because of the relationship between intensity on one hand, and cardiovascular fitness and weight control on the other." Echoes exercise expert Carol Rhodes, "You can enjoy light exercise such as golf and casual walking; just don't confuse these activities with those designed for cardiovascular benefit. Light exercise simply doesn't stress the heart muscle sufficiently to improve cardiac fitness, and it doesn't necessarily lead to weight loss. In fact, that's one of the prime reasons people give up. They exercise at too low an intensity, don't get the results, and quit. You have to raise your heart rate to get benefits."

Research shows that the most effective exercise is done at a sustained moderate-to-vigorous pace. If you're walking, make certain that you keep up a "brisk walk"—that your stride is aggressive, your arms are pumping and you may even break a sweat on your upper lip. Brisk walking means covering three and a half to four miles in an hour, certainly not a leisurely pace.

While matching your pace to an effective level of intensity, do not subscribe to the "no pain, no gain" school of exercise. Unless you're a competitive athlete, "going for the burn" may cause you to exercise too hard or too fast, which can lead to injury or exhaustion. Either way, you get nowhere.

> **THE TALK TEST**
>
> If your forehead feels dewed but you can still carry on a conversation with a fellow exerciser, your pace is probably just about right. If you can't exercise and carry on a conversation at the same time, you're probably exercising too strenuously.

But how to know what's the best pace for you—that "in between" place we call the training zone? One way depends on monitoring your heart rate during the activity by checking your pulse. (Physicians have traditionally measured heart rate by timing the pulse at the wrist, on the thumb side. The neck pulse is easier to find, but you have to remember not to press too hard, as this may produce a marked slowing of the heart rate and an underestimation of the true exercise intensity.)

Practice taking your pulse when you're not exercising. Once you've found your pulse, count it for 10 seconds. Be sure to count the first beat as zero. Then multiply the count by six to calculate your pulse for one minute.

Once you're comfortable taking your pulse, you should determine your maximal heart rate, a limit on how fast the heart is capable of beating during exercising to exhaustion. Ideally, it should be measured during a medically supervised exercise stress test; however, a widely accepted formula is also used:

220 − your age in years = maximal heart rate

Maximal heart rate is largely determined by age as opposed to physical fitness. This means a fit 40-year-old will have an estimated maximal heart rate of 180, while that of a sedentary 24-year-old will be 196. The 40-year-old may be more fit, but being older he'll have a lower maximal heart rate.

You never want to exercise at your maximal heart rate, so the next step is figuring out what your actual training zone should be. The American Heart Association defines it as being between 70% and 85% of maximal heart rate. The estimated target heart rate zone for a 50-year-old, for instance, is between 119 (70%) and 145 (85%) beats per minute.

HOW MUCH IS ENOUGH?

Dr. Barbara Ainsworth, a noted exercise researcher, suggests thinking of exercise in terms of a U-shaped curve. The worst place to be is at the start of the curve, doing nothing. As you begin exercising, you move down the curve and start getting some of the health benefits. The base of the curve represents a wide range of physical activity, and added health benefits can come from increased activity. But doing too much exercise does not produce extra benefits. Indeed, as you move back up the curve on the opposite side, too much exercise can be harmful.

Here's a quick guide:

■ Cardiovascular benefits are apparent once you expend more than 500 calories a week in exercise.

■ Optimal improvements generally occur when you expend between 2,000 and 3,500 calories a week.

■ When more than 3,500 calories a week are burned in exercise, benefits may taper off and the incidence of injury may increase disproportionately.

The table below offers a quick way to estimate maximal heart rate and target heart rate zone for healthy individuals by age group. Because of the variability in maximal heart rate, individual ranges may differ by 10 to 20 beats per minute, or more. An exercise stress test can determine your true maximal heart rate—another good reason to make an appointment with your doctor before starting an exercise program.

HEARTBEATS PER MINUTE

AGE	ESTIMATED MAXIMAL HEART RATE	ESTIMATED TRAINING HEART RATE ZONE
20	200	140 to 170
25	195	137 to 166
30	190	133 to 162
35	185	130 to 157
40	180	126 to 153
45	175	123 to 149
50	170	119 to 145
55	165	116 to 140
60	160	112 to 136
65	155	109 to 132
70	150	105 to 128
75	145	102 to 123
80	140	98 to 119

Once you've determined the parameters of your training zone, use them as a guideline for how hard you should be exercising. Wait until you're 5 or 10 minutes into the exercise, then stop and locate your pulse on the side of your neck or on the thumb side of your wrist. If your pulse rate is below the lower training heart rate limit, you probably need to increase effort; if it's above, you can ease off a bit. An alternative way to determine your exercise heart rate is to use an accurate heart rate monitor to track exercise intensity.

There is no magic to being at the upper end of the zone. In fact, musculoskeletal and cardiovascular complications are more likely to occur at such intensities. Research shows that less intensive activities such as low-impact aerobics are highly effective. Also, remember that your training heart rate, which is geared to age, does not change as you lose weight and get in better shape. What will change is the amount of effort needed to reach the zone. People who are overweight and out of shape have an easier time reaching it than those who are slimmer and in shape. As level of fitness improves, the pace or workload may have to be increased for the activity to achieve the appropriate heart rate range.

The disadvantage of this approach to estimating your training zone is that the formula doesn't always reflect how hard you are working aerobically. There are variations in age-predicted maximal heart rate, usually plus or minus 10 to 20 beats per minute. In addition, extremes in environmental conditions (e.g., hot, humid weather) can throw off results. Even greater errors in estimation can occur in persons with heart disease (all of whom should check with their doctor about an appropriate exercise heart rate) or in those taking certain cardiac medications (such as beta-blockers) that can restrict the maximum heart rate.

An alternative way to monitor your exercise intensity is to use the Rating of Perceived Exertion scale, or the Borg RPE scale. Based on the simple concept that the mind is an excellent judge of how much work the body is doing, the RPE scale grades exercise levels based on the individual's overall feeling of effort and physical fatigue, from rest (6) to maximal exertion (20). These ratings correspond well with metabolic responses such as heart rate and oxygen consumption.

BORG RPE SCALE	
6	No exertion at all
7	Extremely light
8	
9	Very light
10	
11	Light
12	
13	Somewhat hard
14	
15	Hard (heavy)
16	
17	Very hard
18	
19	Extremely hard
20	

Here's how to use it. After you've been exercising for 5 or 10 minutes, ask yourself the question "How hard am I working?" If it feels "extremely light" or "very light," the intensity is probably too low to be effective. You'll need to increase the level of intensity to reach your training zone. Conversely, if your response is "very hard" or "extremely hard," you are probably working too vigorously. Your breathing is labored and you have difficulty sustaining the activity. You should back off a bit on your effort. The training zone is generally described as a perception of intensity somewhere between "light" and "hard"—ideally, "somewhat hard." At this level of intensity you are neither breathing too easily nor out of breath, allowing you to sustain it over a period of time.

> **MYTH ALERT!**
> **SUGAR DOES *NOT* RAISE**
> **YOUR ENERGY LEVEL**
>
> Eating sugar before physical activity can actually do more harm than good, driving the body's sugar into storage. Extra sugar doesn't give extra energy. Think of it as filling up your gas tank to drive your car around the block. It's just not necessary.

T = **Time.** You need to exercise in your training zone for a minimum of 20 to 30 minutes, depending on the intensity. *This is only a minimum* and may not be a long enough time for you to achieve optimal cardiovascular benefits. People who wish to further improve their personal fitness, reduce their risk for chronic diseases or prevent unhealthy weight gain may benefit by exceeding this duration (i.e., 45 to 90 minutes per day).

According to the American College of Sports Medicine, moderate-intensity exercise in 10-minute increments can provide appreciable benefit for general health as long as it adds up to at least 30 minutes per day of physical activity. The Harvard Nurses' Health Study as well as other studies found that shorter exercise bouts provide some cardiovascular benefit as well; however, most cardiac experts still recommend a continuous session of vigorous exercise for at least 20 minutes for cardiovascular benefit.

Time spent exercising is particularly important for weight control. Nonstop exercise for at least 20 minutes helps to rev up metabolism and increase fat-burning. During the first few minutes of exercise, glucose is the primary fuel. As the activity continues past that point, utilization

**MYTH ALERT!
EVEN MARATHON
RUNNERS ARE NOT
IMMUNE TO HEART
DISEASE**

One sad but notable example: the author and distance runner Jim Fixx, who died of a heart attack while jogging one cold winter morning in Vermont. Still, physically active people are at a lower overall risk. Above all, exercise needs to be balanced with healthy eating, stress management and no smoking to create a lifestyle package more likely to ward off, stabilize and possibly even reverse coronary disease.

of body fat increases, especially at mild to moderate intensities. Thus, the more time spent in continuous aerobic exercise, the greater the opportunity to burn body fat.

Also, be sure to leave enough time in your schedule for warm-up and cool-down, such as stretching or the same aerobic activity done at a lower intensity. For example, if you use brisk walking during the endurance phase, you should conclude the warm-up period with slow walking. Similarly, brisk walking serves as an ideal warm-up for jogging. These warm-up and cool-down activities are *not* part of the 20-to-30-minute minimum duration.

Weight Training

The American Heart Association once counseled people with heart disease to refrain from weight training (also called resistance exercise). No longer. The AHA now acknowledges that weight training builds and tones muscles, increases the ability to burn body fat and strengthens bones. It reduces the heart rate and blood pressure responses to standardized lifting tasks, thus decreasing the demands on the heart during daily activities such as carrying groceries or lifting moderate-to-heavy objects. It helps to maintain or increase lean body mass, which may allow the body to burn more calories throughout the day. In addition, resistance training decreases HbA1c in men and women with diabetes. It also modestly reduces both systolic and diastolic blood pressure. Finally, new studies have shown that muscular strength is inversely associated with all-cause mortality and the prevalence of metabolic syndrome, independent of aerobic fitness levels.

Before you start a weight training program, get an OK from your doctor. This is particularly important if you have coronary heart disease,

REDUCING THE RISK OF EXERCISE

Compared with risk at other times, the risk of cardiovascular complications appears to increase transiently during vigorous physical exertion. This seems to be particularly true among infrequent exercisers or occasional weekend athletes with known or hidden heart disease who exercise too strenuously. On the other hand, the net effect of regular physical activity is a lower overall risk of dying from cardiovascular disease.

■ Regular exercise seems to reduce the risk of an exertion-related fatal cardiovascular event, such as a heart attack while jogging.

■ If you're an infrequent exerciser, stick with a moderate-intensity activity such as walking.

■ Novice exercisers should consider appropriate medical screening before starting. This is critical for those with major coronary risk factors, signs or symptoms of heart disease, or people with known heart, lung or metabolic disease.

Recommendations to reduce the incidence of strains, sprains and cardiovascular complications during exercise programs include the following steps:

■ *Obtain good supervision.* Competent exercise professionals can reduce the rate of exercise-related injuries or complications.

■ *Warm up and cool down.* Avoid sudden strenuous exertion and abrupt cessation of vigorous exercise.

■ *Start gradually.* If you plan to take up jogging, start with a brisk walking program and gradually progress to slow jogging over several weeks. Give yourself time to build up a tolerance to exercise. Don't expect to walk briskly for an hour your first day out.

■ *Exercise regularly.* Don't try to cram all your exercise into one day per week.

■ *Avoid high-intensity activity.* As a general rule, exercise should feel no more than "somewhat hard." Remember, if you can't carry on a conversation during exercise, you're probably working too hard.

high blood pressure, heart valve problems, congestive heart failure, a weight problem or a strong family history of heart disease.

A good weight training program includes exercises for every major muscle group, including arms, chest, back, legs and abdomen. Free weights, machines, rubber tubing and calisthenics are effective. Do not overlook your own body for resistance—push-ups and leg raises, for example.

Be sure to get good instruction before you start your program. Look for an instructor who has been certified by the American College of Sports Medicine, the American Council on Exercise or the National Strength and Conditioning Association. The instructor should know your goals and personalize the program based on your needs. It is also important to learn how to perform the exercises effectively. Form is critical to your success, as is proper breathing (exhale when you lift).

Progress in strength training depends on the number of times a week you train, the amount of weight you lift and the number of times you lift it. Although the traditional routine involved performing each exercise three times (three sets of 10 repetitions per set), research has shown that one set provides nearly the same improvement in muscular strength and endurance. Consequently, for the average person beginning a strength training regimen, single-set programs performed a minimum of two times per week are recommended over multiple-set programs.

Such regimens should include 8 to 10 different exercises at a load that permits 8 to 12 repetitions per set for healthy, sedentary adults or 10 to 15 repetitions per set for cardiac patients and for healthy individuals who are older than 50 years of age. The American College of Sports Medicine recommends biceps curls, triceps extensions, chest presses, shoulder presses, pull-downs, abdominal crunches, lower-back extensions, quadriceps extensions, leg curls and calf raises.

Flexibility Exercises

Stretching, the fourth component of a balanced exercise program, is essential for maintaining (or improving) your joint range of motion and function and for enhancing muscular performance. Without a specific program to maintain flexibility, many middle-aged and older adults become hampered by stiffness in the hamstrings, shoulders and back.

It's simple to do. Starting slowly, gently stretch the muscles of each major muscle group for about 10 to 30 seconds to the point of mild discomfort. At least four repetitions per muscle group should be performed a minimum of two to three days per week. Be sure to keep your breathing rhythmic and steady. Make certain not to bounce. At no time should you feel pain.

Stretching (as well as activities that incorporate stretching, such as yoga and tai chi) is a great way to get your muscles ready for more strenuous exercise. But it has other benefits as well. Over time, stretching can keep you from losing flexibility (a consequence of aging) and may even make you more flexible. Increased flexibility reduces the risk of musculoskeletal injury from varied activities and can help you to perform exercise more efficiently.

Many good books, audiotapes and videotapes are available on stretching, yoga and tai chi. In addition, classes are often offered at YM/YWCAs and other community recreation centers.

It's Never Too Late

A PROVOCATIVE STUDY BY DR. BENJAMIN LEVINE AND ASSOCIATES at the University of Texas Southwestern Medical Center suggests that cardiovascular fitness can be reclaimed. Doctors worked with a small group of men who were originally studied 30 years earlier. At that time, these men demonstrated an above-average level of cardiovascular fitness. But, not surprisingly, the men became less physically active over time. Their cardiovascular fitness eroded and their body fatness increased.

For six months, researchers had them exercise in a training routine that included walking, jogging and cycling. By the end of the study, they were exercising pretty rigorously for about 4.5 hours a week. Measurement of their aerobic capacity showed that 100% of the cardiovascular decline that had taken place over 30 years had been reversed. The men returned to the same level of cardiovascular fitness they had enjoyed three decades earlier!

"The message here is very clear. No matter what your age might be, it's your current fitness level, not your past fitness level, that really dictates how fit you are," says Dr. Miriam Nelson, an exercise expert at Tufts University.

HOW TO BURN
150 EXTRA CALORIES A DAY*

ACTIVITY	MINUTES
Washing/waxing car	45 to 60
Washing windows/floors	45 to 60
Volleyball	45
Touch football	30 to 45
Gardening	30 to 45
Walking 1¾ miles (20 minutes/mile)	35
Bicycling 5 miles	30
Dancing (fast)	30
Pushing a stroller 1.5 miles	30
Raking leaves	30
Walking 2 miles (15 minutes/mile)	30
Water aerobics	30
Swimming laps	20
Basketball	15 to 20
Jumping rope	15
Running 1.5 miles (10 minutes/mile)	15
Shoveling snow	15
Stair-walking	15

*These values are estimates for a 154-pound person.

Time for Action

HARVARD RESEARCHER DR. JOANN MANSON once observed, "If there were a magic potion that could make you feel great and could cut your risk of getting heart disease, cancer and diabetes in half, people would be willing to spend hundreds, even thousands of dollars for it." And then she dropped the other shoe: "But it's already available and virtually free—regular physical activity." The fact is, most of us know that exercise is good for us. If you want proof, just look at the soaring sales of exercise equipment and gym memberships every January. So why is it that New Year's commitments to lose weight and get in shape begin to waver after only a couple of weeks?

Some of the reasons are understandable. An exercise program is voluntary and time-consuming. Additionally, not all the health benefits of exercise are readily apparent: a definite demotivator. But somehow—and this is the fact we ought to be focusing on—almost half the people who start an exercise program stick with it. What's their secret? Well, it's not just willpower, which is why we devote the rest of this section to tips for incorporating physical activity into your daily routine and making it an integral part of your lifestyle. Pick the Heart Savers that make the most sense for you, and then stick with them for 90 days.

Just three months. Research suggests that's the critical time period— all you'll need to get hooked on exercise for a lifetime.

Don't Wait till Wednesday

HEART 43 SAVER

Right about now you're probably muttering, "How in the world do they ever expect me to fit all these 'things' into my day?" And it's true—finding the time for relaxation, meditation, exercise and eating right may feel like an insurmountable task all by itself. Part of the solution is a sense of perspective. Think about this: There are plenty of people who had no time to exercise on Monday, had a heart attack on Tuesday and found time to exercise on Wednesday.

■ **Imagine yourself healthy and fit.** Becoming healthy is a journey, not a one-time experience. Set the tone for your journey before you pack your bag. Take the time to think about the benefits of change. We know one woman who lost 100 pounds—20 pounds five different times! She had resolve, that's for sure, but she didn't have a clear picture of what it would mean to change her bad habits *forever*. "When I saw losing weight as a problem, I failed," she recalls. "Then one day my daughter said she was afraid my weight would make me get sick and die. That's when I saw weight loss as an opportunity for better health, with a real benefit for both of us." Next time out she lost 20 pounds and kept them off.

■ **Define your goals.** Do you want to be less anxious? Lose weight? Increase your stamina? Remember, this is a journey. If you don't know where you're going, you won't know if you're on the right road, let alone if you've arrived. Likewise, be specific—"I'm going to lose 20 pounds," not "I'm going to lose some weight"—and realistic about how long it will take to reach your destination. If you expect to lose 20 pounds in two weeks, you won't get there.

■ **Slow down.** The problem for most people is that they want to make all the healthy changes at once. Right now. That's overwhelming and a recipe for failure. The fact is that you *do* have to devote a lot of time to staying healthy, but when you think of the change as evolutionary rather than revolutionary, your chances for success go way up. Walk slowly today and know that tomorrow you can walk more briskly.

■ **Plan for progress.** Take at least a week to think about your program *before you do anything*. Perhaps you need to manage stress. Choose a handful of stress-management Heart Savers—maybe keeping a journal, practicing deep breathing, doing yoga. Outline your plan. Will you set aside 10 minutes for journaling before you go to bed at night? Five minutes right after lunch for deep breathing? A yoga class that meets twice a week? Put your plan into action for two or three weeks before deciding how to refine your stress management program.

Meanwhile, you can start planning your exercise routine. Read through the exercise Heart Savers and outline a plan. Get up earlier so you can walk with a friend for 30 minutes three mornings a week; take the stairs at work; make an appointment to work with a weight-training instructor. When you're ready, put the plan into action, again taking the time to live with it before you figure out how to refine it.

You get the picture. Strive for balance. Focus on successes—and be proud of yourself.

Q & A

O ver the years, exercise critics have rhetorically asked, "Fitness for what?"

Now sobering new studies provide this compelling response: "Fitness for life!"

44 Take the Mirror Test

Think about your present activity level for just a moment. Then think about how it would feel (and may have felt in the past) to be strong and flexible, to have endurance, to be confident in your physical abilities. As one physical therapist counsels, "Forget the sophisticated tests. Just take off your clothes and stand in front of a mirror. Don't judge and don't feel guilty. Simply make an honest assessment of where you are now."

Are you carrying a few more pounds than you should? Have you lost muscle tone? Now visualize yourself as you would like to be: stronger, leaner, healthier. A great motivator is a constant vision of what you might look and feel like once you've achieved your goals.

45 Just Do It!

A program of regular exercise starts with a conscious decision. Make the decision now to "just do it." Commit it to paper: write down what you want to accomplish, which exercises you plan on doing to meet your goal and when you'll do them. Above all, TAKE ACTION! Remember the law of inertia: a body at rest tends to remain at rest; but a body in motion tends to remain in motion.

The ability to give yourself a command and follow it is imperative in order to achieve the life of your dreams. Discipline! Gymnast Peter Vidmar once said: "To be an Olympic champion, I had to do only two things: work out when I wanted to and work out when I didn't."

The form of exercise is not important. Do something you enjoy—walk, bike, swim, go to an aerobics class or use an exercise machine. As Confucius taught, "It does not matter how slowly you go, so long as you do not stop."

46 Get an OK from Your Doctor

Too often people use a concern about a medical condition as an excuse not to exercise. If you're a man over 45 or a woman over 55, ask your doctor for a checkup, including an exercise stress test. This is particularly important for people at increased risk for heart disease (those with symptoms of heart disease and/or two or more major risk factors, such as high blood pressure, elevated cholesterol, cigarette smoking, overweight or sedentary lifestyle) and those with known heart, lung or metabolic disease, especially when vigorous exercise is contemplated. Your doctor can help you decide which exercise is best for you and monitor your progress over time.

47 Start Slow and Steady

Don't expect to go overnight from lounging in a reclining chair to running road races. It takes a minimum of six to eight weeks, depending on age and condition, to begin to notice a difference. Another good rule of thumb according to Dr. Steve Van Camp, a cardiologist in San Diego and a past president of the American College of Sports Medicine, is that it takes about one month to get in shape for every year you've been out of shape.

If you push yourself too hard at the beginning, you can injure yourself. And nothing takes the steam out of an exercise program faster than muscle soreness and stiffness, strains and sprains. Start by picking an exercise of light-to-moderate intensity such as walking. A pace of two to four miles per hour works fine. Begin to integrate two or three 15-minute workout intervals into your day. Once your body gets used to this routine, gradually increase your workout time. Build slowly and steadily to a 45-minute walk, four or five times a week.

Always pay attention to how you feel. Be alert to chest pain, unusual shortness of breath, heart palpitations (irregular or racing pulse rate) and lightheadedness. If any such symptoms occur, discontinue training and seek medical attention.

48 Have Fun

The best exercise is one you'll keep doing. There are hundreds of activities to try: ballroom dancing, rowing, martial arts, skating, handball, volleyball . . . even playing Frisbee. Select an activity that's enjoyable, not a punishment. Think about your personality. Are you an extrovert who loves group activities or an introvert who needs time alone to recharge your batteries? Or you may be an introvert who wants to socialize more or an extrovert who needs more time alone. Do whatever sport or exercise you love. Don't force yourself to jog if you dread it. Advises Dr. Carl Foster of the University of Wisconsin at La Crosse, "Try different forms of exercise until you find something you like so much that you'd do it even if it weren't for your health."

49 Work Toward a Goal

If cardiovascular fitness is your goal, an aerobic workout three or four times a week is generally effective. But if weight loss is your primary aim, it takes more. Plan to do some type of aerobic exercise—walking, jogging, stationary bike, aerobic dancing— on a daily basis. Then look for ways to incorporate a little "extra" into your days: shooting hoops with your kids, dancing to the radio, taking the stairs or parking the car farther away from the store when shopping.

50 Take Time to Stretch

Stretching may not be as flashy as aerobics or strength training, but it's an important part of a complete exercise program. By stretching major muscle groups, especially those involved in whatever exercise you're doing, you'll maintain flexibility while preventing injuries.

Until recently, exercise experts recommended stretching before and after a workout. But that's changed. Instead of doing a warm-up stretch when your muscles are cold, the experts now say you should simply ease into your exercise gradually. If you're going to take a run or a brisk walk, start slowly and gently, increasing your pace only after your muscles are warmed up. It still makes good sense to stretch *after* your workout, when your muscles are warm, to reduce the risk of injury.

But stretching does more than end a workout; it keeps you flexible. After age 30, the body's connective tissues—the muscles, tendons and ligaments—start to shorten, tighten and lose elasticity. Stretching can help you stay limber and improve your range of motion by actually lengthening muscles and tendons. As a result, it can offset age-related stiffness, improve athletic performance and optimize functional movement in daily life. Stretching makes everything easier, from bending to tie your shoes to getting out of a chair or car to pulling up a zipper in the back of a dress.

The American College of Sports Medicine recommends making flexibility training a priority in your exercise program. While brief stretching bouts are better than nothing, to get maximum flexibility benefits you'll have to stretch the major muscle groups two to three days a week.

Join a Group

A commitment to others strengthens resolve. Let's suppose you've made a decision to walk at seven A.M. If you're doing it by yourself, you might just turn over when the alarm goes off, grab some extra sleep and miss your walk. But if you've made a pact to walk with two friends, chances are you'll get up in time to meet them. Joining an aerobic dance class or doing weight training with a friend can also be more fun than going it alone. And you'll find that social interaction often provides the incentive needed for those times when your interest sags.

SPEAKING FROM EXPERIENCE

The act of writing something down makes it real. After my bypass surgery, when I got started on a program of exercise, it was a bit hit-and-miss. Some days I'd have the time and do it. Some days I wouldn't. But exercise was too important to treat so casually. What I did was take my calendar and write at the top of it, "I will exercise every morning." Then I marked out one hour a day as a meeting with "Mr. Nike." Everything else in my life worked around those hours of blocked time. Thanks to "Mr. Nike," I was able to develop the exercise habit. But it started with a written contract with myself.   **—J.P.**

Make a Contract

Commit yourself *in writing* to exercise for six weeks—not an eternity but just long enough to see some results. Plan your activities a week or two in advance. What exercises will you do? Where and with whom? Then mark your schedule on a calendar as if it were a doctor's appointment. Try to exercise at the same time each day so that you develop a routine.

Be careful not to procrastinate by searching for the "right" time. In fact, any time you can and will exercise is the right time—it's up to you, your schedule, your interests and, some would say, your biorhythms. If you're a "morning person" who can't wait to get going, there are many advantages to early morning exercise; it makes you more alert, provides a sense of control that lasts all day and is usually easier to schedule. Some people prefer to do their exercise at noon because it helps them dissipate morning stress and control luncheon appetite. People who exercise before dinner often like the feeling of tension release.

Keep an Exercise Journal

Positive feedback reinforces behavior, which is why keeping an exercise journal (or a computer record) is so valuable. As you watch your minutes and miles build, you'll feel enormously satisfied. A notebook will also keep you honest; in the absence of a written record, people often take credit for more exercise than they actually do.

SAMPLE EXERCISE LOG
GOAL: Exercise 5 days a week

DATE	TYPE OF EXERCISE	HOW LONG?	HOW FAR?
4/1	Walking	51 minutes	3 miles
4/3	Aerobics class	45 minutes	
4/4	Walking	51 minutes	3 miles
4/6	Spinning class	45 minutes	
4/7	Walking	51 minutes	3 miles

Pick a goal for yourself. Write down your accomplishments so that you see them every day. Perhaps it's walking a cumulative 50 miles in a month. As you get closer to your goal, you'll feel a renewed commitment. When you reach it, reward yourself with theater tickets or a new pair of exercise shoes. Then create a new goal and go after it the same way.

Don't Be a Fool for Frauds

Sales of quick-fix weight-loss gadgets and gimmicks have skyrocketed, while sales of diet pills and supplements rose to more than $5 billion in 2009. Don't be a sucker, particularly when so many of these products are not only ineffective but potentially dangerous.

■ **Spot reducing.** Basing their claims on the false notion that it's possible to "burn off" fat from a particular part of the body, deceptive advertisers promise that you can "take inches off your waist, thighs or buttocks without vigorous exercise or dieting and in just minutes a day." Think about it: If spot reducing worked, people who regularly chew gum would have skinny faces!

180

■ **Effortless exercise.** Many years ago, researchers examined the weight-reducing claims made for mechanical vibrating belts. One study showed that the average caloric cost of a 15-minute period of abdominal vibration was 11 calories more than an equivalent period of seated rest (or about ⅓ of an ounce of fat). The investigators concluded, "The vibrator is not to be taken seriously as a device to assist in fat reduction or shifting of fat deposits within the body."

■ **Weight-reducing clothing.** Special weight-reducing garments rely on dehydration and tissue compression. Measurements may be temporarily reduced, but these losses are exclusively water weight.

■ **Electrical muscle stimulators.** Ads for some electric muscle stimulators say they provide the same effects as "3,000 sit-ups or 10 miles of jogging while lying flat on your back." Some of these units have a legitimate purpose in physical therapy; nonetheless, the Food and Drug Administration considers muscle stimulators that are promoted or used for "body shaping and contouring" to be misbranded and fraudulent. In addition, these devices have been known to burn the skin and deliver electric shocks. They can be especially hazardous to pregnant women, heart patients with pacemakers and people who have epilepsy.

Walk Briskly

Brisk walking, also called "power walking," is one of the easiest and most effective aerobic activities. It can be done anywhere, virtually by anyone, and takes no great expertise. In addition, the chance of injury is low. Walking does not jar joints or strain muscles as much as jogging does. And if you allow for gradual conditioning, walking is especially appropriate for novice exercisers and overweight people.

A generally accepted standard for cardiovascular and weight-control benefits is 12 miles of brisk walking per week. This equates to four 45-to-51-minute walks per week of three miles each. If you need to lose a great deal of weight, you might consider a more frequent schedule.

Intensity counts. Brisk walking is just that—brisk! It's not a casual stroll. Practice good form. Walk with a straight spine and a high center

GET THE MOST OUT OF WALKING

■ **Keep up a good pace.** Every minute you shave off your time helps. A 150-pound person, walking for one hour at a brisk pace of four miles per hour four days a week, will, when compared with someone walking at a moderate pace of three miles per hour, burn enough extra calories to lose an extra six pounds in a year.

■ **Use good technique.** Bend your arms at a 90° angle and swing them back and forth, not side to side. The palms of your hands should not swing lower than your hips or higher than your sternum. Arms should stay close to the torso. Pumping your arms to chest level with each stride has the effect of propelling your body forward (rather than side to side), elevating your heart rate and metabolism even more. It's not necessary or even wise to hold or swing hand weights, which can cause arm or shoulder soreness or injury, but your arms should be fully engaged if you want to lose weight and attain cardiovascular fitness.

■ **Practice interval training.** Walk at your normal brisk pace for five minutes, then push it a little harder for the next five, then revert to your normal pace. Or walk using telephone poles (or blocks or fire hydrants) as your guide—go faster from one pole to the next, then ease up to the following pole, then go faster again.

■ **Consider using rubber-tipped walking poles.** Not only do they help reduce stress on the joints, but they also work upper body muscles that are unaffected by normal walking. And that means you'll expend more energy. Researchers at the University of Wisconsin at La Crosse estimate that if you normally burn 400 calories walking, you can burn 500 calories using walking poles—without walking any faster.

of gravity. Don't lean forward too much. Keep your chin up, shoulders back. With your arms swinging upward to shoulder level, your stride should be purposeful. Think of the pace as one you would use if you were late for a doctor's appointment. And that may be faster than you think. As University of Florida research associate Dr. Glen Duncan explains, "Studies show that most people think they're pushing themselves harder than they really are when walking for exercise. So it's important to concentrate on keeping your heart rate up for maximum benefit."

Although you don't need any special gear, make certain you have a pair of comfortable, sturdy shoes that have arch supports and that elevate the heel one-half to three-quarters of an inch above the sole of the foot. Clothing should not be binding.

Start by picking a pleasant place to walk (outdoors in good weather; inside at a YM/YWCA, health club or mall in bad weather). Begin by walking slowly as a warm-up, then increase your pace over a 5-to-10-minute period and gradually swing your arms faster. This action forces your legs to keep pace with your arms. Pumping your arms frees your hips for longer, faster steps. After about 10 minutes, you should be walking in full stride at your aerobic pace. You should feel "dewed," but your breath should be steady. You should never feel breathless. Keep up this pace for 45 minutes, then cool down by gradually slowing your pace over an additional 5 to 10 minutes.

Take One Step and Then Ten Thousand

HEART SAVER 56

If walking turns out to be a good form of exercise for you, consider buying a pedometer. These instruments are easy to use, can be worn on your belt and cost on average between $12 and $30. The basic models just count steps, but the newer electronic versions convert steps to miles and calories burned and include a built-in stopwatch.

Use the pedometer to gauge the level of your normal activity. Inactive people take between 2,000 and 4,000 steps per day; moderately active people, between 5,000 and 7,000 steps per day; active people, at least 10,000 steps per day (roughly 5 miles or 500 calories). For individuals who have a significantly higher BMI, the gross caloric cost per mile is greater than 100 (about 120 to 150 calories per mile) and in proportion to their body weight. As one dedicated walker explained, "Ten thousand steps a day keep the doctor away."

Set a goal: 5,000 steps, 7,000 steps, whatever's right for you. You'll find that the pedometer can provide the motivation needed to go for that extra walk when you're short of your goal.

Run When You Could Have Walked

Jogging and its faster cousin running are two of the best calorie- and fat-burning exercises, and a top-notch cardiovascular workout. They require no particular skill and they're convenient, practical indoors or out. People without orthopedic problems or medical conditions such as overweight or high blood pressure should give running a try, though no one should jog or run without clearance from a physician.

In addition, runners should recognize that pavement pounding can lead to overuse injuries. According to the Centers for Disease Control and Prevention, one-third of people who run at least six miles per week sustain injuries, usually in their knees, ankles and shins. The running surface should be soft, as on a dirt track or park trail.

One benefit of jogging or running is speed—it takes less time than walking to accomplish cardiovascular and weight benefits. The accepted

TRY SNOWSHOEING

If you live in a northern climate or can get to the mountains, snowshoeing is a terrific way to have fun and improve your fitness. It takes you into beautiful, serene settings that calm your mind while exercising your body. And it's easy.

Start by renting or buying snowshoes; they retail for about $75 to $300 a pair. You may also want to rent or buy poles; they'll help your balance and ensure a good upper-body workout as well. Wear warm socks and waterproof boots; wearing gaiters over your shoes will keep snow from getting in. If you're just learning, start out by walking on level ground. (Many areas set aside for snowshoeing have marked trails.) Once you feel sure of yourself, you can go anywhere—up the mountain, into the woods, around the lake.

There are two things that need your attention when snowshoeing. First, drink plenty of water. Staying hydrated will keep your energy up, which is essential for an activity that burns 400 to 600 calories an hour, depending on your speed. Second, if you get off the trail, pay attention to direction so that you can find your way back. An easy way, of course, is to retrace your steps.

minimum for cardiovascular fitness is
9 miles spread over four days per week.
Greater cardiovascular and weight control
benefits accrue with more mileage, perhaps
12 to 15 miles per week.

Essential exercise gear is minimal,
but what you use must be of good quality.
A bad pair of shoes can ruin a good
pair of legs. They must be specifically
designed for jogging or running with firm
support for your arches and heels. The heel area should have about
one inch of padding to cushion the shock of your foot hitting the
ground. Clothing should be comfortable and offer protection from
the weather. Dress for warmth in the winter by wearing several layers
of light clothing rather than one or two heavy layers. The extra layers
trap heat, and it's easy to shed clothes if you get too warm. Make sure
the layer closest to your skin is made of a synthetic material (or silk)
designed to wick away moisture and keep you dry. In cold weather,
wear gloves and, very important, a hat, since a great deal of body heat
escapes from your head.

If you're new to running, it's a good idea to alternate walking
with very slow jogging, and to slow to a walk whenever you become
breathless. This will give you time to get your legs into shape. Gradual
progress is the key to success. Over time, increase the ratio of jogging
to walking until you're jogging on a nonstop basis. Begin your workout
with a brisk walk for 5 to 10 minutes. As you start to jog, slowly increase
your pace. Remember, cardiovascular and weight benefits are a function
of time and intensity. Stay in your training zone for a minimum of 20
minutes nonstop; longer is better. Pay attention to your form. Relax
your upper body; keep your back straight and let your arms swing
slightly; avoid overstriding; and make sure your weight is on your heel,
not your toes, when your foot hits the ground. When you're finished,
spend another 10 minutes cooling down, using a slow jog, then a brisk
walk, then a slower walk.

A JOGGING ALTERNATIVE?

Did you know that walking 3.4 miles per hour on a treadmill at a 14% grade is the energy equivalent of jogging 6 miles per hour on level ground?

EXERCISE INCREASES CARDIOPROTECTIVE
HDL CHOLESTEROL LEVELS

A recent analysis of 25 studies concluded that regular exercise resulted in an average increase in HDL cholesterol of nearly 3 points. The minimum amount of exercise required to boost "good" HDL cholesterol levels was 120 minutes a week.

Be a Road Warrior

58

If you travel as part of your job, you know that airport lines, unfamiliar hotel rooms, meetings, eating on the run and time changes (to say nothing of the business at hand) make it easy to skip your exercise routine. After a hard day, it's also easy to relax in a bar or with HBO and skip your workout. But that won't help you with your fitness goals or with your stress.

These days, it's not that hard to get a workout at your hotel if you have the resolve to do it. Find out from your travel agent if your hotel has a workout facility or a pool; if so, be sure to pack your exercise clothes or swimsuit. If the hotel doesn't have an exercise room, find out if it's affiliated with a local gym or health club where you can get a one-day pass for free or for a small fee.

SPEAKING FROM EXPERIENCE

My lectures take me out on the road a lot, so I choose hotels with exercise facilities and make sure I use them. It takes a certain amount of discipline to climb off an airplane and onto an exercise bike, but I find that sticking to my routine refreshes me and de-stresses my day. If it's good weather, I might just go out for a walk. It's a great way to see a new area, particularly in a big city. You can cover a lot of ground in a city like New York or Chicago with a 45-minute walk, and it's great fun to people-watch, window-shop and be a tourist on the move. **—J.P.**

If you're strapped for time or no workout room is available, most hotel rooms have enough floor space to allow you to do some basic exercises—stretching, push-ups, sit-ups—before starting your day. (Packing a jump rope is a great idea.) Many hotels also have VCR or DVD machines in the room, a perfect way to use a favorite exercise video.

Banish Negativity

59

Here are some things you should never say to yourself:

- **"It's too hard."** If you exercise at the right pace, you won't get tired, sore and out of breath. Starting out slowly and attaining fitness over time takes the "work" out of exercise.

- **"I don't have the time."** An effective daily exercise session takes no more than 45 to 60 minutes, including warm-up and cool-down. The American College of Sports Medicine recommends 30 minutes or more of moderate-intensity activity and 20 minutes or more of vigorous activity. It's certainly possible to find that time just from the hours spent in front of the TV set and/or the computer. Recognize that the effects of exercise are cumulative. Three 10-minute moderate-intensity exercise bouts confer the same benefits as one 30-minute session. (Although two separate 10-minute sessions of vigorous activity are acceptable, most experts recommend one continuous session lasting at least 20 minutes.) It might be helpful to think about physical activity in terms of banking. You don't have to put a dollar bill in your piggy (exercise) bank each time. Four quarters deposited over time add up to the same amount.

A MOTTO TO LIVE BY

Over time, even ordinary effort can produce extraordinary results.

- **"I'm too tired."** Low aerobic fitness often leads to chronic fatigue. When fitness improves, muscles can extract more oxygen from the bloodstream, thus providing a boost to your energy. Gardening, for example, requires a relatively constant supply of oxygen. People who are not aerobically fit may use their entire aerobic capacity, while those who are aerobically fit may use the same amount of oxygen but have a greater "energy reserve."

Here's what you *should* say:

- *"Exercise will help me lose weight and keep it off."*
- *"My muscles will have shape and tone."*
- *"I'll feel more confident."*
- *"I'll meet new people with similar interests."*
- *"My cholesterol and blood pressure will improve."*
- *"I'll feel less stress."*
- *"My heart will get stronger."*

Drink Up

Be sure to drink water before, during and after each workout. Studies suggest that being properly hydrated before exercising in a warm environment can boost your performance and reduce the likelihood of exertional heat stroke, a medical emergency characterized by a markedly elevated body temperature, dry skin, nausea and even unconsciousness. Heat stroke can also be lethal, as it was for Korey Stringer, an All-Pro tackle with the Minnesota Vikings who died after working out in withering heat.

Spring for a Lesson

Exercising with good form and technique maximizes effectiveness and minimizes injury. Check with your local YM/YWCA, community center or gym, or with university- or hospital-affiliated exercise programs to find an exercise professional or personal trainer who has a college degree in physical education and/or is certified by one or more of the prominent organizations in the health/fitness industry: the American College of Sports Medicine, the Cooper Institute, the American Council on Exercise and the National Strength & Conditioning Association. Each has established rigorous knowledge and proficiency standards for exercise professionals, as well as certification programs.

Don't hesitate to ask about the credentials of your exercise instructor or personal trainer.

Make Exercise a Family Affair

One widely cited study showed that a male participant's adherence to an exercise program is directly related to his wife's attitude toward it. Of those men whose spouses had a positive attitude toward the exercise program, 80% demonstrated good to excellent adherence; in contrast, when the spouse was neutral or negative, only 40% showed good to excellent adherence.

Let family members know what you want to accomplish, how you intend to use exercise as a means to that goal and how they can contribute by providing support. Ask for a commitment from them to match your own.

Take a Seat

Both outdoor and indoor biking strengthen the muscles of the back, abdomen and legs, tone the buttocks and thighs, and provide cardiovascular conditioning if done at a sufficient pace or intensity. You can burn a significant number of calories, depending on the terrain, exercise duration and how fast you ride—without the joint and muscle stress often incurred by running or jogging. (People with neck and/or back conditions, however, may find that biking aggravates their problem.)

Outdoor biking can provide cardiovascular benefit, as can indoor biking; either activity can elevate your heart rate into the training zone. To achieve cardiovascular fitness, you'll have to bike outdoors for an estimated 24 miles a week at an aerobic pace (more if you want to lose weight). Start at a slow pace for 5 to 10 minutes to warm up your leg muscles, then progressively increase your speed until you find a comfortable, rhythmic pace within your training zone. Stay in the zone for at least 20 minutes, then pedal slowly for 5 to 10 minutes to cool down.

Aerobic exercise should be continuous, so stoplights and coasting can be problematic. Look for a bike path or a straight stretch of road that will allow you to keep pedaling. And never ride without a protective helmet.

GET THE MOST OUT OF BIKING

If you want the most bang for your buck in the shortest amount of time, take a spinning class. Like aerobic dance, spinning is performed in a group setting with an instructor and music. Everyone uses a stationary bike. The instructor takes the class through a workout/ride at a variety of intensities—sprint, ease-up and added resistance to simulate hills.

The instructor calls for changes in resistance that generally provide nonstop pedaling in your training zone for a minimum of 20 minutes. (Most classes provide about 30 minutes of aerobic work in a 45-to-50-minute class.) Group dynamics, upbeat music and the challenge to keep pace with your instructor combine to increase the intensity and therefore the effectiveness of this biking exercise.

At the same time, you get to control resistance on the wheel of your bike. When the instructor says, "Go to medium resistance," the response is different for each participant. For newcomers, it might mean a setting of 3 or 4; for veterans, it will be closer to 8 or 9. So, go at whatever pace is right for you to achieve your training zone.

Indoor stationary biking lets you exercise at a steady pace while simultaneously reading, watching TV or listening to music. It's a particularly good activity if you need to squeeze exercise into a busy day—and you won't get wet or too hot or cold. On an indoor bike, the way to elevate your heart rate into the training zone is to increase tension (resistance), speed, or both. One problem is that too much tension can take too much out of your legs, which may lead you to give up on biking altogether. Some stationary bikes require a simultaneous pumping action of the arms, potentially enhancing the aerobic benefits. Spinning classes represent another popular alternative.

According to Dr. Thomas Dickson Jr., an orthopedic surgeon who specializes in sports medicine, it's a mistake to think that if you pedal in a harder gear, you'll give yourself a better aerobic workout. Increased resistance will make it harder to pump (not good for the knees), but will also reduce the number of revolutions per minute. A greater benefit is derived from riding in a gear that allows for 60 to 100 rpm.

Indoor bikers should follow the same basic program as outdoor bikers. Pedal slowly with low-tension resistance to warm up. After 5 to 10 minutes, increase the tension slightly until the training zone is reached. A cool-down period should follow at least 20 minutes of continuous cycling at an aerobic pace.

64 Plan a Fitness Vacation

Why not get your heart pumping by going skiing, backpacking, hiking, kayaking or scuba diving? Bike the San Juan Islands, hike the English coast, dive in Maui, or spend a week exercising and eating right at a health spa. The choice is yours to make. It doesn't have to be expensive or exotic to be fun and effective. The important thing is to get yourself out of your daily routine. A vacation that challenges you both physically and mentally will increase your physical fitness, relax your mind, reduce your stress and open your heart to your place in nature.

65 Lift Those Weights!

First off, have a certified professional develop a program tailored to your needs. This should include the following:

- Establishing goals
- Determining how much weight you should lift
- Teaching you the correct technique, using free weights, machines, or resistance tubing and bands
- Setting up a program that covers all muscle groups, including abdominal muscles

The key is to build muscle gradually. Start with relatively light weights that you use 20 minutes twice a week. Don't worry about getting through your entire routine. Add weight gradually over time and adjust the load until you can perform the entire routine. The traditional recommendation is 8 to 15 repetitions per set, three sets of each exercise. But recent research has shown that one set of each exercise can be nearly as effective for novice exercisers. This is great news for nonathletes who

TRY PILATES

Designed to engage the core muscle groups (abdominal, back and inner thigh) in precise movements that stretch and strengthen the body, Pilates exercises (named after Joseph Pilate, who developed the technique in the 1920s) are performed on a mat or on specialized equipment using springs as resistance. Deborah Schneider, a Pilates coach, explains the increased popularity of this exercise nationwide: "People go to Pilates for strength. They use it as an alternative to the more traditional jumping up and down of aerobic exercises."

want increased muscular strength and endurance but don't want to spend a great deal of time on this type of training.

Don't be afraid to start slow. Numerous studies have shown that a three-month weight training program in previously sedentary adults can increase strength by 25% to 100% or more.

Use Your Groceries

66

Make weights out of empty plastic bottles filled with sand or rice, or do a few reps with some big cans of soup.

Disguise Your Exercise

67

Not everyone is comfortable with high-tech gym equipment, and many of us are simply unable to make it to a weekly aerobics class. But we can still be more active during the day. Here's how:

- **Get off the bus or subway a stop earlier and walk.** Experts suggest that this can often add one to two miles to your daily routine. Over a year, it can easily amount to a weight loss of 8 to 12 pounds!

- **Walk to a coworker's desk instead of e-mailing or calling.** Small increases in metabolism throughout the day can, over time, have a beneficial effect on reducing body weight and fat stores.

- **Take the long way to and from the water cooler or restroom.** This supports a key strategy to help people achieve their weight-loss goals, becoming more active in their daily lives.

- **Walk at least 15 minutes during your lunch break.** This simple practice alone can enable you to expend an additional 400 to 500 calories each week.

- **Use a computer workstation that allows you to walk and work.** In recent years, pioneering research studies at the Mayo Clinic have investigated the impact of walking slowly while performing common deskwork. The investigators coined this newly discovered component of energy expenditure as *non-exercise activity thermogenesis* (NEAT), which involves physiological processes that produce heat and burn calories. NEAT includes the energy expenditure of daily activities that are not considered planned physical activity or structured exercise of a person's daily life. Preliminary studies suggest that by walking slowly (one mile per hour) at a computerized workstation, you can literally double your energy expenditure in the course of an eight-hour workday. Steelcase Inc. now markets a work treadmill that combines an office workstation with a treadmill so workers can burn extra calories while earning a paycheck.

- **Stop circling!** Forget about driving around in search of the "closest" possible spot to the shopping mall, movie theater or doctor's office. Park your car at the farthest end of the parking lot and walk to your destination.

- **Find the stairs!** Forget about the elevator or escalator and move from floor to floor the old-fashioned way, burning calories and building strong leg muscles while you do. One study at an at-work stair-climbing program showed it to be a feasible method of increasing aerobic fitness.

- **Get up!** Conveniences such as TV remotes and drive-through windows allow us to stay glued to our seats for hours on end. Try "losing" the remote control. Walk the dog more often. Walk the golf course instead of riding in a cart. Use a bike for short trips.

- **One at a time!** Unloading grocery bags from the car is another way to burn calories and maintain muscular fitness. To get added exercise out of your groceries, bring the bags in from the car one at a time.

■ **Clean up!** Vacuuming, dusting, mopping the floor and gardening are not only ways to keep your house in shape, but also a great opportunity for you to increase activity in daily living.

68 Buy Shoes That Fit

Wait until the end of the day (when your feet are largest) to shop for athletic shoes. Be sure to wear athletic socks, since they can move you into another size. Check that the soles are firm and the arch support good. Recognize that the "first step" in starting an exercise program is buying the right pair of shoes.

69 Don't Neglect Your Arms

So you're walking, jogging or bicycling three or four times a week and you think your exercise program is ideal. Think again. You aren't achieving "total fitness" or "fitness for life." You need aerobic exercise for the upper body as well.

Why arm exercise? The benefits of exercise are largely specific to the muscles that have been trained; in other words, lower extremity training, like walking or jogging, results in improved fitness for your legs but not your arms.

Specially designed bicycles called arm ergometers (they have "levers" instead of handlebars), rowing machines, wall pulleys and light dumbbells are all good for conditioning the upper extremities. Several commercially available devices are noteworthy because they combine arm and leg exercise. One ergometer offers a workout for the arms, using only the bicycle's arm levers; for the legs, using only the pedals; or for both, using the levers and pedals simultaneously. Simulated cross-country skiing machines also provide total body conditioning.

Remember, real-life activities seldom involve jogging in circles or foot pedaling for extended periods. If you'd like to improve your golf drive or tennis slam, or perform household chores or manual tasks without breathlessness or fatigue, include arm training in your personal exercise program.

Feel the Beat

Here's one that demands no prior knowledge or experience, as long as you're willing to just jump in and try (and perhaps feel a little silly until you get the moves down). Aerobic dancing is easy, fun, upbeat—and a great way to burn calories, exercise the whole body and, when done three to four times a week, achieve cardiovascular benefits. You can take a class that includes steps (or not), at either high- or low-impact levels. Normally, a class will last 45 to 60 minutes with stretching and slow movements to warm up and cool down, sandwiching at least 20 minutes of nonstop aerobic activity.

A word to men: Aerobic dancing is not just for women. A study in *The Physician and Sportsmedicine* reported on a group of men aged 33 to 72 who attended aerobic dancing classes three times a week for 45 minutes each session. After six weeks, they had lost weight, lowered resting heart rate and reduced blood cholesterol levels.

Like any aerobic activity, aerobic dance must be done with some intensity and for a long enough period of time to be effective. But effectiveness also rests on the talent of the instructor and the value of the routines. When selecting a class, be sure to find out from the sponsoring agency whether or not the instructor is properly qualified. Sit in on a class before joining. Make certain that warm-up, dancing and cool-down are part of every session and that the proposed intensity matches

GET THE MOST OUT OF STEP AEROBICS

If you're looking to increase intensity, take a step aerobics class. Stair-climbing can increase fitness, burn additional calories and increase metabolism (besides reducing cardiac risk), and all of that holds true for dancing that uses six-to-eight-inch steps. Some of these classes are high impact; if you're just starting out, pick a class that is appropriate for your physical condition. But the increase in effectiveness can be enormous. A 150-pound person will burn up about 280 calories in a 45-minute aerobics class. That same person will burn almost 450 calories in a 45-minute step class.

your ability to perform. Also, check out the floor. Stay away from concrete (and linoleum or hardwood over concrete), which has no "give." The best floor is cushioned hardwood.

And finally, wear loose clothing and shoes specifically designed to offer support during side-to-side movement. Aerobic dancing shoes absorb shock, stabilize the foot and minimize twisting. Never use worn-out shoes or exercise barefoot.

71 Switch Gears to Boost Metabolism

Sustained exercise at a relatively constant intensity enhances endurance, but interval training with its work-rest periods, varied exercise intensities or both may be especially well suited to novice exercisers and heart patients.

Whichever type you do is fine; however, if weight loss is one of your fitness goals, interval training may be more effective in boosting total calories burned because it transiently increases metabolic rate over several exercise bouts. Instead of walking for 45 minutes at a steady pace, walk for 10 minutes at your normal pace, then walk or jog at a higher level of intensity for another 5 minutes. Follow this alternating pattern for an additional 30 minutes. Some walkers and joggers make a music tape, alternating fast and slower songs to match various speeds.

72 Visit the Mall

Exercise indoors when temperatures are extreme—freezing cold or blistering heat—or anytime the weather is simply unpleasant. Being miserable is not part of an exercise routine. If you don't belong to a gym, walk at your local shopping mall. Many malls open their doors early just for this purpose.

Mix It Up

Nothing saps exercise resolve faster than boredom, unless it's injury. To avoid both, cross-train. Someone who only runs, for instance, will have strong calves but may have relatively weak abdominal muscles, limited strength in the upper extremities, and weak quads and shins. To avoid injuries such as shin splints or pulled hamstrings, vary your routine. Likewise, if all you do is walk, there will come a time, no matter how much you love it, when walking will feel like a job. Instead, sign up for new classes, try different exercises and experience the enthusiasm and success of a more challenging routine.

Make Machines Work for You

First things first. Get instruction so that you know how to perform the exercise effectively without hurting yourself.

Next, be sure to vary the machines you use so that you don't overtrain and strain certain muscles. As you get stronger, try to devote more time—45 to 60 minutes for an effective workout.

And finally, take a look at how you can subtly increase the intensity of your exercise. If you program a treadmill to a 5% grade, for example, you will burn an extra 150 calories at a pace of three miles per hour in 60 minutes.

SPEAKING FROM EXPERIENCE

Patients often ask me if just walking and jogging are enough. I vividly recall the response of Dr. Herman K. Hellerstein to a similar question. "There are very few occupations that require sustained walking or jogging," he replied. "Examples included mail carriers, protective service personnel, police officers and their fugitives." Most exercise programs are improperly designed to enhance a person's capacity to perform activities required for daily living. The inclusion of dynamic arm exercise, resistance training and stretching in a physical fitness program should serve to maximize the training benefits to real-life situations. **—B.F.**

EXERCISE TIPS FOR DIABETICS

Numerous studies have shown that aerobic exercise programs improve blood sugar control; however, insulin-dependent diabetics should take the following precautionary measures:

- **Obtain proper medical clearance.** Before starting a vigorous exercise program, individuals over 35 who have had type 1 diabetes for more than a decade or type 2 diabetes should have a medical exam, possibly including an exercise stress test, and be closely screened for complications such as eye problems, kidney disease, poor nerve function, small-vessel disease or heart disease.
- **Wear proper footwear and practice good foot hygiene.** Diabetics, especially those with impaired nerve conduction in their feet, should use cushioned shoes (gel or air soles). It's crucial to look closely before and after exercise for blisters and persistent foot infections that could progress to gangrene.
- **Monitor blood glucose** when starting an exercise program. Diabetics who take insulin or oral medications should check their blood glucose before, during and after exercise if taking insulin or oral medications.
- **Exercise at about the same time each day.** Strenuous or unplanned activity may cause blood glucose levels to drop too low. Exercising late in the evening also increases the risk of hypoglycemia (low blood sugar). Because exercise has an insulin-like effect, exercise-induced hypoglycemia is the most common problem experienced by exercising diabetics who take insulin (and, to a lesser extent, oral hypoglycemia medications).
- **Inject insulin in body areas not affected by exercise.** Injecting insulin into active working muscles increases the likelihood of hypoglycemia. To alleviate this potential problem, an inactive injection area like the abdomen should be used before walking, jogging or bicycling.

- The *treadmill*, a fine alternative to walking or jogging (particularly in inclement weather) allows you to exercise while on an incline, thus increasing the workload and aerobic effect. A study published in the *Journal of the American Medical Association* compared calories burned at a given level of perceived exertion for six different indoor exercise machines. The treadmill evoked the highest caloric expenditure as compared with the other machines.

- **Avoid exercising when insulin is reaching its peak effect.** Glucose levels may decrease markedly during peak insulin action. Thus the action of various insulin preparations should be discussed with a physician in relation to exercise timing. A particularly good time for working out is 15 to 45 minutes after meals, when blood sugar levels are relatively high, rather than before meals, when these levels may be low.

- **Consider ingesting 20 to 30 grams of additional carbohydrate** before exercise if glucose level is below 100 mg/dl. A carbohydrate-rich snack—for example, 6 to 12 ounces of fruit juice or 6 to 8 saltines—should do the trick.

- **Avoid exercise when diabetes control is poor.** Guidelines from the American College of Sports Medicine suggest that exercise should be avoided if the glucose level is greater than 300 mg/dl or greater than 240 mg/dl if ketones are present in the urine.

- **Know the signs and symptoms of hypoglycemia.** Diabetics who have heart palpitations or who feel confused, unusually weak, tired, shaky, anxious, visually disturbed, or dizzy during or after exercise should immediately eat or drink some simple form of sugar. Unrecognized and untreated, these symptoms could lead to unconsciousness or convulsions. To reduce the likelihood of hypoglycemia, a decrease in your insulin dosage or an increase in carbohydrate intake may be necessary before or after exercise. As an additional precaution, exercising with a partner is recommended.

- **Watch for high blood sugar (hyperglycemia),** which can lead to ketoacidosis, commonly called diabetic coma. Symptoms such as excessive thirst, frequent urination, blurred vision, weakness, itchy, dry skin or a fruity odor or breath may result from taking too little insulin, extreme inactivity, overeating, infection or emotional upset. Urine or blood glucose levels should be checked on a regular basis.

- The *indoor cross-country skiing machine* is another excellent calorie-burner, although it's harder to master unless you're familiar with cross-country skiing. If not, go easy and just take your time.

- *Stair-climbers* and *stair-steppers* allow for a great workout in a short period of time. They're good calorie-burners and generally carry a low risk for injury, although some people with back problems may find that machines of this type worsen their condition.

- *Indoor rowing machines* strengthen arms and legs and provide cardiovascular fitness. They're great calorie-burners, especially because these devices engage a large muscle mass. However, people with neck and back conditions should be very careful on them.

- The *elliptical exercise trainer* provides a combination of jogging and stair-stepping, and may include arm levers as well. This machine can give you a low-stress but highly aerobic workout, exercising the upper and lower extremities.

Balance Your Diet

Know What You Eat

FROM THANKSGIVING DINNERS TO SUPER BOWL SNACKS, food embodies pleasure, home, love, tradition and entertainment. It can also have an enormous influence on our physical well-being—eating a balanced diet is one of the smartest things we can do to manage cardiac markers, ward off disease and maximize good health.

Unfortunately, the American diet has become progressively unbalanced. We're eating more animal foods, fast foods, convenience foods and restaurant meals, all of which have made for a diet too rich in fat, sugar, salt and calories. At the same time, we're eating fewer fruits, vegetables, beans and whole grains—foods rich in complex carbohydrates, fiber and antioxidants. And to top it off, we're eating more, *period*. The increase in portion size of common foods is a main contributor to overeating and the current obesity epidemic. As economist John Kenneth Galbraith once said, these trends combine to make America one of the "most overfed and undernourished" countries in the world. According to the U.S. Department of Agriculture, on any given day:

- 3% of Americans will eat a hot dog, ham or luncheon meat.
- 25% will consume a hamburger, cheeseburger or meat loaf.
- 41% will eat a doughnut, cookies or a piece of cake.
- 23% will consume at least one serving of steak or roast beef.
- 41% will down two glasses of whole milk.

Of course, there is no one American diet. Anyone who has enjoyed crab cakes in Baltimore, tacos in Los Angeles or prime rib in Kansas City knows that favorite foods differ from one end of the country to the other, reflecting regional preferences and ethnic traditions. But there is a common American diet pattern. From Boston to San Diego, Seattle to Miami and every place in between, the basic diet is sweet, salty and full of fat.

The Centers for Disease Control and Prevention estimates that almost two-thirds of our calories come from fat, sugar and alcohol, with the remaining calories left to meet our major nutritional needs. This is a poor ratio. What business or sports team could succeed with only one-third of its people pulling the oars for everyone?

As stated in the Surgeon General's Report of 2010, the American diet is linked to an increased risk for coronary heart disease, cancer, high blood pressure, type 2 diabetes, stroke—and the nation's leading ailment, obesity. The report also links our diet to the less threatening but serious problems of gout, osteoarthritis and gallbladder disease.

Says former surgeon general C. Everett Koop, "As diseases of nutritional deficiency have diminished, they have been replaced by diseases of dietary excess and imbalance—problems that now rank among the leading causes of illness and death in the United States. After smoking, food choices can influence long-term health prospects more than any other factor."

A Dietary Snapshot

HEALTH EXPERTS CONSIDER THE CONTEMPORARY AMERICAN DIET to be seriously out of balance. But it wasn't always that way. A comparison of foods consumed in 1910, when the Department of Agriculture first started to keep figures on the food supply, with those consumed today shows a dramatic shift.

- Early in the last century, dietary fat made up just 27% of calories eaten. Today, because of our reliance on meat, dairy products, fried foods, snack foods and fast foods, that figure has risen to 37%, with the average family of four consuming more than 400 pounds of fat per year. The predominance of animal foods has led to a high consumption of saturated fats, a leading factor in the development of heart disease. Moreover, the prevalence of foods containing trans fats—mainly stick margarine, commercially baked goods, chips, crackers and fast food—has contributed to higher cholesterol levels and inflammation.

- In 1910, the average adult consumed some 70 pounds of refined sugar. Today, thanks to high-fructose corn syrup, that figure has risen to 156 pounds, or more than one-third of a pound of sugar each day; it's even worse for children and adolescents. They consume, on average, about 275 pounds of sugar a year. "America's sweet tooth is out of control," says

A DAY IN THE LIFE OF AN AMERICAN TEEN

Dr. Theresa Nicklas, a pediatric nutrition expert, recorded the dietary intake of one 17-year-old boy over a 24-hour period: "For breakfast, he had a fast-food egg-and-bacon sandwich and orange juice on the bus to school. Many of his friends left the school campus for lunch at a fast-food place, but he ate lunch at school: chicken nuggets, baked potato with butter and cheese, two rolls, a canned pear and whole milk. His other choices were pepperoni pizza or a cheeseburger with fries. His afternoon snack took place at a deli: a chicken sandwich globbed with mayonnaise, and a bag of potato chips. Dinner at home was two fried pork chops, another baked potato and two slices of bread. The fact that he didn't eat a single green vegetable in a 24-hour period, and only a little fruit, doesn't surprise us. Unfortunately, this today is more the rule than the exception."

dietitian Bonnie Liebman of the Center for Science in the Public Interest. "Sugar now accounts for about 24% of calories eaten in the American diet." This dramatic increase bears much responsibility for a steady rise in the number of overweight Americans, and for those with elevated triglycerides and metabolic syndrome.

■ Americans consume an estimated two to four teaspoons of salt daily—about 15 pounds a year! About 75% comes from packaged foods and foods eaten away from home, whereas 25% comes from the salt shaker. According to the American Heart Association, the recommended level is no more than 2,300 milligrams of sodium daily, or about one teaspoon of salt. The overeating of salt and sodium has helped to make high blood pressure a cardiac marker for more than 72 million people.

■ Today, Americans eat 150 more calories per day than they did 20 years ago. These extra calories could add up to a 15-pound weight gain in one year. It's easy to overeat when cookies are the size of pancakes, muffins are bigger than baseballs, and sodas are large enough to drown in. "Supersizing" has vastly expanded the calories in a typical fast-food meal. Even *The Joy of Cooking* has given in to the trend; recipes that used to feed six now feed only four. According to the latest National Health and

Nutrition Examination Survey (NHANES), which periodically reviews American eating habits, even those who are choosing healthy foods and avoiding high-fat, high-sugar items are still eating too much.

- With the rise in affluence over the last 100 years, animal foods and refined foods have been systematically substituted for fruits, whole grains, beans and vegetables. It is estimated that 25% of adults do not consume even one serving a day of vegetables. And for those who eat vegetables, French fries constitute one-quarter of all vegetables eaten. Since complex carbohydrates are critical to successful weight control, their waning popularity has worsened the national obesity problem.

Why Do We Eat This Way?

Clearly, most people understand that the modern American diet can be hazardous to cardiovascular health. But only 34% of American adults describe themselves as being "health-conscious" in terms of their eating habits. Why, then, do so many of us eat so poorly?

While a number of factors influence food choices, none is as important as our contemporary way of life. Modern society is stressful and pressure-packed, often driving us to choose what we eat on the spur of the moment and without thought to health. "And when you add in what choices are available, the problem is compounded," says Dr. Kelly Brownell, an obesity expert at Yale University. "Modern society is a toxic environment for making healthy food choices," Dr. Brownell explains. "Everywhere you turn there is an opportunity to eat poorly, backed up by an advertising industry that encourages overeating. In the lab, if you take a rat and toss food from the 7-Eleven into its cage, if you throw in candy bars, throw in Cheetos, throw in marshmallows, things like that, you duplicate such a toxic environment, and as a result you'll get an enormously obese rat."

Eating competes with many other activities in our fragmented schedules. Says registered dietitian Evelyn Tribole, "People are no longer inclined to shop, cook or make food choices based on good nutrition. They often eat on the run and settle for what is available, quickly, from restaurants, take-outs and food stores. Many have simply traded nutrition

TOO MUCH OF A GOOD THING

America has an abundance of food. It's available everywhere, and for the most part, it's cheap. Until the middle of the last century, cyclical food shortages resulting from bad weather and crop failures were a way of life. Refrigeration and rapid transport of food products had not yet been perfected. As a result, people often didn't get enough to eat. (Indeed, records show that many men who enlisted in World War II were so undernourished that they had to be fed for a period of time before starting basic training. Today, a significant number of recruits flunk the army's induction physicals as "too fat to fight.") Diseases of insufficient nutrition such as rickets and scurvy were not unusual.

Today, most of us can eat what we want when we want it. But abundant food does not equate to a healthy diet. Eating too often and too much subjects the average American to diseases of excess.

for convenience." At four P.M. on any given day, 70% of Americans do not know what they'll be having for dinner that night. But it starts with breakfast. In about half of families, one or more people skip breakfast regularly. Nancy Clark, a sports nutritionist, says, "People tell me they don't have time for breakfast. What they don't realize is that by skipping this meal, they can become ravenous later in the day, make all the wrong food choices and overeat." According to a 2009 Harris poll, 46% of adults in the United States eat out at restaurants more than twice a week. Unfortunately, many are fast-food meals, which typically average 1,050 calories, 41 grams of fat, 2,150 milligrams of sodium and virtually no complex carbohydrate foods.

With family meals diminishing, the consumption of junk and snack foods is on the rise. The typical American consumes more than 25 pounds of snack foods each year. To put that into perspective, consider the fact that we pay about $2 billion a year for every sports ticket in the country— pro, college and high school. But we spend the same amount on just five candy products: M&M's, Snickers, Reese's Peanut Butter Cups, Milky Ways and Hershey's Kisses. In addition, our portions dwarf those of past generations, with "supersizing" (for a few pennies more) in fast-food restaurants, pizza promotions (two for the price of one), and all the "giant" candy bars, oversize bagels (4 to 7 ounces) and jumbo soft drinks (32 to 64 ounces) currently available. Restaurant servings of 22-to-38-ounce steaks and fish are commonplace. In some movie theaters, a "medium" popcorn now contains 16 cups—and many people order it buttered.

Time for a Change

Dietary habits are a significant factor in managing cardiac markers, particularly lipids, weight, blood pressure and diabetes, but what most of us choose to eat bears little resemblance to what we should eat for good health. Rather than choosing foods for their nutritional value, we base our dietary decisions on convenience, advertising, taste and cravings. As stated by Laura Shapiro in *Newsweek*, "We've handed over our appetites to the food companies. Our relationship to food is not based on anything that makes sense. It's not based on our bodies, it's not based on family life and the family sitting down to the table, it's not based on what is good for the planet. There's no relationship with the body and the soul and the heart."

"The diet we eat today was not planned or developed for any particular purpose," echoes Dr. Mark Hegsted, a longtime leader in the formation of U.S. nutrition policy. "It is a happenstance related to the productivity of our farmers, the marketing activities of our food industry, particularly fast food, and the pace of life."

The evidence is clear. The modern American diet is linked to an imposing list of chronic diseases and debilitating conditions. That's why more than 17 major health organizations and initiatives, including the American Heart Association, the National Cancer Institute and the National Cholesterol Education Program, have called for changes in the way we eat. As Dr. Hegsted explains, "The risks associated with eating the American diet are demonstrably large. The question to be asked, therefore, is not why we should change our diet, but why not?"

The indictment of the American diet is serious, valid and understood, but this has not moved people to take action. For most of us, the chronic stress of everyday life keeps us eating too much, too often and too many harmful foods—particularly fast foods, junk food and snacks. That's why we use stress management techniques (including exercise) as a vehicle for dietary compliance. People who handle stress effectively are less responsive to anxiety, depression, anger and "the blues" as eating cues. People who exercise regularly feel better about themselves and expect success in making healthy eating changes.

What Makes a Heart-Healthy Diet?

MORE THAN 80 MILLION AMERICANS HAVE CARDIOVASCULAR DIS-ease, which is responsible for more than 800,000 deaths a year. According to the American Heart Association, more than 50% of the population over age 40, and more than 75% of those over age 60, have coronary artery disease. Genetic makeup certainly plays a role with some people. But the most significant reason for the epidemic of heart disease in the United States rests with our unhealthy lifestyle. Too many people are physically inactive, smoke, live with chronic stress and eat a poor diet. In particular, there is a strong relationship between diet, the creation of cholesterol-rich deposits on coronary artery walls and the development of atherosclerosis. What kind of diet, then, should we eat to minimize risk and maximize cardiac health?

For many, the first step is to do what Julia Child once suggested: "Get over the fear of food." Food is not the enemy. Indeed, the food you eat is essential for healthy living. It not only supplies fuel for your body, but also provides the raw materials from which muscle, bone, skin, hair and other tissues are made. Moreover, your diet supplies nutrients that are needed to manufacture hormones and enzymes that control the function of every cell in your body. And finally, a healthy, balanced diet can improve virtually all cardiac markers, while a poor, unhealthy diet can turn those same markers into significant coronary risks.

Unfortunately, the typical American diet is far from healthy. But it doesn't have to be that way. There is great consensus today on the part of the American Heart Association, the American Dietary Association, the surgeon general and other authoritative sources about what constitutes a healthy diet. In particular, the most recent Dietary Guidelines for

Americans issued by the Department of Human and Health Services and the Department of Agriculture set out some simple, effective principles for healthy eating.

Eat the right carbohydrates:

- Eat nutrient-rich foods with vitamins, minerals and fiber such as vegetables, fruits, beans, legumes and whole-grain products.

- Minimize or avoid refined carbohydrates such as cookies, cakes, crackers and other commercial baked goods.

Eat the right fats:

- Moderate total fat content. But when you do eat fats, choose healthy liquid oils such as olive oil and canola oil. In particular, eat fish and other foods containing omega-3 fatty acids.

- Avoid foods with saturated fat and trans fat.

- Consume fat-free or low-fat dairy products with calcium and vitamin D.

- Choose lean meats and poultry without skin.

- Cut back on foods containing dietary cholesterol.

Eat less sodium:

- Cut back or avoid processed foods with high levels of sodium.

- Eat more potassium-rich foods like fruits and vegetables.

Eat less sugar:

- Watch out for foods and beverages with added sugar and other sweeteners like high-fructose corn syrup, which can increase calories in your diet and contribute to overweight and high triglyceride levels.

- If you drink alcohol, do so in moderation.

But the science of healthy eating, as outlined in the above recommendations, goes just so far. You have to put that science into action every day in order to derive benefits. And that's where experience comes in. The Piscatella family has eaten a heart-healthy diet for more than three decades, and that practical application of the science is reflected in the recommendations in this section. For example, we place a high degree of emphasis on palatability. Knowing what to eat and what to avoid is basic, but that's not all there is to it. If you serve healthy food that doesn't taste good, no one will eat it. That's why we advise an eating pattern based on the Mediterranean diet, a delicious and healthy way of eating that you can practice for a lifetime.

We also believe that a great part of the healthy-eating solution lies in eating foods that are whole (not processed) and plant-based. But no food should be forbidden. Everything from red wine to red meat has its place within the context of healthy eating.

And lastly, don't diet. If any of the pop diet programs had worked over the past 60 years, we'd be a nation of skinny folks. We are not. Don't fall into that trap.

The Right Carbohydrates

Carbohydrates have been demonized for the past few years in many popular diet books. And to a certain extent, the reasons for concern are valid. But such books often only present part of the story. Eaten in excess, some carbohydrates certainly can be categorized as harmful. But other carbohydrates are viewed as perhaps the healthiest foods on the planet. So, whether they're harmful or beneficial depends on the type of carbohydrates you choose.

Foods and beverages rich in *refined* (or simple) carbohydrates are high in calories and low in fiber, carry few nutrients, are usually rich in sweeteners and break down quickly in the body. Examples are cookies, cake, doughnuts, soft drinks, sugar and white flour. Such foods cause blood sugar to increase rapidly, resulting in more insulin production and the ready conversion of calories into body fat. If not actually "dangerous," such sugary, refined carbohydrates should be minimized or avoided by anyone interested in heart health, particularly if weight loss is a goal.

As a society, we made a huge mistake a decade or so ago in our response to the recommendations of the American Heart Association and others to reduce fat intake. The science suggested that our high-fat way of eating had a lot to do with dramatic increases in heart disease and obesity, and we responded to the call by cutting fat intake. Unfortunately, we became caught up in "fat mania" and replaced fatty foods with refined carbohydrates, particularly those carrying "low-fat" or "fat-free" labels. These foods may have been low in fat, but they were not low in calories, particularly when eaten to excess. Says Nancy Ernst of the National Cholesterol Education Program, "The experts said nothing about calories, and neither did the food industry. Food manufacturers were extremely aggressive in promoting high-sugar, no-fat products that translated into weight gain." The "low-fat" label on a blueberry muffin was an excuse to eat two. Pretty soon the extra calories turned into excess body fat and we developed a national obesity condition. Refined carbohydrates certainly bear much responsibility for this result.

Foods rich in *complex carbohydrates,* on the other hand, have never been a health problem. Full of great nutrients like fiber, vitamins, phytochemicals and antioxidants, they promote good health, reduce the risk of heart disease and diabetes, and aid in weight control. The Harvard Nurses' Health Study, with some 95,000 participants, found that those who ate whole grains and five servings a day of fruits and vegetables lowered their risk of heart attack by 35%. Examples of such foods are fruits, vegetables, nuts, whole grains, beans and legumes. Considered just about the healthiest of foods, complex carbohydrates are the basis of a heart-healthy food plan.

So, it is not the carbohydrates you eat that can expand your waistline and penalize heart health, it is the *type* of carbohydrates eaten. That's why foods rich in complex carbohydrates should make up about 55% of total calories (some experts suggest 45% for those with metabolic syndrome.) The Dietary Guidelines for Americans issued by the Department of Human and Health Services and the Department of Agriculture recommend daily consumption of the following:

- Five servings or 2½ cups of vegetables
- Four servings or 2 cups of fruit
- Six servings of grains (including three servings of whole grains)

such as whole-grain breads, cereals, pasta, rice and beans

While this might sound like a lot of food, in reality it is not. One serving from the grain group is one slice of bread, or half a cup of cooked cereal, rice or pasta, or one cup of ready-to-eat cereal. A serving from the fruit group is one medium piece of fruit or one-half cup of dried fruit, while a serving from the vegetable group is one-half cup. Meeting these recommendations is not that hard to do, and it's important. Studies throughout the world suggest that people who habitually consume a diet rich in plant food have a low risk of coronary heart disease both because of what they *do consume* (fiber, soluble fiber, antioxidants, vitamins, monounsaturated fats and other nutrients) and because of what they *do not consume* (a lot of saturated fat from animal foods and trans fat from convenience foods.)

Carbohydrates and Heart Health

In the 1940s and '50s, pioneer researcher Dr. Ancel Keys of the University of Minnesota conducted a classic study involving three groups of Japanese subjects, each residing in a different environment and eating a different diet. The first group lived in Japan and ate a traditional Asian diet: lots of vegetables, fruit, legumes, soy products, rice and fish, and little meat. They had a low incidence of heart attacks. The second group lived in Hawaii and ate a mixture of Asian and American foods, which meant fewer fruits, vegetables and grains, and more meat and butter. They had a greater incidence of heart attacks. The third group lived in Los Angeles and ate a totally Americanized diet, from steaks to ice cream. Their intake of fruits, vegetables and grains decreased substantially, and these individuals had the highest incidence of heart attacks.

More recent studies have reaffirmed the benefits of plant foods. The Atherosclerosis in Communities Study found that eating whole grains reduced the risk of heart failure. The Harvard Physicians' Health Study came to the same conclusion: Unrefined foods high in complex carbohydrates and fiber are cardioprotective and can help to control blood pressure and weight. This is now a recommendation in the Step I, Step II and Therapeutic Lifestyle Changes (TLC) diet of the National Cholesterol Education Program.

In addition, the deeper the color of the food, the more effective the protection against heart disease, cancer and other chronic diseases. This is because deeply colored fruits and vegetables, especially green, red and

WHAT WE KNOW VS. HOW WE LIVE

Despite all the relevant published studies and a general awareness on the part of the public, only one in five Americans eats the recommended daily servings of fruits and vegetables. Some 20% eat no fruit at all, and 15% rarely eat a vegetable other than potatoes. Amazingly, according to the American Medical Association, doctors do no better when it comes to fruits and vegetables.

yellow ones, have the most vitamins and minerals, and the plant pigments themselves are high in antioxidants. This doesn't mean you should quit eating light green grapes or white potatoes. But experts recommend including some "darks"—such as spinach, prunes, red grapes, kale, cherries, raisins, carrots and oranges—every day.

Plant foods also contain mass but not a lot of calories, which is useful in filling you up, not out. Foods that need a lot of chewing, like apples or carrots, take a long time to eat and therefore provide sufficient time (about 20 minutes) for satiety to be attained. These foods also absorb water in the digestive system, thereby helping to create a feeling of fullness and satisfaction that keeps you from overeating.

In addition, complex carbohydrates are usually rich in fiber, which aids in weight loss. Fiber passes through the digestive system intact, so not all calories consumed stay with the body. High-fiber foods also produce satiety, which means you're more likely to feel full for a longer period of time. Says registered dietitian Joan Slavin, "There is strong evidence that people who eat high-fiber diets are less likely to be obese."

THE GLYCEMIC INDEX

According to some dietary experts, using the glycemic index (GI) is a good way to differentiate between refined and complex carbohydrates, particularly for those with type 2 diabetes. Refined carbohydrates (called high-GI foods) break down quickly and increase blood sugar rapidly. Complex carbohydrates (called low-GI foods) break down more slowly and do not cause blood sugar to rise.

When your diet consists predominantly of high-GI foods, it can lead to carbohydrate cravings and an increase in appetite—potentially resulting in unwanted weight gain. These foods can cause large fluctuations of both blood sugar and insulin levels, leading to a vicious cycle of overeating.

In addition, the blood sugar spikes produced by high-GI foods can cause your body to produce higher levels of insulin, a hormone that responds directly to what you eat. Insulin regulates fat metabolism and controls blood sugar levels. Blood sugar is the basic fuel that all cells in the body use to make energy. In an optimal state, the body maintains the blood sugar level in a fairly narrow range: not too low (hypoglycemia) and not too high (hyperglycemia). This stability is important because imbalances, particularly hyperglycemia, can cause serious health problems.

It is estimated that about 33% of the American population is resistant to the action of insulin. In other words, their bodies have to produce more insulin than is healthy just to maintain normal blood sugar levels. This condition is called *insulin resistance*. People diagnosed with insulin resistance are generally overweight and often have low energy levels, difficulty losing weight, mood swings and increased muscle loss. In addition, it has been shown that people who have insulin resistance are at an increased risk of developing diabetes and heart disease. For these reasons, it is important to control your insulin levels by eating low-GI foods (complex carbohydrates) and avoiding high-GI foods (refined carbohydrates).

LOW-GI FOODS	HIGH-GI FOODS
Apples	Candy
Berries and cherries	Cookies
Barley	Juices with added sugar
Grapefruit	White potatoes
Legumes (lentils, beans, peanuts)	Chips (potato and corn)
Nuts (almonds, walnuts, soy nuts)	Sugar
Oatmeal (unsweetened)	Most breakfast cereals
Green peas	Sweetened soda
Tomatoes	Sweet snacks
Unsweetened plain yogurt	White bread and bagels

The Right Fats

Dietary fat plays an important role in promoting good health. Fat in the foods we eat is used in the transportation of important fat-soluble vitamins in the body. And polyunsaturated fats (mostly vegetable oils) supply the body with linolenic acid, an essential fatty acid. Without fat in the diet, we wouldn't be able to absorb vitamins A, D, E and K. Fat also provides the body with a concentrated source of energy. At nine calories per gram, fat packs more than two times as many calories as the same amount of protein and carbohydrates. And finally, fat also provides satiety, an important element in appetite control.

So it's clear that fat is fine when it's a healthy type and consumed in the proper amount. From a nutritional standpoint, the daily requirement for fat can be fully satisfied by consuming one tablespoon of vegetable oil. The average American, however, eats eight times that amount: between 800 and 1,000 calories in fat every day, the equivalent of one full stick of butter. It is this overconsumption of fat that constitutes a health issue.

For a long time, "eat low-fat" was the dietary mantra of the American Heart Association. "Eat a diet with no more 30% of calories from fat," they said. And some doctors went further, calling for maximum fat levels of just 10%. But there has been a change in thinking. "It's a myth that one low-fat diet is best for everyone," says nutrition expert Dr. Wayne Calloway. "In fact, research shows that for some, cutting fat too much could reduce protective HDL cholesterol and even increase their risk of heart disease." This thinking is reflected in the most recent American Heart Association guidelines that allow for up to 35% of calories from fat, as long as you restrict saturated and trans fats in favor of healthy oils and eat an otherwise healthful diet of fruits, vegetables, legumes, whole grains, fish, nuts and low-fat dairy products.

▪ **Reduce saturated fat for cholesterol control.** With regard to type, most of the fat in our diet should come from monounsaturated and poly-unsaturated oils. From the standpoint of cardiac health, olive oil is the best, followed by canola oil. The new guidelines call for no more than 10% of calories from saturated fat (please note that the American Heart Association limits it to 7% of calories) and trans fats should be kept as low as possible (no more than 1% of calories). Saturated fat causes a rise in both total and LDL cholesterol. In the Seven Country Study (Finland, Greece, Italy, Japan, the Netherlands, the United States and Yugoslavia), Dr. Ancel Keys observed some 12,000 men in the 40-to-49 age range and found that cultures in which saturated fat made up a high percentage of calories demonstrated elevated cholesterol and a high incidence of coronary heart disease. Thus the Finns, who ate 20% of their calories as saturated fat, had cholesterol levels that averaged 265. The Japanese ate only 5% of their calories as saturated fat and had correspondingly low levels of cholesterol, averaging just 165. A key finding was that the heart attack rate for Finnish men in the study was six times greater than for Japanese men of the same age.

More recently, the Framingham Heart Study, the MRFIT Trial and the NIH Cholesterol Study, among others, have found that reducing saturated fat lowers cholesterol, especially LDL cholesterol. Says Dr. Virgil Brown, a past president of the American Heart Association, "The goal for saturated fat intake is about 7% of calories, no more. Unfortunately, most people consume about 13% to 18% of calories as saturated fat, and for some as much as one-third of total calories eaten. That's a big reason why heart disease is still our number one killer."

> **A RULE OF THUMB**
>
> S aturated fat is the fatty part of food that generally stays hard at room temperature. Both mono- and polyunsaturated oils tend to stay liquid at the same temperature.

Animal foods are a primary source of saturated fat—the visible fat on red meat, poultry skin, bacon drippings, cheese, lard and butter. A second source of saturated fats is "tropical oils"—palm oil, palm kernel oil and coconut oil. Studies show that diets rich in these saturated oils elevate LDL cholesterol and increase the risk of heart attack. Unfortunately, tropical oils are used freely in processed foods because they're relatively cheap. They're found in nondairy creamers, soups, potato chips, salad dressings and crackers—in so many processed foods that on average each American consumes over seven pounds of tropical oils annually.

■ **Avoid cholesterol-raising trans fat.** When polyunsaturated oils are hardened or stiffened into a solid or semisolid state in a process called hydrogenation, a chemical change takes place that produces trans fatty acids, or trans fat. There is much evidence that trans fat can raise total and LDL cholesterol, reduce HDL cholesterol and promote coronary inflammation. In the Harvard Nurses' Health Study, women who ate lots of foods rich in trans fat had a 66% higher risk of heart disease than those

SUPERMARKET SAVVY

Supermarket shelves are loaded with products claiming zero trans fats. But that "zero" on the label isn't necessarily a true zero. According to FDA guidelines, products containing less than 0.5 grams of trans fat per serving can list "zero grams trans fat" on their nutritional label. As a result, just one "zero grams trans fat" serving could contain as much as 0.49 grams of trans fat. For example, Shedd's Spread Country Creek regular soft margarine has 0.44 grams of trans fat per serving. (By comparison, Smart Balance Buttery Spread regular margarine has just 0.07 grams of trans fat.)

Over the course of three meals, just one serving of "zero grams trans fat" at each meal can add up to almost 1.5 grams of trans fat for the day. That doesn't sound like a lot, but the American Heart Association recommends a daily trans fat intake of less than 2 grams. So, you could be consuming almost 75% of your daily limit in "zero grams trans fat" foods.

Instead of relying on advertising, check out the ingredients listed in the Nutrition Facts. If you see ingredients referred to as "partially hydrogenated" or "shortening," you've found trans fat. Avoid these foods.

who did not. A recent article in *The New England Journal of Medicine* found that increasing trans fats in the diet leads to a 29% overall risk of coronary disease.

Companies like using trans fats because they're inexpensive and give foods taste, texture and a long shelf life. Margarine is a good example of how hydrogenation can alter the health characteristics of a food product. As a healthful alternative to cholesterol-raising butter, margarine seems ideal; it's made from polyunsaturated oil (usually corn or safflower oil), which lowers cholesterol. And that holds true as long as the oil remains liquid, in the form of soft, tub-type margarines, spray and squeeze-type margarines, or "diet" margarines. But when hydrogenated into stick form, margarine can raise blood cholesterol. So, if you're concerned enough about your cholesterol to avoid butter and other saturated fats, it makes sense to also avoid stick margarine and other hydrogenated food products. Watch out for solid shortening, crackers, potato chips and other processed foods, commercially prepared baked goods (cookies, muffins, pies and cakes) and fried fast foods such as chicken nuggets and French fries.

The American Heart Association recommends that you consume less than 1% of your total calories from trans fats. So, if you eat 2,000 calories a day, no more than 20 calories should come from trans fats—that means less than 2 grams a day. Trans fats are now on nutrition labels, which is helpful in identifying foods to be avoided.

■ **Reduce total fat for weight control.** Too much fat in the diet can produce an overabundance of calories leading to overweight and obesity. Unfortunately, high-calorie fatty foods—processed meats, baked goods, fast foods, snack foods such as potato chips and chocolate bars, salad oils, whole milk products, and packaged foods and meals—are central to the American diet. Frying is a favorite method of cooking, while fatty sauces and gravies are routinely used as flavor enhancers.

For most of us, gaining weight takes place over a period of time. A few more calories taken in, a few less expended, cause body fat to accumulate. As few as 50 extra calories a day—a single chocolate-chip cookie—can add 350 calories a week. That doesn't sound like much, but it equates to a gain of 5 pounds in a year, or 52 pounds in a decade.

Because of the caloric density of fatty foods, a high-fat diet produces a lot of calories. Fat contains more than twice as many calories as the same amount of protein or carbohydrate: one gram of fat has 9 calories; one gram of protein or carbohydrate has 4 calories. That's why a small package (1.74 ounces) of M&M peanut candies contains 250 calories, while an entire pound of apples has just 240 calories.

■ **Reduce dietary cholesterol.** People get cholesterol in two ways. The body, mainly the liver, produces varying amounts, usually about 1,000 milligrams a day. Foods also can contain cholesterol. Animal foods (especially egg yolks, meat, poultry, shellfish and whole- and reduced-fat milk and dairy products) contain it. Foods from plants (fruits, vegetables, grains, nuts and seeds) don't contain cholesterol.

At one time, dietary cholesterol was thought to be the greatest contributor to elevated blood cholesterol, but that thinking has changed. Saturated and trans fats are now seen as the main culprits in raising blood cholesterol. Says Dr. Ernst Schaefer of Tufts University, "Reducing saturated fat consumption by 50% may lower blood cholesterol twice as much as a similar drop in dietary cholesterol."

Still, consuming too much dietary cholesterol is a cardiac risk. That's why the American Heart Association recommends that you limit your average daily cholesterol intake to less than 300 milligrams. If you have heart disease, limit your daily intake to less than 200 milligrams. (Typically, the average American man consumes about 337 milligrams of cholesterol a day; the average woman, 217 milligrams.)

■ **When you eat fat, make it the right kind.** Many healthy diet patterns—such as the Mediterranean diet—include healthy oils. Like carbohydrates, fats can be divided into good and bad. The best choices are monounsaturated and polyunsaturated oils, as they can help to lower LDL and total cholesterol when used in place of saturated and trans fats. Monounsaturated fats include olive oil and canola oil (the two "best" oils of the group), olives, peanuts, peanut butter, avocados, almonds, cashews and almond oil. Studies in the United States and Canada indicate that these oils reduce LDL and total cholesterol, reduce the risk of blood clot formation and minimize decreases in protective HDL cholesterol. The next best choice is polyunsaturated oils, which are effective in reducing cholesterol when substituted for saturated fats. Polyunsaturated vegetable

CALORIE FOR CALORIE, FAT IS MORE FATTENING

There are marked differences in the body's metabolic response to fats as opposed to carbohydrates or proteins. Some of the calories we consume are utilized immediately as fuel. Those not used right away are converted to body fat for future use; this requires energy, and some of the calories being converted are burned in the process. But not all foods call upon the same amount of energy for calorie conversion. Studies at the University of Massachusetts Medical School found that 23% of the calories in carbohydrates are burned off when converted to body fat. So, if you eat 100 calories of plain potato, 77 calories are available to be stored as body fat. But dietary fat burns just 3% of calories in the conversion process. Eat 100 calories of butter and 97 of them are available to become body fat!

oils, in order of preference for heart health, include safflower, soybean, sunflower, corn, cottonseed and sesame oils.

■ **Maximize omega-3 fatty acids.** Research suggests that omega-3 fatty acids can boost protective HDL cholesterol, lower triglyceride levels and reduce blood clotting, all of which lessen the risk of heart attack. Sources of omega-3s include fish and seafood, leafy green vegetables, tofu, nuts (primarily walnuts and almonds) and flaxseed. The Family Heart Study, a long-term study of 4,600 people, found that a relatively small increase in omega-3 consumption greatly reduced coronary risk.

Fish and seafood are perhaps the best sources of omega-3s. "Fish is very hard to beat as a food item," says Dr. William Castelli, former director of the Framingham Heart Study. "There's something special about fish and fish oil that is extremely beneficial and protects against cardiac disease. In fact, I think people who have had a heart attack or know they have a cholesterol problem would be crazy not to eat fish at least twice a week."

Fish oil is a great source of omega-3 fatty acids and therefore instrumental in reducing the risk of heart attack by lowering cholesterol. It also reduces triglycerides, prevents clotting and promotes the health of coronary artery walls. In its latest dietary guidelines the American Heart Association recommends that everyone eat at least two three-ounce servings of fatty fish (salmon, mackerel, sardines, pompano and tuna) each week. One major study, published in the *New England Journal of Medicine,* concluded that eating "as little as two fish dishes a week, about 7.5 ounces of fish total, may cut the risk of dying from heart attack in half."

A study at Brigham and Women's Hospital in Boston found that men who eat oily fish regularly are greatly protected from heart attacks and in particular from sudden cardiac death. Results from the Nurses' Health Study found this to be true for women also. As reported in the *Journal of the American Medical Association,* "the more frequently a woman ate fish, the less likely she was to suffer a heart attack or die of any cardiac cause."

Research suggests that fat in many nuts and seeds are rich in omega-3s. That's why the recommendation is to eat one serving of nuts and seeds on most days. A study at Hershey Medical Center, affiliated

OMEGA-3s ARE A-1

Although our bodies don't manufacture omega-3s, we're fortunate in our ability to get them from food. Besides fish, leafy green vegetables, nuts, flaxseed, canola oil and tofu can provide us with these heart-healthy fatty acids.

with Pennsylvania State University, suggests that when included as part of a balanced diet, nuts can reduce LDL cholesterol and lessen coagulation, potentially helping to reduce cardiac risk. Good ways to include nuts in your diet include adding a serving of chopped walnuts (about a jigger, or one to two ounces) to your morning oatmeal and mixing a serving of almonds with raisins for an afternoon pick-me-up snack.

Flaxseed, traditionally known as linseed, is a wonderful source of omega-3s. Many experts suggest adding about two tablespoons of ground flaxseed to your daily diet. Sprinkle it on yogurt, cereals and salads or add it to applesauce and casseroles. Unheated flaxseed oil also works well.

Some new types of margarine, made from plant sterol esters, have a cholesterol-lowering effect similar to that of oat bran. Clinical trials have shown drops in total cholesterol of 10% and LDL cholesterol of 14%.

Dr. Walter Willett of the Harvard School of Public Health suggests that good fats should go at the base of the food pyramid, along with complex carbohydrates. Bad fats—saturated and trans fats—should join refined carbohydrates at the top of the pyramid.

Less Sodium

For most of us, salt is something we sprinkle on our food even before we've tasted it, or it's an ingredient of a favorite recipe. In fact, about 35% of our daily sodium is consumed in condiment form. But most of the rest comes from processed foods such as tomato sauce, soups, canned foods and prepared mixes, and from restaurant foods, especially fast foods. The average person snacks on about 21 pounds of potato chips, pretzels, popcorn and other "salty" foods every year. A McDonald's Big Mac with a large fries has about 1,440 milligrams of sodium.

Says Dr. Jeremiah Stamler of Northwestern University Medical School, "Over 95% of men and 75% of women eat more than a teaspoon of salt daily. In fact, the average person consumes two to four teaspoons of salt a day, which translates to 4,000 to 8,000 milligrams of sodium, or a yearly consumption of about 15 pounds per person." The present guidelines advise limiting daily sodium intake to no more than 2,300 milligrams a day, or about one teaspoon of salt. New guidelines may bring that number to 1,500 milligrams a day.

Excessive salt intake has been linked to stroke, kidney and thyroid disease, edema and, in particular, hypertension. Numerous studies show that hypertension, or high blood pressure, is rampant in high-salt societies such as those in Japan and the United States. But in low-salt societies, as in New Guinea and parts of Brazil, hypertension is virtually nonexistent.

Not everyone with an excessive sodium intake is susceptible to hypertension; in many people the excess is promptly excreted no matter how much is consumed. But in about 10% to 30% of the population, there exists a genetic predisposition to high blood pressure. For these people, a diet rich in salt (and sodium) can trigger hypertension and increase cardiac risk. Because there are no tests for sodium sensitivity, it's just prudent to err on the conservative side and moderate salt and sodium intake.

Recent studies suggest that in addition to cutting back on sodium to avoid or manage hypertension, you should be sure to get the proper amount of potassium in your diet. Experts recommend at least 4,700 milligrams of potassium every day. Good sources include tomatoes, beans, fish, bananas, nuts, oranges, melons, dark leafy vegetables and dairy products.

Less Sugar

The American "sweet tooth" is getting bigger. In the early 1800s, each person consumed about two pounds of sugar a year. Today, the average adult eats and drinks more than 600 calories a day from sugar, or about 150 pounds a year. We eat it by the spoonful from the sugar bowl, and we consume huge amounts more from soft drinks, cookies, salad dressings and candy. About 70% of all added sugars and sweeteners come in the form of liquid high-fructose corn syrup. With sugar accounting for 24% of calories consumed in the United States, we now eat more sugar in a week than our forefathers did in an entire year.

This level of consumption is a significant contributor to the twin epidemics of obesity and heart disease. Foods rich in sugar, such as commercial baked goods and soft drinks, can provide a great amount of calories in a small amount of food/beverage. A 12-ounce can of orange soda, for instance, has almost 12 teaspoons of sugar and 175 calories. Many sugary foods such as candy bars are also rich in fat, producing a double whammy on weight-control efforts. Moreover, most of these foods provide little fiber and mass, so there is no signal that you've had enough to eat. This is particularly true of sugar-rich beverages. Says Dr. Richard Mattes of Purdue University, "Liquid calories don't trip our satisfaction mechanism."

Foods that are rich in refined sugar contain "empty calories" with little or no nutritional value. They take up space in your diet that could otherwise be filled with nutritious foods rich in vitamins, minerals and fiber.

A diet with too much sugar can increase weight, elevate triglycerides and promote metabolic syndrome, increasing the cardiac risk from these important markers.

DRINKING SUGAR

About 65% of young girls and 74% of young boys consume sugar-sweetened drinks each day. These drinks are the leading source of added sugars in the diets of today's American kids. Overconsumption may increase the likelihood of childhood obesity. An astonishing 7.1% of American calories come from sugared water.

The Truth About . . .

Fiber

Often called roughage, bulk or bran, fiber is a nondigestible component of plant foods. (Think in terms of whole fruits, raw vegetables, whole grains and cereals, beans and high-fiber snacks such as nuts.) Fiber aids in weight control because it passes through the digestive system intact, which means that not all calories consumed stay within the body.

The typical American diet is too low in fiber, providing only about 11 grams of fiber per day per person, far short of the American Dietetic

Association's recommendation of 20 to 35 grams per day. Most adult men should shoot for 30-plus grams of fiber a day; women, 20 grams. For an idea of how much this is, remember that 28 grams equals one ounce, so your daily fiber intake does not have to be unreasonably large. But you can overdo a good thing. More than 50 or 60 grams of fiber a day may decrease the amount of vitamins and minerals your body absorbs.

Research shows that *soluble* fiber can reduce total and LDL cholesterol. As it moves through the digestive system, soluble fiber forms a gel that interferes with the absorption of cholesterol and is particularly effective in reducing cholesterol in people with levels over 200. Soluble fiber is found in oat bran, oatmeal, barley, rice bran, fruits (apples, oranges, strawberries, prunes), vegetables (carrots, corn, broccoli), and beans and peas (lentils, navy and pinto beans). Psyllium, sold commercially as Metamucil, also contains soluble fiber.

Studies conducted by Dr. James Anderson at the University of Kentucky showed that participants reduced their cholesterol by 13% to 19% by consuming one cup of oat bran, or about three bowls cooked, per day. (Eating three bowls of oat bran is not a dietary recommendation; we should get our soluble fiber from a variety of foods.) Similar results were reported in a study at Harvard University. This is important information in light of evidence that a 1% reduction in cholesterol produces a 2% to 3% lowering of heart attack risk.

Soluble fiber is not a magic pill. (One woman reportedly sprinkled oat bran on ice cream, thinking it canceled out the fat.) Instead, understand that maximum benefits occur when foods rich in soluble fiber become part of an eating plan that is healthful overall. How much soluble fiber do you need? Experts are not certain, but the consensus is that consuming three grams a day—about the amount in one and a half cups of cooked oat bran—is sufficient to elicit a cholesterol-lowering response.

Soy Protein

Soy protein, found in products such as soybeans, soy milk and tofu, has been found to have a positive impact on LDL cholesterol and other cardiac risk factors. The cholesterol-lowering properties of soy were first seen in studies on Asian populations that exhibited lower cholesterol and far less heart disease than western populations. It was initially thought that dietary fat content—low among Asians, high for westerners—was the key factor. But upon further investigation researchers found that what Asians were eating—rice, vegetables, whole grains and particularly soy—was just as important as the fat they were not eating.

Subsequent studies seemed to confirm soy's effectiveness. An analysis of 38 clinical studies demonstrated that substituting soy products for animal foods could lower LDL cholesterol by as much as 8%. As a result, in 2000 the American Heart Association concluded that "it is prudent to recommend including soy protein foods in a diet low in saturated fat and cholesterol."

The evidence of soy's efficacy was so compelling that the Food and Drug Administration approved a health claim for soy protein and coronary heart disease. The FDA suggested that "25 grams of soy protein a day, as part of a diet low in saturated fat and cholesterol, may reduce the risk of heart disease." The link between soy protein and heart-disease protection seemed strong enough that the FDA allowed foods with at least 6.25 grams per serving to carry this health claim on their label. (Studies showed that it would require up to four servings of such products to yield the cholesterol-lowering benefit.)

But, once again, science marched on. Because of their belief that health claims should be based on sound evidence that indicates an unambiguous relationship between a food substance and the health benefit indicated in the manufacturer's health claim, the American Heart Association recently undertook a reevaluation of the evidence on soy protein and cardiovascular disease and came to a different conclusion. The majority of current research suggests that a very large amount of soy protein, more than half the daily protein intake, may lower LDL cholesterol (usually in people with very high cholesterol) by a few percentage points *when it replaces dairy protein or a mixture of animal proteins.* However, this reduction is very small relative to the large amounts of soy protein consumed. Furthermore, there are no evident beneficial effects of soy protein consumption on HDL cholesterol, triglycerides, lipoprotein(a) or blood pressure.

"Thus," says the American Heart Association, "the direct cardiovascular health benefit of soy protein is minimal at best." Nevertheless, while soy may not be the magic bullet for cholesterol we once thought it was, consuming soy protein as a substitute for animal foods rich in saturated fat is still a smart move for heart health.

Alcohol

Moderate alcohol consumption, such as a glass of red wine with dinner, is associated with a reduced risk of heart disease and stroke. Says Dr. R. Curtis Ellison at the Boston University School of Medicine, "It's now commonly accepted in the medical community that alcohol can reduce the risk of atherosclerosis, the gradual 'silting up' of arteries that can lead to a heart attack or stroke." Even the American Heart Association acknowledges that moderate alcohol consumption may be cardioprotective.

Alcohol works to improve cardiovascular health by causing HDL to increase and LDL to decrease. Anytime you can get that movement—HDL going up, LDL coming down—it's good for your cardiac health. Alcohol also decreases the blood's propensity to clot and aids in dissolving clots that have already formed.

YES OR NO?

Should everyone drink alcohol? Of course not. But if you do drink alcohol, moderate intake can be beneficial in terms of cardiovascular health. Excessive alcohol consumption, on the other hand, is linked to overweight, high blood pressure, accidents and liver disease.

Most doctors advise abstinence from alcohol during pregnancy.

Many alcoholic beverages, including red wine and beer, contain powerful antioxidants that are even more potent than the antioxidants found in citrus fruits, soy foods or black tea. (Antioxidants comprise a broad array of naturally occurring compounds that aid in protecting cells against inflammation by reducing the damaging effects of oxidation.)

And finally, recent studies have found that people who consume alcohol in moderation show signs of less arterial inflammation when compared with nondrinkers and heavy drinkers. In particular, moderate drinkers have significantly lower levels of C-reactive protein, a marker of inflammation.

Dr. Arthur Klatsky, a cardiologist with Kaiser Permanente in Oakland, California, conducted some of the early research on alcohol in the 1970s. Using the computerized health records of more than 100,000 people, Dr. Klatsky looked for factors that significantly affected the risk of heart disease. "We found that moderate drinkers, those who consume from one to three drinks per day, have a lower risk of dying from heart disease than either those who abstain altogether or those who drink heavily," he says. "In fact, nondrinkers and heavy drinkers seem to have heart attacks at the same rate. Light drinkers, on the other hand, have a decreased rate."

Subsequent population studies by the World Health Organization, the American Cancer Society and Oxford University in 21 countries validated Dr. Klatsky's findings. But until recently it was not known whether or not a reduction in stroke risk also occurred in moderate drinkers. As reported in the *New England Journal of Medicine*, a study of more than 22,000 men found that just a single glass of wine or beer a week was associated with a 20% reduction in the risk of ischemic stroke, which is caused by clots that reduce blood flow to the brain. Of interest is the fact that men who had only one drink a week had the same risk reduction as men who had one drink a day.

Does the type of alcohol consumed make a difference? This question first came up in response to what became known as the French Paradox: Why it is that the French seem to be able to consume large amounts of food high in fat and cholesterol and still have one of the industrial world's lowest rates for cardiovascular disease? Was red wine the key to health?

Actually, while some experts believe red wine to be superior to white wine and spirits, studies on beer and whiskey show that it is alcohol, and not a particular type of alcohol, that provides increased heart attack and stroke protection. Says Dr. John Trevithick of the University of Western Ontario, "Our study found that beers have as many antioxidants as red or white wine, which ties in with other studies. The key, of course, is consuming beer in moderation."

Vitamins and Antioxidants

For the past decade or so, it was believed that certain vitamins and antioxidants were extremely beneficial to cardiac health. As such, certain vitamins and antioxidants—beta-carotene, vitamin C, vitamin E, folate and vitamins B_6 and B_{12}—were recommended in food as well as in supplement form. It was thought that antioxidants in particular could counteract oxidation, which plays an important role in the development of atherosclerosis. A number of early studies suggested that antioxidants could block LDL oxidation and curb the earliest stages of plaque formation.

But new science presents a clearer perspective. Many of these vitamins and antioxidants may be protective when consumed in foods, but the same is not true when taken as supplements.

A good example is vitamin E. Early studies showed that taking vitamin E supplements helped to lower heart attack risk. But a number of more recent studies show that vitamin E supplementation not only was ineffective for heart health, but taking too much might be harmful to your health, including raising the risk of heart attack and heart failure. The Physicians Health Study II and other studies suggest that there is little evidence to support the efficacy of vitamin C, beta-carotene and folate in supplement form. A study reported in the *Journal of the American Medical*

LUTEIN: A POWER-PACKED ANTIOXIDANT

Researchers have found that the antioxidant lutein is potentially more beneficial than beta-carotene in preventing thickening of blood vessel walls. An 18-month study by Dr. James Dwyer at the University of Southern California found that participants with the lowest blood lutein had carotid arteries four times thicker than those with the highest levels. The working theory is that lutein prevents LDL cholesterol from sticking to artery walls.

While its effects are still being investigated, early indications are that lutein may also protect eyesight, reduce cancer risk and combat arthritis. Good sources include kale, collard greens, spinach, broccoli, Brussels sprouts and corn.

Association on folic acid and B vitamins came to the same conclusion. Indeed, work by Dr. Greg Brown at the University of Washington indicates that antioxidant supplements may blunt the benefits of statin drugs and niacin, used to lower LDL and raise HDL in heart patients.

Does that mean that vitamins and antioxidants are ineffective? No, of course not. But it means that the form in which you consume such vitamins and antioxidants is of great importance. That's why the American Heart Association doesn't recommend using antioxidant vitamin supplements, but instead recommends that one eat a variety of nutrient-rich foods daily from all the basic food groups. This is in line with numerous studies that have found the disease-fighting role of vitamins and antioxidants to be extremely effective when they come from whole foods. A study at the University of Texas, for example, showed a 30% decrease in the risk of heart disease in men whose daily intake of vitamin C equaled that found in one or two oranges and who consumed an amount of beta-carotene equal to that found in two carrots. The Harvard Nurses' Health Study showed that those who ate at least five servings a day of fruits and vegetables lowered their risk of heart attack by 33%.

Clearly, whole foods should be the primary source of your cardio-protective vitamins and antioxidants. Eat a sweet potato for beta-carotene, a red bell pepper for vitamin C, dry roasted almonds for vitamin E, and fortified ready-to-eat cereal for folate. Then, if you wish, you can use supplements as . . . well, supplements.

An exception to the above is vitamin D. New research has linked low levels of vitamin D with an increase in cardiovascular risk. In a study of 1,739 offspring from Framingham Heart Study participants, researchers found that those with low levels of vitamin D had twice the risk of a cardiovascular event such as a heart attack, heart failure or stroke in the next five years compared with those with higher levels of vitamin D. According to Dr. Thomas Wang of Harvard Medical School, "The higher risk associated with vitamin D deficiency was particularly evident among individuals with high blood pressure."

A study of more than 3,000 participants in Germany had similar results. Those with the lowest levels of vitamin D experienced the highest level of cardiac mortality. Says Dr. Harald Gobnig of the Medical

University of Graz (Austria), "The evidence linking low vitamin D to heart attacks is overwhelming."

Sunlight is the best provider of vitamin D. Experts say as little as 15 minutes of direct sunlight several times a week will get you your recommended dose. However, people who live in the northern tier of the United States during the winter probably do not get enough exposure. A study in Boston showed that as many as 35% to 40% of residents have a vitamin D deficiency.

Unfortunately, it is difficult to get enough vitamin D through a normal diet since few foods naturally contain it. Eating eggs, fatty fish and vitamin D–fortified foods, such as fat-free and low-fat milk and dairy products, cereals and certain brands of orange juice can help.

Supplementation may also be effective in this case. Check with your doctor. And remember, get some exposure to the sun and eat foods rich in vitamin-D first. Then use supplementation if warranted.

Water

Even with all the so-called "designer" water being carried around, Americans are still drinking nowhere near the recommended six to eight glasses (two quarts) of water a day. In fact, most of us are dehydrated.

An adequate intake of water is necessary for good overall health. But if weight control is a goal, there are a number of reasons to drink more water:

■ **It contains no calories.** You can drink water all day long and not have it contribute extra calories to your diet. But reach too frequently for a cola (144 calories), a beer (regular, 150 calories; light, 90 calories) or a glass of apple juice (120 calories), and those liquid calories will add up.

WHAT ABOUT COFFEE?

The best research suggests that *moderate* daily consumption of coffee (2 cups) does not penalize heart health. One reason is that coffee is loaded with disease-fighting antioxidants.

■ **It's filling.** In analyzing why many people are not successful in restricting calories to lose weight, experts found that dieters weren't getting enough food to feel satiety. They felt deprived and dissatisfied, and soon reverted to their old way of eating. Water (along with complex carbohydrates) helps to maintain satisfaction without adding calories. An adequate intake not only keeps the stomach full, but actually decreases hunger pangs.

■ **It can help you to cut down on snacking.** When your body is dehydrated, your brain receives a message that your body needs more water. But this message may be interpreted as a hunger cue. So instead of having a glass of water, you might have a snack. Surveys of American eating habits show that as water has been replaced as the drink of choice by diet soda, iced teas and specialty coffees, snacking habits have skyrocketed. But staying hydrated, experts say, often prevents snacking and overeating.

Portion Size

Much of the problem with the way America eats today can be traced to portion size. We simply eat too much, period. Look at the difference in caloric intake from the 1970s to now:

DAILY CALORIES CONSUMED

	MEN	WOMEN
1970s	1,877	1,542
Today	2,612	2,450

It's easy to understand why obesity rates have risen as well. A big reason for this change is "portion distortion," with pancake-size cookies, bagels that look like life rafts and soft drinks resembling small swimming pools. Says Dr. Denise Bruner, past president of the American Society of Bariatric Physicians, "Plate size is part of the problem. Dinner plates used to be 10.5 inches in diameter at sit-down restaurants; now they're closer to 12.5 inches, resembling small hubcaps. As a result, an 8-ounce serving of pasta has evolved into a 16-ounce serving simply to fill the larger plate."

And fast-food restaurants have kept pace. Five years ago, the standard was a 3.5-ounce hamburger, two ounces of French fries and an 8-ounce soft drink. "Supersizing" has expanded the average meal to a 5-ounce hamburger, four ounces of French fries and a 20-ounce soft drink.

Portion distortion is also going on at home. Studies show that two-thirds of Americans eat everything on their plates, no matter what the size. Indeed, new research suggests that when people are given larger portions, they eat 30% more food before feeling full.

The root of the problem, according to experts, is that many people do not know what a normal portion is. The USDA Handbook #8, published in 1963, was the first to list "standard portion sizes" for a variety of foods. For the next dozen or so years, food products pretty much came in those sizes. Then, after some marketing genius decided to increase portion size, a dietary culture of monster muffins and giant bagels began to evolve. "People are currently taking in more calories because of big portions that no longer reflect a single serving," says Robyn Flipse, R.D. "It isn't that we want to eat multiple servings. It's just that people no longer know what one serving looks like, and this has played a critical role in the ever-expanding American waistline."

For example, the USDA defines one portion of bread as "one ounce." But a large bagel today can weigh about 4 ounces—the equivalent of four pieces of bread. The single portion for a muffin is 1.5 ounces, but often one muffin will contain three or four portions.

What are we to do? Experts suggest following the eating style practiced in Okinawa. The people of this Japanese island, who live long and healthy lives, govern the amount they eat according to a practice called *hara hara bu,* roughly translated as stopping when you're 80% full. Some ways to make this work include:

- **Serve and put away food.** It's hard to take seconds if the food is already off the table.
- **Use smaller glasses and plates.**
- **Make snacking a hassle.** If ice cream is not in the house, you probably won't drive to your local 7-Eleven at 10:00 P.M. just to satisfy your craving.
- **Focus on your food.** Turn off the television, put away the newspaper and enjoy what you're eating.

SPEAKING FROM EXPERIENCE

After writing and lecturing on healthy eating for more than three decades, I've learned that putting a cardioprotective diet together involves more than reading the latest data in the field of nutritional science. We cut out all dietary fats, only to find that some types are beneficial to the heart. We threw out all carbohydrates, only to learn that complex carbohydrates are at the core of healthy eating. And we overreacted to oat bran, treating it like arterial Drano. Single-idea messages don't work. We need a sense of perspective and balance.

There is no such thing as a bad food. All foods are good, including chocolate, Brie, ice cream and Oreos—as long as they're part of a balanced diet. Eating well is about enjoyment and health. This is where my recommendations depart from low-fat and high-fat extremes. Some experts feel that a diet extremely low in fat—no more than 10% of calories from fat—provides optimal cardiovascular protection. But while that may be so, I found such a diet to be very restrictive—it proposes no meat, poultry or fish, and just one cup of nonfat milk a day. Also, I was constantly worried about my next meal: finding the right ingredients, using correct cooking methods, requesting changes when ordering in a restaurant. And, because the diet is so low in fat, I was constantly hungry.

The other extreme, of course, is the high-protein, low-carbohydrate eating plan. Centering food choices on increased meat and whole-milk dairy products and then eliminating all pasta, bread, fruits and most vegetables is supposed to help with weight loss. And for some people it may (although their weight loss is likely of fluids, not body fat). But for others, such a diet may simply provide a means of eating fewer calories. Remember, what proponents of this style of eating call "high-protein"—a bacon cheeseburger, for example—most nutritionists call "high-fat." And fat satisfies. Suppose you're trying to eat no more than 1,000 calories a day to lose weight. If you ate all those calories as fruits and vegetables, chances are you'd be hungry all day and might end up eating more than your calorie goal. But if your 1,000 calories came mostly from meat, the fat content of these foods would probably keep you satisfied for a longer time, helping you get through the day without eating more than your calorie goal. The result would be a diet higher in fat but lower in total calories.

This manner of eating makes little sense to me and other people concerned with heart health. Many of the recommended foods are rich in saturated fat, which increases harmful LDL cholesterol. And while the diet rightly counsels fewer *simple carbohydrates* (commercially baked goods, for example, usually rich in sugar, trans fats and white flour), it also calls for a reduction or elimination of *complex carbohydrates*—fruits, vegetables and whole grains. Where, then, am I to get cardioprotective fiber, soluble fiber and antioxidants?

My advice is to base your diet on foods high in complex carbohydrates and fiber, in particular vegetables, fruits, whole grains and beans. Eat lean meat and poultry, and be sure to eat fish at least twice a week. Watch portion control. Be sure to get a good supply of antioxidants and vitamins from your food. Attempt to fit more soy products into your diet. When it comes to fats, olive and canola oils should be the first choices. Stay away from stick margarine and food products with trans fat. Use nonfat and low-fat dairy products. Enjoy alcohol in moderation. Drink plenty of water.

But most important, give yourself time to make permanent changes. That's where stress management and regular exercise can help as precursors of dietary change. Remember, the process is evolutionary, not revolutionary. **—J.P.**

Time for Action

THE TRADITIONAL APPROACH to managing diet was based on exclusion. It concentrated on what you couldn't have, such as high-fat foods that might cause cholesterol to rise. Many doctors even provided patients with a listing of so-called "bad" foods. Red meat, chocolate, ice cream . . . all were banned.

While deprivation might work initially, the pendulum eventually swings to bingeing. Anyone who has attempted to give up ice cream knows the scenario. The craving hits and you eat a peach, then another, and then another. But the ice cream craving is still there, stronger than ever. So you have a little taste. Now you feel like a total failure. You've eaten a forbidden food! You're just a weak-willed wimp (one patient exclaimed, "I have the backbone of a chocolate éclair!"), so you eat more ice cream—and lose hope that you'll ever be able to eat "right."

It's time for a fresh approach to diet based on inclusion, focused on foods that you *should* eat, particularly plant foods.

SPEAKING FROM EXPERIENCE

People often ask whether they need to be vegetarians to have healthy diets, but not everyone can manage a vegetarian diet correctly. Some young women, for example, proclaim themselves to be vegetarians and then eat cereal three times a day. That's a terrible idea. Other vegetarians have a diet rich in cheese and simple sugars. That's no good, either. Certainly, a vegetarian diet rich in complex carbohydrates can have a very positive effect on cardiac health, but there is evidence that eating some lean protein can make you feel full longer and keep you from overeating a high-carbohydrate meal.

The secret is not necessarily to eliminate animal foods, but to eat these foods less often. Basically, we need to rethink meat and potatoes. In the traditional American meal, meat has been the star of the show and whole grains, vegetables and fruit have been the bit players. It's time to reverse the roles. **—J.P.**

Give Up Dieting

75

HEART SAVER

The most common New Year's resolution is to lose weight. Things usually start out well: an orange stands in for a candy bar, whole-grain cereal for a doughnut, a turkey sandwich for a double cheeseburger. But by January 15 most dieters have started to settle back into their old eating patterns. This is a tough lesson to learn. If you want ongoing success, you must first get rid of the concept of "dieting"—a short-term weight reduction program during which you shed excess pounds rapidly by decreasing caloric intake. In this context, there is often no relationship between diet and habit.

> **DIETING IS . . .**
>
> ". . . the all-consuming obsession with the food you shouldn't have eaten yesterday, but did; the food you have eaten today, but shouldn't have; and the food you shouldn't eat tomorrow, but probably will."
> —Sandra Bergeson,
> *I Hate to Diet Dictionary*

You'll form a habit only when you make permanent changes to your diet pattern over the long run. That's why the question is not "How do I want to eat for the next week?" The question to ask is "How do I want to eat for the rest of my life?" It's not as scary as it sounds, if you base your decisions on the following time-tested standards:

- **Sound nutritional science.** Contrary to the claims of infomercials and full-page ads for pills, powders, magic drinks, the latest crash-diet book or "effortless" exercise equipment, there are no slimming supplements or quick-fix solutions for losing weight. Remember the line from *Jerry Maguire:* "Show me the money!" Apply that to your health decisions and say, "Show me the science!"

- **Moderate and realistic expectations.** If your new diet forbids favorite foods and indulgences, depends on your spending long hours in the kitchen and involves complicated record-keeping, it will not work. It's about moderation, not undue sacrifice.

- **A reasonable timetable.** Take time to institute important changes. There is no need to do everything at once. If you're drinking whole milk, for instance, and want to move to fat-free milk, don't think it will happen overnight. Take five or six weeks to move gradually from whole to 2% milk, then to 1% and finally to fat-free. The gradual reduction of fat will allow your taste buds to adapt.

76 Decide to Lose Fat, Not Pounds

Most people rely on the bathroom scale as an arbiter of weight. Up a few pounds and it's like a little death. Down a few and it's better than winning the lottery. But a scale can tell you only what you weigh, not how much of that weight is fat-free muscle and bone, and how much is body fat. Suppose two people each weigh 150 pounds. One person is 140 pounds of muscle and 10 pounds of fat, while the other is 100 pounds of muscle and 50 pounds of fat. Do you need more proof that not all weight is created equal?

The real goal, then, is to lose body fat. A good starting point is an estimate of your own body fatness. This can be determined in most fitness centers, many sports medicine clinics and universities, and some physicians' offices, using one or more of the following methods.

■ **Water immersion.** This technique, in which you're weighed on a hanging scale immersed in water, is based on the principle that bone and muscle tissue are denser than water, whereas fat tissue is less dense. Therefore, a person with higher body fat weighs less in water than a person of the same weight who has more lean body mass.

■ **Skinfold measurements.** Popular in health clubs, this technique uses calipers to pinch folds of tissue in areas such as your stomach above the waistline, your hips and the backs of your arms. Since the amount of subcutaneous fat is proportional to the overall amount of body fat, the sum of the skinfold measurements can be plugged into a formula to estimate relative body fatness. The technique doesn't measure fat embedded between muscle fibers, however, and the formulas are population-specific, accurate only when the subject is matched to the correct equation, based on age, gender and ethnicity.

■ **Electronic impedance.** This test involves passing a small electrical current through the body and measuring the impedance, or opposition to current flow. Since fat-free tissue is a good conductor of electric current, whereas fat is not, the greater the resistance to current flow, the higher the proportion of fat tissue. Similarly, infrared beams, which travel faster through muscle than through fat, can be used to assess body composition.

■ **Dual energy X-ray absorptiometry.** Clinical settings commonly use this method (sometimes referred to as DXA or DEXA), which not only measures body composition but also detects osteoporosis.

If you don't want to bother with the foregoing tests, you can estimate your body fat at home using the charts below, developed by Dr. Jack Wilmore for his book *Sensible Fitness.* Men should measure their waist (at belly-button level) and then line up that number on the body weight scale. Draw a line from girth to weight. Note where the line crosses the percent body-fat line. In this example, we have a 180-pound man with a 35-inch waist. His body-fat content is about 18%. Women should measure their hips at the widest point, then line up that number on the height scale. In this example, a woman with 37-inch hips who stands five feet four inches (64 inches) has just under 26% body fat.

Now compare your body-fat percentage with the following guidelines for age and gender. Remember, it's not the loss of pounds that makes a difference, it's the reduction of body fat.

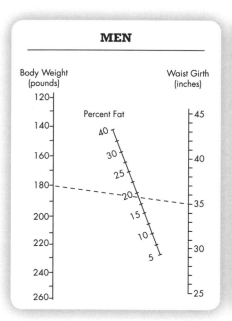

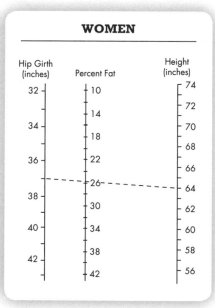

RECOMMENDED BODY-FAT PERCENTAGE

AGE	MEN	WOMEN
20 to 29	12%	19%
30 to 39	16	20
40 to 49	18	23
50 to 59	19	26
60 and over	20	27

Now that you know how much body fat you need to lose (translated into inches off your waist or hips), you can set realistic and attainable goals. Don't expect to lose 50 pounds or drop two collar or dress sizes in 30 days. It took months, perhaps years, to gain the extra weight, so you can't expect to lose it overnight. Instead, set short-term goals: the challenge of trimming 5 pounds seems more doable than losing 25. And

YO-YO DIETING

Erma Bombeck once wrote, "One-third of the country is on a diet. Another third just fell off a diet. And the remaining third is going on one next Monday." Statistics say she was right, but data also suggest that about 97% of crash dieters not only regain the lost weight within one year but actually put on extra weight. This is particularly true when caloric intake falls to under 1,200 calories a day for men and 900 for women.

Large weight losses do occur with fasting or on near-starvation diets, but approximately 60% of the loss can come from the body's "lean" weight (water, muscle and organ tissue). This happens with the so-called "high-protein/high-fat, low-carbohydrate" diets. By eliminating carbohydrates, which retain fluids, these diets merely act as short-term diuretics. Scale weight goes down because of fluid loss.

But scale weight and fluids will reappear. To make matters worse, some of these diets are so low in calories that they may result in the utilization of muscle tissue as fuel. Since muscle is an effective calorie burner, this may make efforts at weight reduction even more difficult.

finally, always keep the "why" behind your goals in mind. If you're over-weight, you're more likely to reduce your body fat if you focus on health benefits such as lowering blood pressure and raising HDL rather than on simple poundage.

Keep a Food Journal

To change the way you eat, you have to know what, when, where and how much you're eating right now. The problem is, we often forget (or choose to forget) what we eat. As one chronic dieter said, "I count calories whenever I sit down to eat. But the food I eat when I'm walking through a mall or clearing the dinner dishes, those are standing calories—and *standing calories* don't count!" Before you start any sort of diet plan, you should write down everything you put in your mouth for at least three days; a five- or seven-day record is better. And that means *everything:* the half an orange left over from breakfast, the handful of gumdrops on your way out the door, the bite of your friend's dessert. Be sure to include salad dressings, coffee creamers and other easily forgotten foods. Use one of the popular calorie counters available at most bookstores to estimate calories and, if you wish, fat.

It's important not to change anything during this time. Don't try to be "good." Just record everything you eat, when you eat it and, above all, *why.* Were you truly hungry or were you eating simply as a response to emotional stress, anxiety or boredom?

If this sounds like a drag, consider the research by Dr. Daniel Kirschenbaum of Northwestern University Medical School, who tracked 38 dieters from two weeks before Thanksgiving to two weeks after New Year's. The participants who wrote down everything they ate managed to lose an average of seven pounds during the holidays, while those who didn't gained three pounds on average. "After a week of writing down foods, most people have a good idea how many calories are in about 75% of what they eat," Dr. Kirschenbaum said. "Keeping a food diary works so well because it focuses you. It makes what you're doing real, reminds you forcefully of your goal and helps you feel more in control."

SAMPLE FOOD JOURNAL

DAY OF WEEK: Tuesday

WHEN/ WHERE	WHY	WITH WHOM	FOOD EATEN	CALORIES	FAT-GRAMS
7:30 A.M. Kitchen	Very hungry	Family	½ cup orange juice	55	0
			Jelly doughnut	225	9
			Coffee w/ 2 tbsp. half-and-half	40	4
10:00 A.M. Cafeteria	Not very hungry; ate for social reasons	Coworkers	Large mocha coffee	390	25
			Cinnamon bagel	195	1
Noon Office	Moderately hungry; worried about presentation	Alone	Tuna sandwich	585	28
			French fries, regular	230	13
			8 oz. 2% milk	120	5
2:00 P.M. Meeting room	Not hungry; anxious about presentation	Managers	Bag of jelly beans	250	0
6:30 P.M. Kitchen	Hungry	Family	5 oz. London broil	300	22
			Baked potato	145	0
			w/ 2 tbsp. sour cream	50	6
			Green salad	15	0
			w/ 2 tbsp. blue cheese dressing	155	16
			Glass of white wine	70	0
8:30 P.M. TV room	Not hungry; social eating	Kids	1 cup corn nuts	375	12
9:15 P.M. TV room	Not hungry; feeling lonely	Alone	½ cup French vanilla ice cream	265	17
Total				3,465	158

242

At the left is an example of a page from a food journal. Keep to the format we've shown here, or modify it to work specifically for you. You'll be surprised how fast the numbers can add up—the totals in our sample journal represent nearly two to three times the recommended daily values for calories and fat. But when you take the time each day to record your intake, the journal will become a tool for managing your diet.

78 Develop a Hydration Plan

Water regulates body temperature, transports nutrients and oxygen, carries away waste, helps to detoxify the kidneys and liver, and dissolves vitamins and minerals. It also helps in maintaining a balanced diet, not overeating, and exercising more effectively. And while milk, juices and soft drinks may do the trick, experts recommend an increase in the intake of water, plain H_2O, to meet daily fluid needs. This may seem like a simple suggestion, but evidence indicates that you may not be drinking enough water on your own. You need a plan:

- Spread out your consumption over the entire day. Don't wait until you're thirsty.
- Drink before you get the urge. If you wait for the signal that you are thirsty, you may already be slightly dehydrated.
- Drink one glass of water with each meal.
- Drink one glass before you exercise and another two glasses afterwards.
- Drink a glass of water when you brush your teeth as part of your morning ritual.
- Keep a pitcher of water laced with fresh lemons in the refrigerator. It's a satisfying alternative to soda pop.
- Carry a water bottle around with you and sip from it steadily throughout the day. Experiment with different-size bottles. A 32-ounce water bottle might seem more overwhelming to finish than two 16-ounce bottles.
- Try different temperatures of water. Some people like their water room temperature, while others like theirs icy cold. Know what you like.

Make a Daily Fat Budget

Reducing dietary fat is great in theory but difficult in practice. Establishing a daily fat budget, as odd as that may sound, will really help you get on the right track. The money analogy works: You have to know how much you can spend before you decide how you're going to spend it. You can calculate your fat budget with the three simple steps that follow.

First, estimate your ideal weight. Unfortunately, most height-weight charts simply allow for too much weight, whether you're a man or a woman. A more accurate way to determine ideal weight is to use the following formula developed by Dr. Richard Freeman at the University of Wisconsin Medical School:

- *Men* get 105 pounds for the first five feet of height. Every additional inch is plus six pounds. Accordingly, a man of six feet has an ideal weight of 177 pounds.

- *Women* get 100 pounds for their first five feet of height. Every additional inch is plus five pounds. Thus, a five-foot-five woman has an ideal weight of 125 pounds.

These recommendations apply only if you have a "medium"-size frame. To find out whether your frame is medium, large or small, measure your wrist just below your wrist bone (toward your hand) with a cloth measuring tape, then use the table below to determine your frame size in inches:

FRAME SIZE	SMALL	MEDIUM	LARGE
Men	Under 7	7	Over 7
Women	Under 6	6	Over 6

If you have a medium frame, the Freeman formula predicts your ideal weight. For a large frame, add 10% to the ideal weight; for a small frame, subtract 10%. Experts like the Freeman formula because it represents an ideal weight that corresponds to a healthy body-fat percentage (see page 238). If your scale weight and your ideal weight are the same, then your body-fat percentage is also in line.

Second, you need to know how many calories you can consume each day to sustain your ideal weight. (Remember, if you weigh 180 pounds but your ideal weight is 150 pounds, you need to eat for 150 pounds, not 180.) According to the American College of Sports Medicine and the American Dietetic Association, you can estimate your daily caloric needs as follows:

LEVEL OF ACTIVITY	CALORIES NEEDED PER POUND PER DAY
Extremely inactive, or sedentary (*Example:* No aerobic exercise in the course of a week)	11
Moderately active, or light activity (*Example:* Aerobic exercise 2 to 3 times a week)	13
Active, moderate exercise and/or work (*Example:* Aerobic exercise 4 to 5 times a week)	15
Extremely active, heavy exercise and/or work (*Example:* Aerobic exercise 6 to 7 times a week)	18

Your level of activity: _____

Multiplying your ideal weight by appropriate calories provides you with the number of calories you need for the day. For example, if your ideal weight is 125 pounds and you are "moderately active," you need 1,625 calories on a daily basis to sustain that weight and activity level.

The third step is to convert daily calories into grams of fat—your fat budget. If you want to lose weight, no more than 25% of your daily calories should come from fat.

GRAMS OF TOTAL FAT PER DAY

TOTAL CALORIES PER DAY	20%	25%	30%
1,000	22	27	33
1,100	24	30	36
1,200	27	33	40
1,300	29	36	43
1,400	31	39	47
1,500	33	42	50
1,600	36	44	53
1,700	38	47	57
1,800	40	50	60
1,900	42	53	63
2,000	44	56	67
2,100	47	58	70
2,200	49	61	73
2,300	51	64	77
2,400	53	67	80
2,500	56	69	83
2,600	58	72	87
2,700	60	75	90
2,800	62	77	93
2,900	64	80	96
3,000	66	83	100

Remember, your fat budget is a maximum for the day. Unless you're extremely active (you run 10 miles a day) or work outdoors in very cold climates, there's no reason to go above 60 grams of fat per day. On the other hand, most health professionals counsel not to go lower than 15 fat-grams daily.

Now Keep to Your Budget!

Start each day with your fat budget number in an "account." As you make food choices throughout the day, the key is to stay within the maximum number of fat-grams—and to consume fewer than your maximum if you want to lose weight. Let's use an example of a woman who consumes 1,800 calories a day. On a 25%-fat diet, she can have a maximum of 50 fat-grams. She's home for breakfast and dinner, but often eats lunch in a restaurant. The sample menus that follow show how she can use her budget to make smarter choices for all three meals as well as for mid-morning and evening snacks. Commentary from registered dietitian Bev Utt accompanies each menu.

SAMPLE FAT BUDGET

FOOD CHOICES	FAT-GRAMS
Starting Balance	50
Breakfast	
Oatmeal, ½ cup	1
Banana, 1 medium	1
Fat-free milk, 1 cup	1
Whole-wheat toast, 1 slice w/ strawberry jam	1 0
Coffee w/ whole milk, 2 tbsp.	1

What Bev Utt has to say: "Breakfast should provide good nutrition without a lot of extra calories or fat. Spending only five grams of fat to get good taste and nutrition makes great sense. By comparison, if she had two scrambled eggs with hash browns, toast and margarine, it would have eaten up 26 fat-grams—over half her budget for the entire day."

Mid-morning Snack	FAT-GRAMS
Apple	1
Large cappuccino w/ fat-free milk	.5

What Bev Utt has to say: "A low-fat breakfast often leaves you a little hungry in the mid-morning, so a snack can be a good thing. She has made a smart choice. The apple is filling and contains fiber, and the cappuccino with nonfat milk provides calcium. Compare this selection with the more typical American morning snack of a cinnamon roll at 9 grams of fat and a large mocha made with whole milk at 25 grams of fat. It's easy to see how high-fat snacking has contributed to America's weight problem."

Lunch	FAT-GRAMS
Premium Grilled Chicken Classic Sandwich (no mayonnaise)	4.5
Side salad w/ nonfat vinaigrette dressing, 1 packet	0 0
1% low-fat milk, 8 oz.	2.5

What Bev Utt has to say: "Up to lunchtime, she's in great shape for the day . . . only 6.5 grams of fat 'spent.' But like a lot of people, she has little time for lunch. McDonald's will have to do. The key, then, is making smarter choices in a fast-food environment. She has eaten a fast-food meal with only 7 grams of fat. Compare her choices with a Big Mac at 29 grams, a chocolate shake at 14 grams and an order of French fries at 19 grams."

Dinner	FAT-GRAMS
Grilled salmon fillet, 4 oz.	12
Wild rice, 1 cup	4
Stir-fried vegetables, 2 cups	1
Pear, fresh, sliced	1
Wine, 4.5 oz.	0
Coffee w/ whole milk, 2 tbsp.	1

What Bev Utt has to say: "Going into dinner, she has spent only 13.5 grams of fat—less than half of her budget. And that's good because Americans usually have dinner as their big meal of the day. She has a tasty, healthy dinner and it's only 19 grams of fat. Plus, much of that fat came from heart-healthy fish oil. Again, when you decide to eat fat, make it a healthy choice."

Evening Snack	FAT-GRAMS
Microwave low-fat popcorn, 2 cups	1

What Bev Utt has to say: "This compares nicely with a cup of cheese combos at 21 fat-grams or potato chips at 10 grams."

TOTAL FAT-GRAMS SPENT   **33.5**

Bev Utt's final comments: "The above examples illustrate how to manage fat and calories yet eat satisfying food—even including lunch in a fast-food restaurant. No one would go hungry on such a day, yet total fat was contained. Do you have to go through life with a fork in one hand and a calculator in the other? No. But remember, if you want to develop the low-fat habit, you must practice it successfully in real-life situations, like eating on the run. Having—and using—a daily fat budget makes it easier."

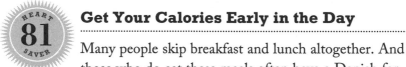

Get Your Calories Early in the Day

Many people skip breakfast and lunch altogether. And those who do eat these meals often have a Danish for breakfast and fast food for lunch. When these people get home in the evening and relax, they tend to become ravenous and eat much more at dinner than they need. The American Dietary Association estimates that over half of overweight women eat 70% of their daily calories after seven P.M. A better way is to take in the majority of calories at breakfast and lunch so they can be burned during the course of the day. *New York Times* columnist Jane Brody offers her perspective: "If you're driving from New York to Los Angeles, does it make more sense to fill the gas tank after you've arrived in Los Angeles or before you leave New York?"

Numerous studies suggest that timing affects caloric utilization. In one study, each of two groups of women ate 2,000 calories a day; the only difference was that the first group received all their calories at breakfast and the second group ate all 2,000 calories at dinner. Every person in the breakfast group lost weight, and every person in the dinner group gained weight. The time-honored advice still holds true: "Eat like a king at breakfast, a prince at lunch and a pauper at dinner." Wake up like royalty.

HOW MANY CALORIES SHOULD YOU EAT?

According to guidelines from the American College of Sports Medicine, the optimal approach to weight loss combines mild caloric restriction (no fewer than 1,200 calories a day) and an exercise program that promotes a daily energy expenditure of more than 300 calories.

Here's another way to think about it. If you want to lose an average of one pound per week (and if you have fewer than 25 pounds to lose), multiply your current weight in pounds by 10. That's roughly your daily calorie level, though it obviously depends on your level of physical activity.

Be Cautious About Dietary Cholesterol

It's frustrating and disillusioning when experts lift the ban on something they once condemned. And for many people, this is a good excuse to stop trying to eat right. There was a time when eliminating foods rich in dietary cholesterol—eggs, liver, shrimp and organ meats—was touted as a means of controlling blood cholesterol. But science marched on, and current research shows that dietary cholesterol has much less impact on blood cholesterol than dietary fat. This means that the fat you cook your egg in may be more significant than the egg itself. "I'd rather eat a poached egg from time to time," says dietitian Bev Utt, "than have an Egg Beaters omelet fried in butter."

Still, it's important to moderate your intake of dietary cholesterol: no more than 300 milligrams per day, and no more than 200 milligrams if you have heart disease, according to the American Heart Association. The best way to do that is to reduce the amount of all animal foods in your diet. Keep in mind that simply replacing large portions of beef with large portions of chicken won't do any good, since the flesh of all animals contains similar amounts of cholesterol—about 100 milligrams per three-ounce portion.

Rough Up Your Diet

We should all be eating 20 to 35 grams of fiber a day, with at least 3 grams as soluble fiber. But most of us don't even come close. A good step in the right direction is to learn which foods are fiber-rich. Be sure to read labels on packaged foods; they'll tell you the amount of dietary fiber in each serving.

Now figure out how to incorporate high-fiber foods into your diet. Center your meals on plant foods rather than animal foods. Serve reasonable portions of meat, poultry or fish, and surround them with larger servings of vegetables, beans, peas, potatoes, rice and fruits. Plan for a cooked vegetable and a salad at dinner.

■ **Have a high-fiber breakfast.** It's easy to get fiber at breakfast: oatmeal, oat bran cereal, other bran cereals and low-fat bran muffins.

Or you can find a whole-grain cereal that contains at least 5 grams of fiber per serving (or mix it with your regular brand). Top it with wheat bran, wheat germ, oat bran, raisins, bananas or berries, all of which are good sources of fiber. It always makes sense to start your day with oats, which, because of their soluble fiber, are allowed to bear a heart-healthy claim. But don't try to get all of your soluble fiber at breakfast. It takes about 1.5 cups of cooked oatmeal or 3 cups of dry oat cereals to get enough fiber to have a cholesterol-lowering effect.

- **Go for fruits and vegetables.** Choose whole fruits with skin. Eat a baked potato with the skin on. Instead of iceberg lettuce, choose romaine or spinach for your salad. Serve hummus, made from chickpeas, instead of sour-cream dips. Eat raw fruits and vegetables whenever possible. Keep fresh and dried fruit on hand for snacks.
- **Eat beans.** Studies show that just 4 ounces of cooked beans a day can significantly reduce your levels of total and LDL cholesterol.
- **Choose whole, unprocessed grains.** Try barley (excellent in hearty soups and as a side dish), bulgur (great to replace rice in recipes and a main ingredient in tabbouleh), triticale (a hybrid of wheat and rye that can also be cooked as a breakfast cereal or as a substitute for rice), whole-wheat couscous, millet, quinoa, amaranth, buckwheat (kasha) and whole-wheat or whole-rye berries.
- **Buy whole-grain breads.** Look for those made from stone-ground flour. The next best choice is 100% whole-wheat or other whole-grain bread such as rye or pumpernickel.

SPEAKING FROM EXPERIENCE

Decreasing fat is important, but increasing fiber is also critical to a healthy diet. A study of 13,000 middle-aged men from seven countries suggests that fiber, not fat, determined how successful they were at managing weight. In fact, the leanest men ate a whopping 40% of calories from fat, far more than is recommended, but they consumed 41 grams of fiber a day. The study concluded that a high-fiber diet can go a long way in canceling out the effect of fat calories, at least in relation to body weight. **—J.P.**

COMMON SOURCES OF FIBER

FOODS	AMOUNT	GRAMS OF FIBER	GRAMS OF SOLUBLE FIBER
Fruits			
Apple, w/ skin	1 medium	3.5	1.0
Apple, w/o skin	1 medium	2.5	1.0
Banana	1 medium	3.0	0.5
Blackberries	½ cup	4.0	1.0
Dates, dried	½ cup	4.4	1.2
Figs, dried	½ cup	8.2	4.0
Orange	1 medium	3.0	2.0
Peach	1 medium	2.0	1.0
Pear, Bartlett	1 medium	4.0	2.0
Prunes, dried	½ cup	6.6	3.8
Raisins, dried, seedless	½ cup	2.3	1.1
Vegetables			
Asparagus	½ cup	1.0	0.4
Beets	½ cup	1.3	0.6
Broccoli	½ cup	1.5	0.5
Brussels sprouts	½ cup	4.5	3.0
Carrots	½ cup	2.0	1.0
Cauliflower, cooked	½ cup	2.0	0.5
Collard greens, cooked	1 cup	5.5	3.0
Green beans	½ cup	2.0	1.0
Potato, w/ skin	1 medium	3.0	1.0
Soybeans, green, cooked	½ cup	4.0	1.5
Spinach	½ cup	1.8	0.6
Squash, winter, cooked	½ cup	1.5	0.5
Sweet potato, w/ skin	1 medium	4.0	1.5
Tomato, fresh	½ cup	1.0	0.0

COMMON SOURCES OF FIBER *(continued)*

FOODS	AMOUNT	GRAMS OF FIBER	GRAMS OF SOLUBLE FIBER
Beans, Peas and Other Legumes			
Baked beans, plain or vegetarian, canned	½ cup	6.5	2.0
Black beans, cooked	½ cup	5.5	2.0
Black-eyed peas, cooked	½ cup	5.5	1.0
Chickpeas, cooked	½ cup	6.0	1.0
Green peas, cooked	½ cup	4.5	1.5
Kidney beans, cooked	½ cup	6.0	3.0
Lentils, cooked	½ cup	8.0	1.0
Lima beans, cooked	½ cup	6.5	3.5
Navy beans, cooked	½ cup	6.0	2.0
Northern beans, cooked	½ cup	5.5	1.5
Pinto beans, cooked	½ cup	7.0	2.0
Breads, Grains and Pasta			
Barley	½ cup	4.0	1.0
Rice, brown	½ cup	2.0	0.0
Rice, white	½ cup	0.5	0.0
Rice, wild	½ cup	1.5	0.0
Rye bread	1 slice	1.5	1.0
Spaghetti	½ cup	1.0	0.5
Spaghetti, whole-wheat	½ cup	2.0	0.5
White bread	1 slice	0.5	0.0
Whole-wheat bread	1 slice	2.0	0.5
Breakfast Cereals			
All-Bran	½ cup	10.0	1.0
Bran Buds	⅓ cup	13.0	3.0
Bran flakes	¾ cup	5.0	1.0
Oat bran	¾ cup	4.5	1.5
Oatmeal	¾ cup	3.0	1.5
Raisin bran	¾ cup	4.8	0.8
Shredded wheat	¾ cup	3.5	0.5

COMMON SOURCES OF FIBER *(continued)*

FOODS	AMOUNT	GRAMS OF FIBER	GRAMS OF SOLUBLE FIBER
Nuts and Seeds			
Almonds	1 oz.	3.0	0.0
Brazil nuts	1 oz.	1.5	0.0
Cashews	1 oz.	1.0	0.0
Peanuts, dry-roasted	1 oz.	2.5	0.0
Pecans	1 oz.	2.0	0.0
Pistachios	1 oz.	3.0	0.0
Sunflower seeds	¼ cup	3.5	0.5
Walnuts, English	1 oz.	1.5	0.0

PASTA, RICE AND POTATOES: IT'S WHAT'S ON TOP THAT COUNTS

One cup of enriched pasta provides vitamins, minerals, about 10% of the USRDA for protein and less than one gram of fat—all for just over 200 calories. But even the healthiest pasta turns into a high-fat, high-calorie dish when it's drenched in Alfredo sauce or served with a pound of sausage. One cup of pasta with a quarter-cup of marinara or red clam sauce and a tablespoon of grated Parmesan cheese has only about 275 calories, or about the same as a cup of low-fat yogurt sweetened with fruit preserves. Also, don't overlook Asian noodles such as soba (buckwheat), udon and saifun (cellophane), which are particularly good in chicken broth with vegetables.

The same principle applies to rice, a low-fat, nutrient-rich food that makes for excellent side and main dishes, particularly when it's whole-grain brown rice. Instead of topping it with butter, butter sauce or gravy, serve it as a side dish with a few drops of sodium-reduced soy sauce or as a main dish covered with beans or stir-fried chicken and vegetables. Watch out for packaged rice dishes that contain added fat; most of them don't need to be made with the butter or oil as suggested in the cooking instructions. And don't be fooled into thinking that a packaged rice dish is fat-free because the Nutrition Facts list fat content as zero. Some manufacturers give nutritional information "as packaged," so that the fat called for in cooking is not reflected.

The best toppings for a low-fat baked potato include nonfat sour cream, low-fat or nonfat yogurt, salsa and fresh herbs such as chopped dill, parsley and chives.

Put More Fish in Your Diet

Because of the protective omega-3 fatty acids found in fish oil, the American Heart Association recommends eating fatty fish at least two times a week. Some types of fish are richer in omega-3 fatty acids than other types. Highest on the list is Atlantic mackerel, with 2.5 grams of omega-3s per three ounces. The figures for three-ounce portions of other fish are shown below.

TYPE OF FISH	OMEGA-3s (GRAMS PER 3 OUNCES)
Herring	1.7
Lake trout	1.6
Salmon	1.2
Tuna	0.5
Pacific halibut	0.4
Channel catfish	0.3
Shrimp	0.3
Dungeness crab	0.3
Swordfish	0.2
Red snapper	0.2
Sole	0.1

Don't Drown Your Fish in Fat

It's very easy to dilute the benefits of fish-eating in a sea of high fat. But that doesn't have to happen:

■ **Be smart about tuna.** Picking up a four-ounce can of tuna packed in water instead of oil can save you 20 grams of fat, or about 180 calories. And if you're making tuna salad, remember that three tablespoons of mayonnaise will add about 300 calories to a sandwich.

- **Use heart-healthy cooking methods** such as grilling, broiling, poaching, barbecuing and microwaving. Avoid frying or deep-fat frying, which can add more than a gram of fat per ounce of fish. If you do fry, use a grill pan or a nonstick pan with a little cooking spray.

- **Skip fatty condiments** such as butter, butter sauce, mayonnaise and tartar sauce, particularly if weight control is your goal. A tablespoon of melted butter is 100 calories; the same amount of tartar sauce is 90 calories. Better choices include fresh lemon and lime, horseradish, tomato salsa, low-sodium soy sauce, flavored vinegars, vinaigrettes, wine and oil-free dressings.

- **Read labels.** Be sure the fish in a frozen meal is not breaded, deep-fried and/or drowned in a fatty sauce.

- **Order smart in a restaurant.** In a sit-down restaurant, ask questions about cooking methods: "Is it fried? Breaded? Batter-dipped and fried?" If so, avoid it. Opt for fish that is baked, broiled, steamed or grilled, without oil or butter. Watch out for condiments and sauces such as drawn butter, cream sauce and cheese sauce.

In fast-food restaurants, make smarter choices. A serving of Baked Cod at Long John Silver's, for instance, has just 4.5 grams of fat, while Wendy's Fish Filet Sandwich will set you back 24 fat-grams.

Become Label-Literate

86

If you live in the real world and buy processed foods, it's necessary to know what's in them. And that means reading food labels. Take for example a sandwich ham advertised as "95% fat-free." What the claim actually means is that fat makes up just 5% of the ham's *weight*. It has nothing to do with the true measurement, the *calories* that come from fat. About 40% to 60% of calories in sandwich ham come from fat, which is a long way from the low-fat claim.

Food labels typically have a section called Nutrition Facts (see the example on page 259). This is where you'll find an accurate description of fat in grams, not percentages, as well as calories and other elements contained in the food.

In particular, take note of the following information:

- **Serving size.** Pay attention to the number of servings in the container. If you buy a bag of chips that contains four servings and you eat half the bag, you'll have to double the calories and fat on the label since you've eaten two servings.
- **Calories.** Watch out for "fat-free" foods. While they contain no fat, they still have calories. And from a weight-control standpoint, all calories count! The label will tell you if the food is too calorically dense for your dietary goals.
- **Fat-grams.** Once you know your fat budget, it's relatively easy to decide whether any particular food "fits."
- **Saturated fat.** If you want to avoid high total and LDL cholesterol levels, buy foods with a low saturated-fat value.
- **Trans fats.** These may be worse for your arteries than saturated fat. If the ingredients list includes hydrogenated or partially hydrogenated oils, you can be sure trans fat is in the food.
- **Fiber.** There's a big difference between two slices of French bread (1.5 grams of fiber) and the same amount of pumpernickel bread (4 grams of fiber)—particularly if you're trying to reach the recommended level of 20 to 35 grams of fiber a day.
- **Sugars.** Remember, 4 grams of sugar equals one teaspoon. Quaker Cap'n Crunch, for instance, lists 12 grams of sugar per serving. Think of it as three teaspoons . . . or one tablespoon.
- **Sodium.** Your goal is to consume 2,300 milligrams or less of sodium a day—or approximately one teaspoon of salt. To give you an idea, a cup of Newman's Own Pasta Sauce, for instance, has 1,400 milligrams of sodium.
- **Dietary cholesterol.** Remember the guideline of no more than 300 milligrams a day.

In addition to Nutrition Facts, food labels contain advertising and descriptive terms. In the past, terms like "light" and "low-fat" could be used virtually any way the packager wished. The FDA now requires such eye-catching nutrition terms to meet specific definitions. Believe us— they make for fascinating reading!

Nutrition Facts

Serving Size ½ cup (114 g)
Servings Per Container 4

Amount Per Serving

Calories 90   Calories from Fat 30

	% Daily Value*
Total Fat 3 g	**5%**
Saturated Fat 0 g	**0%**
Trans Fat 0 g	**0%**
Cholesterol 0 g	**0%**
Sodium 300 mg	**13%**
Total Carbohydrate 13 g	**4%**
Dietary Fiber 3 g	**12%**
Sugars 3 g	
Protein 3 g	

Vitamin A	80%	*	Vitamin C	60%
Calcium	4%	*	Iron	4%

*Percent Daily Values are based on a 2,000-calorie diet. Your daily values may be higher or lower depending on your calorie needs:

	Calories	2,000	2,500
Total Fat	Less than	65 g	80 g
Sat Fat	Less than	20 g	25 g
Cholesterol	Less than	300 mg	300 mg
Sodium	Less than	2,400 mg	2,400 mg
Total Carbohydrate		300 g	375 g
Fiber		25 g	30 g

Calories per gram:
Fat 9   Carbohydrate 4   Protein 4

OLD TERMS, NEW MEANINGS

WHAT THE LABEL SAYS	WHAT THE LABEL MEANS
Free	The product contains no or only negligible amounts of calories, cholesterol, fat, sodium or sugar.
Calorie-free	Less than 5 calories per serving.
Cholesterol-free	Less than 2 milligrams cholesterol and 2 grams or less saturated fat per serving.
Fat-free	Less than 0.5 grams fat per serving.
Sodium-free	Less than 5 milligrams sodium per serving.
Sugar-free	Less than 0.5 grams sugar per serving.
Low	May be used on foods that can be eaten frequently without exceeding the dietary guidelines for fat, saturated fat, cholesterol, sodium, sugar and/or calories.
Low calorie	40 calories or less per serving. *(When it comes to meals and main-dish items like frozen dinners and entrées, this guideline translates into about 120 calories or less in 3.5 ounces of food.)*
Low cholesterol	20 milligrams or less cholesterol and 2 grams or less saturated fat per typical serving. *(A main dish or meal labeled "low cholesterol" has about 60 milligrams of cholesterol per 10 ounces.)*
Low fat	3 grams or less per 100 calories. *(Watch out for milk products, which have been exempted from the "low fat" regulation. So, "2% milk" will be termed "low fat" even though it contains 5 grams of fat per serving.)*
Low saturated fat	1 gram or less saturated fat per serving. *(A main dish can usually make this claim if less than 10% of its calories come from saturated fat.)*

OLD TERMS, NEW MEANINGS *(continued)*

WHAT THE LABEL SAYS	WHAT THE LABEL MEANS
Low sodium	140 milligrams or less sodium per serving. *(This translates into about 400 milligrams of sodium in a typical 10-ounce main dish, or 600 milligrams in a 16-ounce meal.)*
Very low sodium	35 milligrams or less sodium per serving.
High	Means the food must contain 20% or more of the Daily Value for a particular nutrient. "Rich in" or "excellent source of" may be used instead of "high."
Good Source	Means that a serving of the food supplies 10% to 19% of the Daily Value for a particular nutrient.
Light or Lite	Can mean a number of different things: ■ If a food contains 50% or more of its calories from fat to begin with, such as sausage or cheese, "light" means that at least half its fat has been removed. ■ If a food is less than 50% fat to begin with, it can be called "light" if either the fat content has been cut in half or the calories have been reduced by a third. ■ For a main dish or meal, "light" means the dish meets the definition of either "low calorie" or "low fat." ■ "Light" can also mean that the sodium content of a low-calorie, low-fat food has been reduced by at least 50%. However, if the sodium is reduced by 50% in a food that is not low in fat and calories, the label must state "light in sodium." ■ "Light" can also refer to color or texture, but the label must say so clearly. It can also be used without explanation when "light" has traditionally been part of the food's name, e.g., brown sugar or cream.

OLD TERMS, NEW MEANINGS *(continued)*

WHAT THE LABEL SAYS	WHAT THE LABEL MEANS
Reduced	Means that a product contains 25% less of a nutrient (such as fat) or of calories than the regular product.
More	Tells you that a serving of food contains 10% more of the Daily Value for a nutrient than the regular food. The label on the calcium-fortified orange juice, for example, could specify that the product supplies "more calcium" than regular juice.
Lean and Extra-Lean	Describe the fat content of certain meats, poultry, seafood and game meats.
Lean	■ Less than 10 grams of fat, 4 grams of saturated fat and 95 milligrams of cholesterol per serving. *(With the exception of many main dishes and entrées, a "lean" food generally has more fat than a "low-fat" food and more saturated fat than a "low in saturated fat" food.)*
Extra-lean	■ Less than 5 grams of fat, 2 grams of saturated fat and 95 milligrams of cholesterol per serving. *(With the exception of many main dishes and entrées, an "extra-lean" food generally has more fat than a "low-fat" food and more saturated fat than a "low in saturated fat" food.)*
Percent fat-free	Used only on foods that meet the "low-fat" or "fat-free" definitions. *Describes the percentage of fat by weight, not the percentage of calories from fat.*

Go Lean

87

We get about one-third of our daily fats from animal foods, and this is hardly a healthy situation. The trick is to modify the meat in our diet, not to eliminate it altogether. Meat is a good supplier of protein, iron and B vitamins; it's particularly effective in repairing muscle tissue broken down by regular exercise. And not all meat is high in fat and calories; ounce for ounce, a slice of apple pie has more than double the amount of fat contained in lean meat.

However, not all cuts of meat are the same. Some favorite meats— T-bone steak, prime rib, New York strip, rib eye, rib roast, brisket, pork spare ribs and lamb roast, for example—can have 20 to 30 grams of fat per 3.5-ounce serving. And few people limit themselves to such small servings.

Fortunately, modern breeding and trimming methods have made leaner cuts available, many containing just 6 to 9 grams of fat and under 200 calories per 3.5-ounce serving. For beef, choose "Select" grade over "Choice" and "Prime." Look for cuts labeled *round* or *loin,* or any of these: tenderloin, London broil, flank steak, club steak, and round, eye of round and sirloin tips.

THE SKINNY SIX

CUT OF BEEF (3.5 OZ.)	CALORIES	GRAMS OF FAT	GRAMS OF SATURATED FAT
Top round, broiled	179	4.9	1.6
Eye of round, roasted	166	4.9	1.8
Round tip, roasted	183	6.9	2.3
Top sirloin, broiled	192	7.1	2.8
Top loin, broiled	205	9.3	3.5
Tenderloin, broiled	208	9.9	3.7

For pork, lamb and veal, the leanest cuts are labeled *loin* or *leg.* Some smart choices include extra-lean canned ham, pork tenderloin, Canadian bacon, pork center loin, fresh ham, lamb loin chop, lamb leg, veal leg and veal loin. Also, most cuts of game, such as buffalo, elk and deer, are lower in fat than either beef or chicken.

HOW TO STRETCH MEAT

If you use meat in chili, casseroles and stir-fries, you can use a lot less. This works particularly well if you substitute grains and beans for part of the meat in many recipes. As an example, you can cook one thinly sliced steak in a stir-fry with crisp vegetables. It will feed four people as deliciously as four steaks but with a reasonable amount of fat and calories.

If you're a meat-aholic, try some of these ideas:

- **Cut down on frequency.** If you're among the many Americans who still eat bacon for breakfast, bologna for lunch and pork chops for dinner, switch to having meat at just one meal each day. Also reduce the number of red meat days to perhaps three a week, if you can. Look for opportunities to use more poultry, fish, beans, grains and vegetables. When you do include meat in a meal, go for the best. Why use up your fat budget on a greasy burger when you could enjoy roasted pork tenderloin?

- **Read labels.** Some deli meats can have 12 grams of fat per ounce, and meat entrées are typically among the fattest of frozen meals since many of them come in "he-man" portions, smothered in fatty sauces and gravies, and surrounded by other high-fat foods. A good rule of thumb to follow is no more than 3 grams of total fat per 100 calories.

- **Use healthy cooking methods.** Roasting, broiling, grilling, baking and stewing allow fat to drip off, whereas frying seals fat in. In general, the longer meat cooks, the more fat it loses, so medium and well-done are preferable to rare.

- **Watch portion size.** A three-to-four-ounce serving of lean meat often contains fewer than 200 calories, but many people simply eat too much, even when a lower-fat cut is chosen. Portion control seems to be particularly difficult for men, who list red meat (especially steak, hamburgers and pizza with meat topping) as a favorite food.

So, what constitutes an appropriate serving of about 3.5 ounces? It's the size of a woman's palm, or an audiocassette (not a video!) or a standard deck of cards.

 ■ **Order smart.** In a sit-down restaurant, ask for meat entrées to be lean, well-trimmed and cooked in a low-fat manner. Order a small piece of London broil, veal or sirloin done to "medium" or "well done," and ask that no butter or oil be used in the preparation. Skip fatty sauces. If you order beef, ask for the "petite," "queen" or "8-ounce" cut rather than the "king" or "16-ounce" portion. Ordering smart in fast-food restaurants and delicatessens is also key. A Jack in the Box hamburger at 280 calories and 12 grams of fat is clearly a better choice than their Ultimate Cheeseburger at 1,010 calories and 71 grams of fat.

Watch Out for Ground Beef

The best way to minimize the fat content is to buy the leanest ground beef available. And that means reading food labels.

In the past, descriptions like "lean" or "extra-lean" were used, but labeling laws have banned such terms. Instead, ground beef must be described in lean-to-fat ratios by weight. Look for meat with a high lean-to-fat ratio. The figures in the chart below refer to four-ounce, medium-broiled servings of ground beef:

% LEAN/% FAT BY WEIGHT	CALORIES	FAT-GRAMS
73% lean/27% fat	291	21
80% lean/20% fat	268	18
85% lean/15% fat	240	14
90% lean/10% fat	199	11
95% lean/5% fat	155	6

Add Soy to Your Diet

Americans tend to think of soy foods as, well, not too good—either a gelatinous goo or dry and tasteless. We need to think again. Today the choices and varieties of soy foods are plentiful. It's not actually that hard, since you can find soy in soybeans, soy milk (available in fortified versions and in several flavors), tofu (soybean curd which comes in different consistencies: firm, soft and silken), sports bars that contain soy, tempeh (a chewy, soft soybean cake), soy nuts (peanut-like), veggie burgers, textured vegetable protein (TVP, a good substitute for ground beef), breakfast cereals fortified with soy, isolated soy protein powder (for adding to shakes and baked products) and soy flour. Grams of protein for common soy foods are listed below.

FOOD	PROTEIN (GRAMS)
Soybeans, cooked/canned, ½ cup	13.0
Soy nuts, ¼ cup	12.0
Soybean burgers, 3.5 oz.	10.0
Soy crumbles, ground, ½ cup	9.0
Tofu, 3 oz.	
Firm	8.5
Silken	6.0
Soy flour, ¼ cup	8.0
Tofu yogurt, 8 oz.	8.0
Soy milk, 8 oz.	6.0
Soybean sprouts, 1 oz.	4.0
Miso, 1 tbsp.	2.0

Remember, soy is not a "magic bullet." It should be eaten as part of a balanced diet, not in lieu of it. And bear in mind that soy foods are most effective for heart health when they are substituted for meat and other products containing animal protein.

Get an Oil Change

Most of us eat too much fat. But what's more to the point is that we eat the wrong *type* of fat, choosing the ones that raise cholesterol over those that lower it. Let's go over the basics. All vegetable oils contain 120 calories and about 14 grams of total fat per tablespoon. They differ primarily in the types of fatty acids in their makeup: saturated, polyunsaturated and monounsaturated. While we tend to catalog an oil as one of the three types, in reality no fat is made up exclusively of one type of fatty acid. See page 268 for an idea of how many fat-grams are contained in a tablespoon of the most common oils.

Monounsaturated vegetable oils are the best choice for your heart. All of them are beneficial, but in the world of cardiac health olive oil rules. It reduces the risk of clot formation within coronary arteries while lowering "bad" LDL cholesterol when substituted for saturated fats.

In the past, monounsaturated oils were viewed as being essentially neutral with respect to cholesterol—not harmful, but not particularly healthful, either. Then the science changed radically when Dr. Scott Grundy of the University of Texas Southwestern Medical Center published his landmark study on the effectiveness of monounsaturated fats in lowering cholesterol levels. "This may explain why populations using olive oil—Italians and Greeks, for example—have fewer heart attacks than do other populations," says Dr. Grundy. Investigation in this area also indicates that canola oil can be instrumental in reducing the risk of coronary heart disease. As Dr. Grundy has observed, "While olive oil may explain the low incidence of heart problems among Mediterranean populations, canola oil may explain it for Asian populations. In both cases, the monounsaturated oils are used as replacements for saturated fats."

FAT-GRAMS PER TABLESPOON OF COMMON OILS

TYPE OF OIL	MONOUNSATURATED	POLYUNSATURATED	SATURATED
Monounsaturated			
Almond	10	2	1
Canola	8	4	1
Olive	10	1	2
Peanut	6	5	2
Polyunsaturated			
Corn	3	8	2
Cottonseed	2	7	4
Safflower	2	10	1
Sesame	5	6	2
Soybean	3	8	2
Sunflower	3	9	1
Walnut	3	9	1
Saturated			
Coconut	1	0	12
Palm	5	1	7
Palm kernel	2	0	11

The next healthiest choice is *polyunsaturated oils.* According to Dr. Margo Denke, a lipids expert at the University of Texas Southwestern Medical Center, polyunsaturated oils reduce LDL

TOO MUCH OF A GOOD THING?

Healthy oils are most effective when they *replace* unhealthy fats. But apparently some people think that if a little olive oil is good, a lot of it must be even better. The rule is *all fats in moderation, even the healthy ones.*

If you're used to making sandwiches with butter on two pieces of bread and switch to soft corn oil margarine to replace the butter, that isn't much of a change. But if you use margarine on one piece of bread and mustard on the other piece, that is a change. Not only have you shifted to a healthier fat, but you're taking in less total fat. Remember, too high an intake of fat, even the healthy kind, can contribute to overweight and increase cancer risk. There is no need to consume large amounts of any fat, whether it comes from a steer or from olives.

---

cholesterol levels when substituted for saturated fats, but this benefit is somewhat blunted by the fact that they also lower levels of beneficial HDL. And when they're hardened into solid fats, as in stick margarine, polyunsaturated oils increase cholesterol-raising trans fats.

Saturated fats and *trans fats* are the worst choices for cardiac health because they cause cholesterol, particularly LDL cholesterol, to rise significantly. In addition to animal foods, sources of saturated fats include palm oil, palm kernel oil and coconut oil. Trans fats are typically found in stick margarine, baked goods, chips and fast food.

See the following tips on how to avoid saturated fats and choose more monounsaturated fats.

- **Reduce animal foods.** Instead of a small salad, a half-cup of rice and a giant steak, switch to a large salad, a full cup of rice, two vegetables and half a chicken breast.

- **Read labels.** Avoid products in which oils have been hydrogenated and foods made with tropical oils. Beware of terms like "all-vegetable oil" and "made with 100% vegetable oil," since they do not identify the oil used in the food. Another favorite advertising term is "made with one or more of the following oils—soybean, cottonseed, palm and/or coconut oil." When you can't tell which oil a food contains, stay away from it. And, of course, watch out for the term "hydrogenated."

■ **Use high-quality oils.** Because virgin or extra virgin olive oil is so flavorful, you may be able to use less and still produce the desired taste with fewer calories.

■ **Try flaxseed.** Since the oil in flaxseed contains high levels of cardioprotective omega-3 fatty acids, many experts recommend adding about two tablespoons of ground flaxseed to your daily diet. Sprinkle it on yogurt, cereal or salads, mix it with juice or add it to baked goods and soups just before serving. Keep ground flaxseed refrigerated. Ready-made flaxseed breads, muffins, cereals and breakfast bars can be found in many stores.

■ **Remember that healthy oils are not magic elixirs.** Despite all their benefits, they do not offset poor dietary choices, smoking and a sedentary lifestyle.

Be Picky About Poultry

91 With the exception of duck and goose, poultry is an excellent substitute for red meat: lower in fat, lower in calories and really tasty. Chicken breasts pan-fried in a nonstick pan are as easy to cook as minute steaks. Roasted and broiled chicken take no more work than a pork roast. Roasted turkey breast is a great alternative to roast beef. And ground chicken and turkey breast can be used as a substitute for ground beef in many recipes, including tacos, chili and spaghetti. But don't be fooled into thinking that all poultry is created equal. One example: half a rotisserie chicken (the kind usually found in the deli department of a grocery store) has about 41 grams of fat and 665 calories.

Below are a few principles that will keep you from making high-fat/high-calorie mistakes.

■ **Select only the leanest cuts.** One simple rule will point you in the direction of the leanest cuts of chicken and turkey: *Choose a skinless white breast.* Unlike red meat, poultry is not marbled with fat; instead, the fat is concentrated just beneath the skin. If you remove the skin before cooking, you'll save about five grams of fat per piece of chicken. If you prefer to cook poultry with the skin on, be sure to remove it before serving. In addition, white meat has about one-third less fat than dark.

The table below will help you see the differences in 3.5-ounce portions of roast chicken and turkey.

POULTRY MEAT	CALORIES	GRAMS OF FAT	GRAMS OF SATURATED FAT
Chicken			
Light meat, skinless	165	3.5	0.9
Light meat, w/ skin	195	7.7	2.1
Dark meat, skinless	205	9.6	2.6
Dark meat, w/ skin	250	15.6	3.5
Turkey			
Light meat, skinless	155	3.2	1.1
Light meat, w/ skin	195	8.2	2.3
Dark meat, skinless	185	7.1	2.4
Dark meat, w/ skin	220	11.4	3.5

■ **Use healthy cooking methods.** Frying a chicken breast in oil, lard, vegetable shortening or grease will offset any low-fat benefit, as will smothering it in fatty gravy. Use cooking methods that allow fat to drip off, such as roasting, broiling, barbecuing, baking, steaming and stewing. If you do fry, use a nonstick pan with cooking spray, flavored vinegar, defatted broth or wine.

■ **Watch out for ground turkey.** Processed poultry products like chicken hot dogs, turkey bacon and turkey bologna often contain dark meat, skin and fat. Consequently, they can be as fat as—or fatter than—their beef and pork counterparts. One of the worst offenders is ground turkey. Some brands contain 13 to 16 grams of fat in a four-ounce serving. Be sure you're buying "ground turkey breast," not just "ground turkey." Made from skinless white meat, ground turkey breast has just 3 to 4 grams of fat per serving.

■ **Read food labels.** While Healthy Choice Grilled Basil Chicken with 6 grams of fat would fit your fat budget, there is little chance that

Swanson Hungry-Man Chicken Pot Pie with 29 grams of fat would work. Look for frozen chicken meals with no more than 3 grams of fat per 100 calories.

■ **Use portion control.** "People have been heavily blitzed with the message to eat less fat," says Dr. Walter Willett, chief of nutrition at Harvard's School of Public Health. "But replacing a 12-ounce steak with the same amount of poultry doesn't make sense. Instead, servings of poultry—or any animal food—should be three or four ounces, surrounded by grains, beans, vegetables, fruit and other foods rich in complex carbohydrates and fiber."

■ **Order smart.** In a sit-down restaurant, order baked, broiled, roasted or barbecued poultry without skin and with any sauces served on the side. In fast-food restaurants, avoid fried chicken, wings or nuggets. (Wendy's Ultimate Chicken Grill Sandwich at 320 calories and 7 grams of fat is quite different from its Chicken Club Sandwich at 540 calories and 25 grams of fat.) At a delicatessen, a turkey sandwich is a great choice as long as you don't ask for it to be larded with mayonnaise, bacon and cheese; instead, order the sandwich with mustard, lettuce and tomato.

92 Don't Pass the Salt

The key to cutting down the amount of sodium you eat is being conscious of how much of it you actually eat. It's easy enough to be careful about table salt and obviously salty foods like pickles, bacon and potato chips. (Salt is sodium chloride. It's the sodium in salt that is a health issue.) But it's much harder when the sodium is a hidden ingredient. And it is hidden—in foods like cheese, peanut butter, bread, cereals and commercial salad dressings and spaghetti sauce. One ounce of corn flakes has nearly twice the sodium found in an ounce of salted peanuts, and two slices of white bread contain more sodium than 14 potato chips.

Here are some ways to steer clear of salt:

■ **Eat more fresh foods** and fewer processed foods. A medium potato contains just 5 milligrams of sodium; processed into potato chips, it has 1,560 milligrams. Fresh peas contain .9 milligrams of sodium per one-fourth cup; the same amount of canned peas, 230 milligrams. A 3-ounce portion of steak has 55 milligrams of sodium; a frozen meat loaf dinner, about 1,300.

■ **Hide the salt shaker.** If you need additional seasoning on your food, use non- or low-sodium spices such as black pepper, garlic or garlic powder, tarragon, chili flakes, chili powder, lemon juice or combinations of your own homemade or commercial dried herbs and seasonings (such as Mrs. Dash and Spike). Avoid soy sauce and similar seasonings that are rich in sodium. If you're a salt diehard, consider using a one-hole shaker.

■ **Reduce salt in cooking.** Question each time that salt is called for in a recipe. Sometimes less salt or no salt will do. If you determine that salt is truly needed, reduce the amount called for by at least a fourth. After a few weeks, reduce the amount by another fourth. Use lemon juice, flavored vinegars, herbs and spices to bring out natural flavors.

■ **Read food labels** and familiarize yourself with the most commonly used advertising descriptions:

> "Low sodium" means 140 milligrams or less per serving.
> "Very low sodium" means 35 milligrams or less per serving.
> "Sodium-free" means less than 5 milligrams per serving.
> "Reduced sodium" means at least a 25% reduction from the regular food.
> "Unsalted" means no salt added, but not necessarily no sodium added.

■ **Learn other names for sodium.** In addition to salt, these include baking soda, baking powder, celery salt, garlic salt, onion salt, kosher salt, rock salt, seasoned salt, sea salt, sodium ascorbate, sodium benzoate, sodium caseinate, sodium citrate, sodium erythorbate, sodium nitrate, monosodium glutamate (MSG), sodium bicarbonate, sodium propionate, sodium saccharin and sodium phosphate.

■ **Order smart.** In a sit-down restaurant, ask that your food be prepared without added salt, garlic salt, sea salt or MSG. At a fast-food restaurant, ask to see the nutritional breakdown of the various dishes. There's a big difference between a Jack in the Box Ultimate Cheeseburger with 1,580 milligrams of sodium and a McDonald's Hamburger at 520 milligrams. And to be on the safe side, make sure your at-home meals are lighter in sodium on days when you eat a meal in a restaurant.

Make Your Mustache Fat-Free

93

Milk is rich in vitamins, minerals, protein and calcium, but some types of milk also come with unwanted baggage—too much heavily saturated fat. The challenge is to choose milk products that are tasty, nutritious and not loaded with excess fat.

■ **Make the best milk choice:** fat-free (also called nonfat and skim). Only 2% of its calories come from fat, yet it has all the calcium, vitamin D and protein benefits of whole milk. Fat-free buttermilk and 1% "light" milk are also good choices. See the breakdown for different types of milk on the facing page.

SPEAKING FROM EXPERIENCE

When we started to change our family diet, my daughter Anne was six and my son Joe was four. They both said there was no way they would drink "blue milk." What we did was mix the 2% milk that they were drinking with fat-free milk, which we wanted them to drink. Over time we increased the nonfat portion and decreased the 2% portion, until finally they were drinking 100% fat-free.

The only problem was, we served it to them in a 2% container, and one day at breakfast Anne asked me, "Dad, is this milk any good?" "It tastes fine to me," I said. "Why do you ask?" "Because the container says it's a year old," she replied.

At that point I told her that she and Joe were drinking fat-free milk. They wanted to go back to 2% milk (on principle, I think), but their taste buds had changed. They now actually *liked* fat-free milk.

The secret is to take small steps. Move from whole milk to 2%, then 1%, and finally to fat-free over a period of four to six weeks.

—J.P.

TYPE OF MILK (8 FL. OZ.)	CALORIES	GRAMS OF FAT	GRAMS OF SATURATED FAT
Whole milk	150	8.1	5.1
Whole chocolate milk	210	8.5	5.3
2% reduced-fat milk	125	4.7	2.9
2% reduced-fat chocolate milk	180	5.0	3.1
1% low-fat milk	100	2.6	1.6
Fat-free milk	85	0.4	0.3

Replacing a cup of whole milk with the same amount of fat-free milk saves 8 grams of fat—the same as two pats of butter! At three cups daily, that's a yearly calorie saving equal to 22 pounds of body fat.

- **Drink milk for calcium.** The National Institutes of Health recommends the following guidelines:

AGE	MILLIGRAMS OF CALCIUM PER DAY
1 to 5	800
6 to 10	800 to 1,200
11 to 24	1,200 to 1,500
Women 25 to 50	1,000
Women 50 to 65 taking estrogen	1,000
Women 50 to 65 not taking estrogen	1,500
Men 25 to 65	1,000
Men or women over 65	1,500
Pregnant or lactating women	1,200 to 1,500

At about 300 milligrams of calcium per cup, fat-free milk is a calcium powerhouse. But remember, other foods can also be good calcium sources: fat-free and low-fat yogurt and cheese, calcium-fortified orange juice and cereals, collard greens, sardines, salmon, kale and soybeans.

- **Drink milk for vitamin D.** Four 8-ounce glasses of milk can supply the recommended amount of vitamin D. Other food sources include eggs, fatty fish and organ meats.

Get Your B's

94

Foods (as opposed to supplements) rich in folate, vitamin B_6 and vitamin B_{12} may be beneficial for cardiac health. Here are some ways to make sure you're getting enough:

- **Choose complex carbohydrates.** Leafy green vegetables like spinach are rich in folate, as are tomatoes, oranges and other citrus fruits, as well as oatmeal. But pound for pound, it's hard to beat legumes such as beans and peas. Pintos, garbanzos, baby limas, blacks, navies and small white beans have 250 micrograms or more of folate, while cranberry beans and black-eyed peas have 350 micrograms.

- **Choose fortified cereals.** Many cereals and other grains are fortified with B vitamins. Some have 400 micrograms of folate in a single cup.

- **Use healthy cooking methods.** According to Dr. Mary Frances Picciano, professor of nutrition at Pennsylvania State University, "Folate is a surprisingly delicate vitamin, and the more a food is processed or cooked, the less folate it's likely to contain." So even if you're eating more than one serving a day of vegetables, if that serving is fried, overcooked, or processed beyond recognition, it's probably not doing much for your folate levels.

The recommendation is for 400 micrograms of folate daily. The USRDA for B_6 is 1.3 milligrams daily for women and 1.7 milligrams for men. For B_{12}, it's 2.4 micrograms daily.

FOLATE

FOOD	MICROGRAMS
Black-eyed peas, 1 cup	350
Cranberry beans, 1 cup	350
Cooked chickpeas, 1 cup	280
Cooked asparagus, 1 cup	262
Cooked spinach, 1 cup	262
Cooked lentils, 1 cup	258
Oatmeal, 1 cup	199
Cooked artichoke, 1 cup	155
Orange juice, 1 cup	109
Cooked broccoli, 1 cup	80

VITAMIN B$_6$

FOOD	MILLIGRAMS
Banana, 1 medium	.48
Avocado, $\frac{1}{2}$ medium	.42
Hamburger, 3 oz.	.39
Chicken, 3 oz.	.34
Fish, 3 oz.	.29
Potato, 1 medium	.20
Cooked spinach, $\frac{1}{2}$ cup	.16
Rice, brown, $\frac{1}{2}$ cup	.16

VITAMIN B$_{12}$

FOOD	MICROGRAMS
Liver, beef, 3 oz.	68
Clams, canned, ½ cup	19
Oysters, canned, 3.5 oz.	18
Tuna, 3 oz.	2
Yogurt, 1 cup	1
Milk, fat-free, 1 cup	.9
Halibut, 3 oz.	.8
Egg, 1 large	.8
Chicken, 3 oz.	.4
Cheese, cheddar, 1 oz.	.2

Move the Cheese

95

Americans are gaga for cheese—to the tune of 30 pounds or so a year for each and every one of us. According to the Stanford Center for Research in Disease Prevention, cheese is the hardest food for us to trim from our diet, particularly for women, who rank it much higher than meat as a "favorite and frequently consumed food," right behind chocolate and ice cream.

The problem is that, while most cheese is a good source of protein and calcium, it can also be a concentrated source of fat, saturated fat and calories. Most regular cheese is about 60% to 80% fat, two-thirds of which is saturated. This means that a typical 1.5-ounce serving, about one and half slices of American cheese, contains as much fat as three and a half pats of butter, or about 14 grams of fat. The key is balance.

■ **Know what you're eating.** Fat content fluctuates greatly with different types of cheese.

TYPE OF CHEESE (1 OZ.)	GRAMS OF TOTAL FAT	GRAMS OF SATURATED FAT
Regular, or full-fat	9 to 11	6 to 7
Reduced-fat, or part-skim	5 to 7	3 to 5
Light	2 to 4	1 to 3
Nonfat	Less than 0.5	Trace

■ **Read food labels.** This is the only way to know how fatty a cheese really is. (Just because the label says a cheese is "part-skim," "low-fat" or "semi-soft" doesn't necessarily mean it's low in fat.) And pay attention to serving size as well. Most labels for cheese use a one-ounce serving size—a pitifully small amount for a cheese lover.

■ **Grate it.** "Stretch" cheese by grating it, then use teaspoons—not cups—to flavor vegetables, salads, soups and pasta. A sprinkle of sharp cheese such as Parmesan, Romano or feta, added at the last moment, will zip up your meals without much added fat.

■ **Try nonfat and low-fat varieties.** Using a nonfat cheese on a sandwich, say, will save you 10 grams of fat and 70 calories. Low-fat is also good, but be careful of cheeses that are "lower in fat." A reduced-fat cheddar, for instance, may have 5 grams of fat per ounce—less than regular, but still a lot.

■ **Make taste an issue.** If you don't like the cheese, you won't eat it, no matter how much fat and calories it saves you. If you can't find a fat-free or reduced-fat cheese that satisfies you, stick with regular cheese—as long as it fits into your fat budget.

Hide the Sugar Bowl

Commonly used in coffee and tea, in homemade baked goods and on cereal and fruit, table sugar contributes about 30% of our total sugar intake. Consider using less or no sugar in drinks or using a sugar substitute. Use fresh or dried fruit on cereal. And when cooking from a recipe, reduce the amount of sugar called for by one-third;

279

normally, there is no change in taste. Apple juice and applesauce are good sugar substitutes in baking. The most dangerous source of sugar is high-fructose corn syrup found in processed foods. It is the primary reason why American adults consume over 150 pounds of refined sugar a year. Here are some other ways to cut back:

- **Limit processed foods.** These foods provide about 70% of the sugar we eat. Some sources are obvious because they taste sweet; examples include breakfast cereals, soft drinks, canned fruit, ice cream, gumdrops and jam. But many processed foods, such as peanut butter, tomato sauce and canned soups, have hidden sugar. Even ketchup has sugar!

- **Read labels.** Remember that 4 grams of sugar equals one teaspoon. So, if the label states that your breakfast cereal has 12 grams of sugar, take a moment to visualize the three teaspoons of sugar you're about to eat.

- **Don't be misled by the names given to ingredients.** When you read the list of ingredients on a food label, watch for high-fructose corn syrup, sucrose, maltose, dextrose, lactose, fructose, malt, corn solids, corn syrup, honey, molasses, invert sugar, raw sugar, maple sugar, corn sweetener, malted barley, date sugar and turbinado. Also, it's advisable to avoid any product whose label lists sugar, under any name, among the first three ingredients.

- **Switch to fresh fruit.** Americans eat almost 25.5 pounds of candy each year. And when we're not snacking on Snickers, we're often indulging in other sugar-rich desserts. But keep this in mind: A four-ounce serving of iced chocolate cake contains about 10 teaspoons of sugar. A much better way to satisfy your sweet tooth is with the natural sugar found in a ripe peach, a crisp apple or an ice-cold watermelon wedge.

- **Stay away from nonfat baked goods.** These items are generally loaded with sugar to boost their flavor. "If you don't have a weight problem when you start eating low-fat muffins, you may have one afterward," says Netty Levine, R.D., at Cedars-Sinai Medical Center in Los Angeles. "They may take out some fat, but they add more sugar, which jacks up calories. And watch out for the portions. That calorie figure on the label is for one serving, but a big muffin may be three or more servings. That could make it a 450-calorie muffin!"

LIQUID CALORIES

Most people who drink soft drinks aren't aware of the incredible amount of sugar—and calories—that can be crammed into a can or bottle.

SOFT DRINK (12 OZ.)	CALORIES	TEASPOONS OF SUGAR	% OF CALORIES FROM SUGAR
Coca-Cola	140	9.75	100
Mountain Dew	165	11.5	100
Pepsi-Cola	150	10.2	100
Shasta Orange	196	12.2	100
Sprite	148	8.2	100

"Liquid calories don't trip our satisfaction mechanisms," says Dr. Richard Mattes, author of a study at Purdue University whose participants ate 450 calories worth of jelly beans every day for four weeks and 450 calories worth of soda every day for another four weeks. On the days they ate jellybeans, the participants consumed about 450 fewer calories of other foods. But on the days they drank soda, they ended up eating 450 calories more than normal.

In a study of participants in the Framingham Heart Study, drinking more than one soft drink per day increased the odds of developing metabolic syndrome.

Whenever possible, skip soft drinks in favor of water. Keep a large pitcher of water in your refrigerator. Or, if you prefer, rely on bottled water. Many people like a mixture of one-third orange juice and two-thirds carbonated water—it tastes like a soft drink but has fewer sugar calories.

■ **Be smart about sugar substitutes.** Even though the FDA condones moderate use of sugar substitutes, we should still be wary of them. Studies show that they encourage us to maintain a taste for very sweet foods, which can lead to overindulgence and weight gain. Also, some people have trouble understanding that a diet cola does not offset the calories in a pepperoni pizza.

Drink Tea

Tea has long had a reputation as a cure for frazzled nerves or blue moods, and green tea is associated with a decrease in cancer risk. Now studies suggest that drinking at least one cup of green or black tea daily could cut your risk of heart attack and stroke significantly.

The benefit may be due to powerful plant chemicals known as flavonoids. Found naturally in tea, flavonoids are powerful antioxidants that may protect blood vessel linings from injury and inflammation. In addition, they have the same anticoagulant property that aspirin has, reducing the ability of blood platelets to stick together.

The findings are fairly dramatic. A study headed by Dr. Michael Gaziano, a heart specialist at Brigham and Women's Hospital, selected 340 men and women who had suffered heart attacks and matched them by age, gender and neighborhood with people who had never had heart attacks. The study then investigated their coffee- and tea-drinking habits for one year. Dr. Gaziano found that those who drank one or more cups of black tea every day slashed their heart attack risk by a staggering 44%, compared with those who did not drink tea.

The same result was found in a study of 805 Dutch men who consumed a diet rich in black tea, apples and onions, all of which contain large quantities of flavonoids. Not only was heart attack risk reduced substantially, but those who drank more than four cups of tea a day cut their risk of stroke by 69% over those who drank less tea. More recently, researchers writing in the *European Journal of Cardiovascular Prevention and Rehabilitation* have found that people who drink green tea have better blood vessel function just 30 minutes later. Such improvement reduces the risk of atherosclerosis.

Such positive results from the research translates into a strong lifestyle recommendation to drink more tea. But let's put it in perspective:

- **Don't imagine that drinking tea will offset an unhealthy lifestyle.** If you really want to maximize the effect of tea, add it to healthy habits. It won't work if you're smoking, sitting on a couch and eating junk foods.

Whole grains are a nutritional bonanza—low in fat, rich in nutrients such as protein, B vitamins and vitamin E, good sources of fiber and low in calories. They're also central to reducing the risk of heart disease. But it can be difficult to incorporate them into your meals throughout the day.

For starters, you can think of whole grains as side dishes rather than just breakfast foods. One cup on average provides 3 to 10 grams of fiber but only about 200 calories. Of course, you may have to wean your family from the more processed versions. One mother told me that her son loved white rice but hated brown rice. She simply mixed them—one-half white, one-half brown—until her son's taste buds adjusted and the family progressed to all brown rice.

In addition, most of us eat only rice, wheat or corn, so I recommend experimenting with other grains such as whole or pearled barley, bulgur and whole-wheat couscous.

Dietitian Bev Utt suggests trying different whole grains in one-dish meals. You might start with couscous, for example, then layer on sautéed peppers, green onions and other vegetables, garbanzo or black beans, and even a small amount of chicken or meat. One-dish meals are a great way to maximize whole grains in your diet.

—J.P.

- **Don't drink herbal tea** if you want the benefit of flavonoids.
- **Don't worry about condiments, temperature or form.** Milk, sugar and lemon do not diminish the effect of flavonoids. Neither does drinking your tea hot or cold. (Some people make a day's supply with three tea bags in 20 ounces of water, cool it in the refrigerator, transfer to a container and sip all day long.) And there is no difference between tea prepared with loose tea leaves, tea bags or granulated crystals.
- **Don't go crazy.** The amount of tea needed to provide a cardioprotective effect is still under debate. Until we know the "threshold" dosage (whether it's one or six cups a day), remember your grandmother's advice: "Moderation in all things."
- **What about caffeine?** Some studies suggest that coffee is a great source of protective antioxidants and, when consumed in moderation, benefits cardiac health. Because both tea and coffee contain caffeine,

moderate consumption is advised. Excessive caffeine can stimulate the heart, produce extra heartbeats, increase heart rate and raise blood pressure. One way to minimize caffeine is by brewing full-leaf tea. Since the smaller the leaf, the stronger the concentration of caffeine, a tea bag made from cut-leaf tea or "dust" will release nearly twice as much caffeine per cup as full-leaf tea. Another way is to shorten the brewing time. A four-minute infusion of black tea will provide 40 to 100 milligrams of caffeine, while a three-minute infusion will provide only 20 to 40 milligrams.

98 Get Your Antioxidants from Food

According to the American Heart Association, "It is preferable to get vitamins and minerals such as beta-carotene, vitamin C and vitamin E in a nutritious diet rather than through supplements. We continue to recommend that Americans eat a variety of foods daily from all the basic food groups."

Beta-carotene is concentrated in very dark green and deep yellow fruits and vegetables. It has no USRDA, but many experts recommend a range of 5 to 30 milligrams daily.

FOODS HIGH IN BETA-CAROTENE

FOOD	MILLIGRAMS OF BETA-CAROTENE
Carrot juice, 1 cup	38
Cooked sweet potato, ½ cup	17
Cooked canned pumpkin, ½ cup	16
Cooked carrots, ½ cup	11
Cantaloupe, ½ medium	8
Raw carrots, ½ cup	5
Mango, 1 medium	5
Cooked spinach, ½ cup	4

Vitamin C is readily found in a variety of fruits and vegetables. The USRDA is 60 milligrams daily; however, research suggests that the optimal level of vitamin C for cardiovascular protection may be 500 to 1,000 milligrams per day.

FOODS HIGH IN VITAMIN C

FOOD	MILLIGRAMS OF VITAMIN C
Cantaloupe, ½ medium	195
Grapefruit, 1 medium	100
Raw red pepper, ½ cup	95
Honeydew melon, 1 cup	92
Papaya, 1 cup	87
Strawberries, 1 cup	84
Kiwi, 1 medium	75
Orange, 1 medium	70
Orange juice, ½ cup	60
Cooked broccoli, ½ cup	58
Cooked Brussels sprouts, ½ cup	49
Raw green pepper, ½ cup	45
Raw tomato, 1 cup	34
Cooked sweet potato, ½ cup	32
Raspberries, 1 cup	31

Vitamin E is the toughest of the antioxidants to get through diet alone. Many sources of vitamin E, such as nuts and seeds, vegetable oils and peanut butter, are rich in fat, so it can be a challenge to balance an adequate intake of vitamin E against the potential for breaking your fat budget.

Although the USRDA for vitamin E is 15 milligrams (22.4 international units) for adults, some experts suggest that a cardioprotective level is 133 to 533 milligrams (100 to 800 international units).

FOODS HIGH IN VITAMIN E

FOOD	MILLIGRAMS OF VITAMIN E
Total cereal, 1 cup	20
Dry-roasted sunflower seeds, 3 tbsp.	14
Granola, ½ cup	8
Almonds, 1 oz.	7
Wheat germ, ¼ cup	5
Peanut butter, 2 tsp.	3
Olive oil, 1 tbsp.	2

Don't overlook vitamin D. Research now suggests that too low a level can increase cardiac risk, while maintaining a healthy level is cardioprotective. Sunshine is the best source of vitamin D, but good food sources include salmon, mackerel, tuna, sardines, milk (nonfat and low-fat are the best choices), ready-to-eat fortified cereals, eggs and cheese.

Know Your Margarines

The dairy section is full of margarine options—so many that it's sometimes hard to know what to buy. Here are a few rules to keep in mind:

- **Avoid stick margarine.** When an oil is hardened to produce a food product, as corn oil or safflower oil is to produce stick margarine, the hydrogenation process increases trans fatty acids. The harder the margarine, the more trans fat it contains. And, remember, trans fats increase blood cholesterol.

CHOLESTEROL-LOWERING SPREADS

Benecol and Take Control contain plant stanol esters, which have somewhat the same cholesterol-lowering effect as oat bran. Benecol is used as a spread as well as in cooking, baking and frying. Clinical trials conducted in Finland and the United States showed it to be effective in reducing total cholesterol and LDL cholesterol levels by an average of 10% and 14%, respectively. Take Control is used as a spread but not in baking or frying. Trials indicate that the use of this plant stanol margarine may lower LDL cholesterol by 7% to 10%. Smart Balance also has spreads made with plant stanol esters.

■ **Choose soft margarine.** Because liquid and tub margarines are not heavily hydrogenated, they are more heart-healthy than stick margarine. Be sure, however, to choose a soft margarine made with a polyunsaturated oil such as safflower oil or corn oil.

■ **Be aware of labels.** Some spreads claiming "zero grams trans fat" can contain up to 0.49 grams of trans fat. Make sure the listing of ingredients doesn't contain the terms "partially hydrogenated," "hydrogenated" or "shortening" in the description.

■ **Choose cholesterol-lowering margarine.** In a recent study from the University of Texas Southwestern Medical Center, 23 families ate butter while another 23 families used cholesterol-lowering margarine. After five weeks the adults on the "margarine diet" experienced an 11% drop in LDL cholesterol.

Dropping total and LDL cholesterol by double digits simply by eating those margarines is indeed remarkable. There are, however, a few things to consider:

■ Study participants who got the best cholesterol-lowering results used plant stanol margarine in place of—not in addition to—other spreads.

■ Be aware of fat and calories. A serving of Benecol (one tablespoon) contains 8 grams of fat and 70 calories. At the recommended amount of three servings per day, that's 24 grams of fat and 210 calories. A serving of Take Control (one tablespoon) contains 6 grams of fat and 50 calories. At the recommended two servings per day, that's 12 grams of fat and 100 calories. If you're restricting dietary fat for purposes of weight loss and cardiac health, be certain that two or three pats of margarine a day will fit into your fat budget.

■ And finally, plant stanol margarine is not a cure-all. Don't eat a poor diet and then try to offset it with cholesterol-lowering margarine. There is no offsetting mechanism when you spread Benecol or Take Control on a croissant.

The bottom line is to keep your perspective. When you choose to eat fat, make the healthiest choice you can, be it olive oil, canola oil or plant stanol ester margarine. Then remember that healthy fats are still fat.

Have a Drink . . . If You Drink

In moderation, alcohol is associated with a reduced risk of heart attack and stroke. But heavy drinking can cause cirrhosis, cancer, birth defects, brain damage and fatal accidents, and can contribute to overweight, obesity and metabolic syndrome. An excessive intake of alcohol can also impair the pumping capacity of the heart. And recent research shows that it can raise levels of C-reactive protein, a harbinger of coronary inflammation.

In other words, if you drink alcohol, be smart about it:

■ **If you don't drink, don't start** simply because of the potential health benefits of alcohol. Exercising regularly, eating right and not smoking all have major health benefits and no downside.

■ **If you do drink, do so in moderation**—which means no more than one to two drinks a day for men, one for women, ideally with meals. This does not mean averaging a drink a day by abstaining on weekdays and binge-drinking on weekends. That pattern is clearly harmful to health.

■ **Understand what constitutes a drink:** 12 grams (one-half ounce) of pure alcohol. This is the amount in 12 ounces of beer, 1.5 ounces of 80-proof liquor or 5 ounces of wine.

■ **If you have a condition that could be aggravated by alcohol,** such as high blood pressure, elevated triglycerides, obesity, cardiomyopathy (a weakened heart) or atrial fibrillation, or if you're taking prescription medications, talk with you doctor about whether or not drinking is safe for you.

■ **Understand that alcohol is not a magic cure-all** for poor lifestyle habits. Not smoking, eating a diet low in saturated and trans fats, and exercising regularly—these should be first and foremost among your lifestyle habits.

■ **Strive for a balanced diet.** While it may be good news to learn that beer contains a potent antioxidant (xanthohumol), the bad news is that you would have to drink 117 gallons of beer a day to obtain its maximum health benefits. Be sure you're getting sufficient antioxidants from multiple food sources.

■ **Determine if you can afford the extra calories** that come in alcoholic beverages, particularly if you're trying to lose weight. Ounce for ounce, alcohol has almost as many calories as fat.

BEVERAGE	CALORIES
Scotch, whiskey, gin, vodka (1.5 oz.)	
80-proof	97
86-proof	105
90-proof	110
94-proof	116
100-proof	125
Brandy, cognac (1 oz.)	65
Liqueurs (1 oz.)	75 to 100
Dry wine (3.5 oz.)	87
Sweet wine (3.5 oz.)	142
Beer, ale (12 oz.)	140 to 165
Light beer (12 oz.)	95 to 105

EAT TO BEAT STRESS

When we feel stressed, we tend to seek out sweet, fatty food that raises our mood but unfortunately also raises our weight. But we don't have to resort to chocolate (the "edible tranquilizer"), ice cream, cookies and cake to boost our serotonin levels. Complex carbohydrates can have the same effect. Dr. Leigh Gibson at University College in London recommends the following foods to fight emotional eating:

- Fresh fruit or fruit canned in its own juice
- Whole-wheat toast with jam
- Multi-grain waffle with light syrup
- Tomato soup
- Sweet potato, or baked potato with light sour cream and chives
- Oatmeal
- Lightly sweetened whole-grain cereals such as Multi-Grain Cheerios

Rewrite Your Favorite Recipes

A trip to the bookstore is often the first step for many people trying to change their diets. They buy a low-fat cookbook, shop for hard-to-get ingredients with unpronounceable names, spend hours in the kitchen and are then disappointed when the family refuses to eat the great new dish they've prepared.

Here's why. We like our own food, our own favorite recipes, better than we like the recipes of other people. *The fact is that most American families prepare 12 recipes 80% of the time.* So instead of worrying about how to create a hundred new low-fat meals, it's more effective to reduce fat and calories in those recipes that already have your family's stamp of approval.

Let's say your family likes to have French toast on Sunday mornings. The traditional recipe calls for mixing whole milk and four whole eggs, dipping bread in the mixture and frying it in bacon fat. How can this recipe be lightened without losing taste? First, you can use fat-free milk instead of whole milk; Egg Beaters, or one whole egg and three egg whites, instead of four whole eggs. Next, instead of bacon grease, use a nonstick pan or griddle with a little cooking spray. Now you can afford to top the French toast with fresh fruit and yogurt, fruit compote, or even a small dollop of soft margarine and a little maple syrup. It will be fantastic.

Eat Your Beans

Beans and other legumes are great sources of complex carbohydrates, fiber, folate, protein, phytochemicals and other nutrients, yet contain little or no fat and no cholesterol. In particular, they contain *soluble* fiber, which is effective in lowering blood cholesterol.

A good way to get enough beans and peas—the most common types of legumes—is to mix them with other foods in your diet. Examples are black beans and rice, white bean and tuna salad, pasta and beans, bean tacos and falafel. Dietitian Bev Utt suggests one-dish meals: "A Tex-Mex salad, for instance, uses greens as a base. Then add black beans, canned corn, green onions and sautéed chicken. I use a light ranch dressing and serve with a warm tortilla."

Add lentils, split peas, black beans or white beans to soups and stews. Use pinto beans with ground beef or textured vegetable protein in tacos and burritos. And add navy, kidney and garbanzo beans to salads. Be adventurous.

Easy on the Mayo

Regular mayonnaise is a fat disaster, with about 10 grams of fat and 2 grams of saturated fat per tablespoon—ounce for ounce, more fat than spareribs. But there are options. "Light" or "calorie-reduced" mayonnaise usually contains half the fat and saturated fat of regular mayonnaise. Examples with 3 to 5 grams of fat per tablespoon include Hellmann's/Best Foods Reduced Fat, Miracle Whip Light, Kraft Light and Weight Watchers Light. "Fat-free" mayonnaise

---

HOLD THE BUTTER

Few foods are so rich in fat that they fall outside the prescription for low-fat eating, but butter is one. Not only is butter rich in fat—a single pat contains 4 grams of fat, a tablespoon almost 11 grams of fat—but over 50% of the fat content is saturated. Ounce for ounce, butter is fatter than prime rib. It's also insidious. A pat here, a spread there—it adds up all too quickly. If you're concerned about calories and cholesterol, the best advice is to avoid butter altogether.

1 teaspoon of butter	=	1 teaspoon of regular mayonnaise
	=	2 teaspoons of French or Italian salad dressing
	=	3 teaspoons of mayonnaise-type salad dressing
	=	3 teaspoons of cream cheese
	=	4 teaspoons of table cream
	=	5 teaspoons of sour cream

---

has less than one-half gram of fat and only a trace of saturated fat per tablespoon. Some good examples are Kraft Free, Miracle Whip Free and Smart Beat Fat Free.

But here's a case where you should let your taste buds guide you. Some people like "fat-free" mayonnaise on their sandwiches, particularly along with a spicy mustard, yet prefer to use "light" mayonnaise when it comes to tuna salad. Also, remember that just because you use reduced-fat mayonnaise, this doesn't mean you can use twice as much.

Be Smart About Snacks

Americans love to snack. On average, we eat snack foods over 200 times a year, and we're eating more all the time. Annual candy consumption, for instance, recently jumped from 19 to over 25 pounds per person.

There is actually nothing wrong with snacking, provided you do some serious thinking about what you choose to munch on. Indeed, it may be healthier (in terms of reduced weight and cholesterol) to eat small meals throughout the day rather than two or three large ones. The problem for most people is what they choose to eat rather than how often they eat.

Most popular snacks are excessive in fat, sodium, sugar and calories. Potato chips, the all-American favorite, get 50% to 60% of their calories from fat. Eating eight ounces of chips is tantamount to adding 12 to 20 teaspoons of oil to a baked potato!

Here are some ways to be smart about snacks:

- **Restock your cupboard and refrigerator.** The first step should be to replace cookies, chips and other high-calorie munchies with healthier, nutrient-packed snacks.

- **Eat more fruit.** Sweet, tart, chewy or crunchy, fresh fruits are one of the best deals around. One hundred calories will get you any of the following:

1 apple	29 grapes	1 cup of raspberries
5 apricots	1 or 2 oranges	2 cups of strawberries
1 banana	1 nectarine	2 or 3 tangerines
½ cantaloupe	2 peaches	10 ounces watermelon
20 cherries	1 pear	⅕ honeydew melon
1 grapefruit	3 plums	

Try fruits in different forms. Frozen grapes, for instance, are a refreshing alternative to fatty snacks. And dried fruits, while higher in calories, are a valuable source of fiber and nutrients.

- **Fill up, not out.** Choose watery vegetables like cucumbers, radishes, celery, zucchini, red and green peppers, cauliflower, mushrooms and broccoli: all are under 10 calories per ounce.

BUY LESS, EAT LESS

Research suggests that buying packaged foods in giant economy sizes can increase consumption by as much as 43%. A smart strategy is to buy big at the store, then repackage the contents into smaller sizes when you get home.

■ **Eat nuts in moderation.** First, let's look at the bad news—the fat and calories—in nuts. The figures in the table below apply to dry-roasted one-ounce portions.

TYPE OF NUT	CALORIES	GRAMS OF FAT	GRAMS OF SATURATED FAT
Almonds	167	14.8	1.4
Brazil nuts	186	18.8	4.6
Cashews	163	13.2	2.6
Filberts/hazelnuts	191	19.1	1.4
Pecans	190	20.0	2.0

On the other hand, let's remember that nuts are artery-friendly: rich in unsaturated fats, vitamin E, omega-3 fatty acids, fiber and B vitamins. Several studies have found that including nuts in the diet may reduce LDL cholesterol. In the Harvard Nurses' Health Study, women who ate more than five ounces of nuts a week experienced a 35% reduction in their heart attack risk compared with women who ate one ounce of nuts a week or none at all.

So, should nuts be part of a heart-healthy diet? By all means, yes, especially if they take the place of chips or a candy bar. Just don't pick up a whole jar or can of them and settle down in front of the TV.

■ **Look for alternatives.** A regular-size Baby Ruth gets its 275 calories from one tablespoon of fat and 8 teaspoons of sugar: a nutritional disaster. So what do you do when the craving hits? Try sweet and smooth snacks like fruit sorbet, frozen grapes, low-fat and nonfat yogurt, ice milk, angel food cake, sherbet, juice and applesauce. If nothing but chocolate will do, go small and eat a mini-bar. You can also cut up a favorite candy bar into bite-size pieces you pop in the freezer. When a craving hits, eat one piece. By the time the candy thaws in your mouth, which can take several minutes, your craving may be satisfied.

RECOMMENDED SNACKS

CARBO-RICH

Low-fat popcorn	Frozen bananas, grapes, berries, mango	Twice-baked potatoes
Chex mix		Raisins
Whole-grain crackers	Veggies and dip (low-fat yogurt, black bean, salsa)	Caramel-covered rice cakes
Cracker sandwiches (low-fat cheese, fruit spread)	Fruit juice popsicles	Cracker Jack
	Cereal by the handful	Pretzels
Fruit dipped in fat-free caramel	Rice pudding	Dried fruits

CALCIUM-RICH

Frozen yogurt	Hot chocolate made w/ fat-free or 1% milk	Veggies w/ nonfat cream cheese
Vanilla pudding		
Light ice cream	Flavored low-fat milks (chocolate, strawberry)	English muffin w/ low-fat or nonfat cheese
Tapioca		
Yogurt		

PROTEIN-RICH

Turkey jerky	Peanut butter on: veggies, crackers, apples, English muffins, cracker bread	Sliced turkey breast
Bean dip on tortilla chips		
Lean meat roll-ups		

OK ONCE IN A WHILE

Sponge cake	Cookies
Fruit roll-ups	Cupcakes

Don't be fooled by many of the so-called "energy bars." The "energy" in most bars is simply calories. Many have the same profile as candy bars. Be sure to read the label.

Traditional potato chips can be among the worst of snacks, with 8 to 10 grams of fat—and about 3 grams of saturated fat—per ounce. Some varieties are available with reduced fat and calories. One ounce of Pringles Original Potato Chips (about 17 chips) contains 160 calories and 11 grams of fat, while the same amount of Pringles Light Crisps has 70 calories and no fat. But if you "can't eat just one" (ounce, that is), it's best not to start.

Cookies, crackers, pretzels and muffins come in low-fat varieties; however, they may not be low in calories or trans fat. A Dunkin' Donuts reduced-fat blueberry muffin may be lower in fat than other muffins, but it still contains 450 calories. A single SnackWell's Devil's Food cookie has 50 calories. Be sure to read labels whenever possible. And be realistic about the size, amount and calories of such snacks.

Popcorn is as American as apple pie and can be a whole lot leaner. A four-cup serving of plain air-popped popcorn has only one gram of fat. Many brands of microwave popcorn have a richer taste than air-popped, yet are genuinely lower in fat. Watch out for ready-to-eat popcorn, such as that sold in movie theaters. A study by the Center for Science in the Public Interest found that a medium-size bucket of movie popcorn could contain as much as 43 grams of fat and almost 650 calories. Hit it with "butter" topping and it climbs all the way up to 71 grams of fat and 910 calories. That puts it in triple-cheeseburger country. Moreover, much of the fat used in this kind of popcorn is saturated.

■ **Drink water.** Research shows that five to eight glasses a day will help to curb snacking tendencies.

Dress Salads Lightly

Which has more fat and calories: a tablespoon of salad dressing or a tablespoon of hot fudge? You're wrong if you picked the hot fudge. Commercial salad dressings are about 90% fat, or about nine grams of fat per tablespoon. To put this in perspective, a single packet of Newman's Own Creamy Caesar Dressing at McDonald's contains more fat than one-half cup of Ben & Jerry's Cherry Garcia ice cream!

A better way to dress a salad is with balsamic vinegar or balsamic vinegar mixed with a bit of olive oil. If you use commercial dressings, be sure to try one of the many "nonfat" (also called "no-oil") and "light" (also called "calorie-reduced") versions. "Light" dressings will save, on average, about seven grams of fat per tablespoon. However, fat-grams

"FAT-FREE" WARNING

Since the 1990s, Americans have embraced nonfat foods with a vengeance, but the average adult has gained eight pounds over this period! "People perceive fat-free food as good and think they can eat as much as they want," says Cathy Nonas, director of the Van Itallie Center for Nutrition and Weight Management at St. Luke's-Roosevelt Hospital in New York City. "But snacking all day can rack up as many calories as eating a meal, without providing any of a meal's nutritional benefits."

When first introduced, many fat-free foods were tasteless and bland (think rice cakes). Food manufacturers then decided to offset flavor loss by increasing the amount of refined sugar. As a result, many fat-free foods now have calories comparable to—and sometimes higher than—their full-fat versions. In addition, when health experts called for a reduction of dietary fat to reduce the risk of heart disease, cancer and obesity, no one expected that an aggressive food industry would grab onto the message with such single-mindedness. "We never said anything about calories, and neither did the food industry," says Nancy Ernst, nutrition coordinator of the National Cholesterol Education Program. "So what's being promoted is high-sugar, no-fat products that do not help weight maintenance and in some cases translate into weight gain."

and calories can add up rapidly even from "light" dressing if you use it too freely. "Nonfat" dressings can be a better choice, although they differ greatly in taste. Experiment.

If you do eat regular or "light" dressing, a good tip is to serve it on the side. Dip your fork into the dressing, then eat the salad. You'll get all the flavor of the dressing while minimizing your fat and calorie intake.

To make matters worse, people simply eat too many fat-free foods. According to Dr. Chris Rosenbloom of Georgia State University, "Research shows that if people are told the food is fat-free or lower in fat, they tend to eat three to five times as much as they normally would if the food contained fat. If I put out a plate of Toll House chocolate-chip cookies, you might eat one or two, maybe 100 or 120 calories. But if I put out a box of fat-free cookies, chances are you'll eat 8 or 10."

Figure Out Fast Food

Quick, cheap and tasty, fast food is almost irresistible. Unfortunately, most of it is laden with excessive fat, sodium, sugar and calories. And it's getting worse. Not too long ago, a McDonald's Quarter Pounder with 410 calories and 19 grams of fat was pretty much king of the hamburger realm. Today, it looks positively lean next to the Double Western Bacon Cheeseburger at Carl's Jr. with 970 calories and 52 grams of fat, or Jack in the Box's Ultimate Cheeseburger with 1,010 calories and 71 grams of fat. Even Taco Bell's Taco Salad in the Shell—a salad!—has 840 calories and 45 grams of fat.

In a perfect world, no one would eat this kind of fast food. But this isn't a perfect world, and sometimes we don't want to cook, or we're running late, or we just want the stuff. Remember: *Haste makes waists.* The best way to handle this reality is to make smart food choices within a fast-food environment:

FAST FOOD	CONTENT
McDonald's Hotcakes (w/o margarine)	340 calories, 9 grams of fat, 2 grams of saturated fat
Subway 6″ ham sandwich (w/o cheese and mayo)	290 calories, 4.5 grams of fat, 1.0 grams of saturated fat
Wendy's Ultimate Chicken Grill Sandwich (w/o cheese and dressing)	320 calories, 7 grams of fat, 1.5 grams of saturated fat
Jack in the Box Chicken Teriyaki Rice Bowl	580 calories, 6 grams of fat, 1 gram of saturated fat

Arby's, Burger King, Wendy's, McDonald's and other fast-food places offer salads with nonfat salad dressing.

Now all you need to do is put all this knowledge into practice. Suppose you're in the mood for a hamburger at lunchtime and you stop off at McDonald's.

MEAL #1

ITEM	CALORIES	GRAMS OF FAT	GRAMS OF SATURATED FAT	GRAMS OF TRANS FAT
Quarter Pounder with Cheese	510	26.0	12.0	1.5
French fries, large	500	25.0	3.5	0
Strawberry shake, 16 oz.	710	20.0	12.0	1
Apple pie	250	13.0	7.0	0
Total	1,970	84.0	34.5	2.5

Meal #1 has a lot of fat, saturated fat, trans fat and calories for the amount of food eaten. But what if you ordered smarter?

MEAL #2

ITEM	CALORIES	GRAMS OF FAT	GRAMS OF SATURATED FAT	GRAMS OF TRANS FAT
Hamburger	250	9.0	3.5	0.5
French fries, small	230	11.0	1.5	0
1% milk	100	2.5	1.5	0
Total	580	22.5	6.5	0.5

Here are some things to watch:

■ **Serving size.** As the number of hamburger patties increases, so does fat. Single hamburgers have about 2 ounces of meat; quarter-pounders, about 3 ounces; triple burgers, 4 or more ounces. Many deli sandwiches are large enough to feed two people.

■ **Add-ons.** Cheese, bacon, mayonnaise or mayo-based "special sauces" often come on hamburgers. Instead, opt for lettuce, tomato, onion, ketchup or mustard. Avoid fatty gravies and sauces on chicken and fish.

■ **Side orders.** A large order of French fries can contain more fat and calories than a quarter-pound hamburger. Coleslaw, onion rings and potato salad are also high in fat and calories.

■ **Chicken and chicken nuggets.** Battered and fried, often with skin on, these items can be high-fat disasters.

■ **Extra cheese.** Two slices of pizza with sausage, pepperoni and extra cheese have about 510 calories, 23 grams of fat and 11 grams of saturated fat. Instead, order a cheese pizza with half the cheese, extra tomato sauce, and load up on vegetables instead of meat. You'll have a pizza your heart can live with.

Don't Go Menu-Mad

Americans eat out on average 233 times a year, or more than four times a week. We obviously find the experience pleasurable. But dining out can pose a serious problem for cardiac health. Restaurant foods generally contain liberal amounts of fat in the form of oil, butter, cream, lard, meat drippings, fatty meat, cheese and cheese sauce. In addition, many items are fried, deep-fried, pan-fried and sautéed. As a result, restaurant meals can be high in fat, calories and saturated fat, as well as salt and sugar. So what can you do to enjoy restaurant food without penalizing your health? Here are a few tips:

■ **Choose to eat healthy.** The operative word is "choose." Make a mental decision to combine good taste and good health.

■ **Know fat content.** Your fat budget represents the maximum amount of fat-grams you can have in a day and still be on a lean, balanced diet. Once you know how much fat comes in an average serving of your favorite restaurant foods, you'll be able to determine if the foods fit your budget.

For example, let's suppose your fat budget is 40 grams of fat and you'd like to go out for dinner at an Italian restaurant. If you know ahead of time that pasta in a marinara sauce, linguine in red clam sauce and even spaghetti with two small meatballs all have under 20 grams of fat, you can budget your eating throughout the day to make any of these selections. But without that knowledge you can make mistakes.

Pasta in a white, pesto or Alfredo sauce can contain 50 to 90 grams of fat.

■ **Don't set yourself up to overeat.** If you skip meals all day long to "save calories" for a restaurant meal, you can be so famished by dinnertime that you succumb to your appetite and overeat. A better plan is to eat breakfast and lunch, but make them lean. This will allow for more calories and fat at dinner, but it will keep you from feeling famished. Be sure to stay hydrated throughout the day so that you'll be a little full when you order. Watch out for alcohol as it can increase your hunger. Be aware of portion sizes. If you order beef, ask for the "petite," "queen" or "8-ounce" cut rather than the "king" or "16-ounce" portion. Avoid buffets and "all-you-can-eat" restaurants. Share desserts. And resist any urge to join the "clean plate club."

■ **Be inquisitive.** Ask questions about how each dish is prepared. Is it made with butter, margarine, cream, oil or animal fat? Is it fried or deep-fried? Is salt or sugar added? Restaurant personnel can be very helpful with regard to meal content and preparation. Also, look for key words on the menu. Avoid foods described as buttery, sautéed, fried, pan-fried, crispy, creamed, au gratin, scalloped, au lait, à la mode, au fromage, marinated, basted or prime. Stay away from béarnaise, beurre blanc and hollandaise, butter sauce, cream sauce, aioli, pesto, or anything served in its own gravy or cheese sauce. Better choices are: steamed, in broth, in its own juice, poached, garden-fresh, roasted, broiled, stir-fried and lean.

■ **Choose your restaurant carefully.** Know where you can get food that tastes great yet won't hurt your nutritional goals. It's harder to order smart in a prime rib restaurant that specializes in oversize portions.

■ **Be aware of portion distortion.** Oversize servings are turning Americans into oversize people. Share an entrée. Push half to the side and ask for a doggie bag. Or order from the appetizer menu.

PORTION PATROL

Be conscious of how much you're eating. In a study at Pennsylvania State University, researchers found that when they served men 2.5 cups of macaroni and cheese, the men ate 1.9 cups. But when they were served a 5-cup portion, they ate 2.5 cups. After the meals, participants rated their fullness the same, regardless of how much they had eaten.

Limit Caffeine

Americans consume about 33 million gallons of coffee a day, equal to 30 seconds of full flow at Niagara Falls. Chocolate ranks number one for women on surveys of "favorite and most frequently eaten" foods. And soft drinks, colas in particular, have replaced water as America's drink of choice. One of the reasons for the popularity of coffee, chocolate and soft drinks is a common component: caffeine. In a society that never rests, it keeps us alert, awake and energized.

CAFFEINE CONTENT

ITEM	MILLIGRAMS OF CAFFEINE
Coffee, 8 oz.	
Drip	150
Brewed	135
Instant	95
Decaffeinated	5
Espresso, 1.5 to 2 oz.	100
Tea, 8 oz.	
Black	50
Green	30
Instant	15
Decaffeinated	2
Chocolate	
Milk chocolate candy, 1 oz.	6
Cocoa, water mix, 8 oz.	14
Soft drinks, 12 oz.	
Coca-Cola	45
Pepsi-Cola	37
Diet Pepsi	35
Dr Pepper	40
Mountain Dew	55

But too much caffeine has a negative impact on cardiac health. It stimulates the heart, forcing it to work harder and in some instances producing extra heartbeats. Caffeine can also increase heart rate and blood pressure and, according to some studies, the amount of fatty acids in the bloodstream. A Johns Hopkins University study of over 1,000 men found that those who drank five cups of coffee a day had nearly three times the risk of heart disease as those who drank no coffee.

Research to date has not conclusively linked heart disease to moderate consumption of coffee, but it seems reasonable that those concerned with cardiac health should avoid overstimulation of the heart by caffeine. That advice also holds true for people desiring weight control. Caffeine can cause blood sugar to drop, producing feelings of hunger that can sabotage good dietary intentions. And finally, too much caffeine may cause insomnia, nervousness and stomach upset.

Should you avoid caffeine altogether? Probably not. But if you drink coffee all day long, eat chocolate frequently or drink soft drinks regularly, it may be prudent for you to examine your dietary habits and consider changes to reduce caffeine intake.

Brush and Floss Your Teeth

Okay, so this one isn't exactly about eating, but it does have something to do with cardiac health. A number of studies show a link between periodontal (gum) disease and an increased risk of heart attack. In fact, it's estimated that a person with periodontal disease is two to three times more likely to have a heart attack than one without periodontal disease.

Here's the theory. Plaque that builds up on the teeth produces chronic inflammation of the gums, causing irritation, redness, swelling and bleeding when you brush. If the plaque isn't removed, the gums separate from the teeth, leaving pockets that fill with bacteria. The most common strain found in these pockets is *Streptococcus sanguis*. When it enters the bloodstream, this bacteria may be a significant causative factor in heart attacks and strokes.

303

Dental bacteria seem to undermine cardiovascular health in three ways. First, infections from dental plaque can cause injury to coronary artery walls. Second, people with gum disease are more likely to produce an inflammatory response that may place them at elevated risk of suffering a heart attack. And finally, gum disease can initiate blood clotting. While cholesterol buildup may narrow the artery opening, a blood clot is what seals the opening, choking off blood flow in narrowed heart or neck arteries, triggering heart attacks or strokes. Researchers at the University of Minnesota, led by Drs. Mark Herzberg and Maurice Meyer, found that *Streptococcus sanguis* produces a protein called PAAP (platelet aggregation associated protein), which forms on the bacteria's outer cell walls. Blood platelets then stick to the protein and begin to clot, blocking arteries and potentially inducing heart attacks.

Given all of the above, it seems prudent to:

- **Brush your teeth** at least twice a day. Electric toothbrushes, rinses and toothpaste help to prevent periodontal disease.
- **Floss** at least once a day.
- **See your dentist** for regular cleaning. People who are genetically predisposed to dental plaque buildup have a 20% chance of developing periodontal disease. If this concerns you, talk to your dentist about a test that can identify those who are at risk.
- **Be sure your diet includes** plenty of complex carbohydrates, especially fruits and vegetables. Reduce sugar and highly refined carbohydrate foods such as baked goods.
- **Consider bone implants** to replace dental bone lost from periodontal disease.
- **Consider aspirin therapy** to ease inflammation and arterial damage and to promote anticoagulation. Be sure to talk to your doctor.
- **Chew sugarless gum** to help fight dental decay. Gum containing xylitol, a sweetener made from birch bark, has been shown to partially suppress the growth of cavity-promoting bacteria in the mouth.

Epilogue

WHEN WE WERE WRITING THIS BOOK, we sometimes found ourselves overwhelmed by the staggering incidence of heart disease in this country. We wanted to help the millions of people afflicted to help themselves. At those moments we remembered this inspirational story from *Chicken Soup for the Soul* by Jack Canfield and Mark V. Hansen.

One at a Time

A friend of ours was walking down a deserted Mexican beach at sunset. As he walked along, he began to see another man in the distance. As he grew nearer, he noticed that the local native kept leaning down, picking something up and throwing it out into the water. Time and again he kept hurling things out into the ocean.

As our friend approached even closer, he noticed that the man was picking up starfish that had been washed up on the beach and, one at a time, he was throwing them back into the water.

Our friend was puzzled. He approached the man and said, "Good evening, friend. I was wondering what you are doing."

"I'm throwing these starfish back into the ocean. You see, it's low tide right now and all of these starfish have been washed up onto the shore. If I don't throw them back into the sea, they'll die up here from lack of oxygen."

"I understand," our friend replied, "but there must be thousands of starfish on this beach. You can't possibly get to all of them. There are simply too many. And don't you realize this is probably happening on hundreds of beaches all up and down this coast? Can't you see that you can't possibly make a difference?"

The local native smiled, bent down and picked up yet another starfish, and as he threw it back into the sea, he replied, "Made a difference to that one!"

PRESCRIPTIONS, PROCEDURES AND PROGRAMS

Drug Therapy

SOMETIMES MANAGING STRESS, exercising more and watching your diet—the front line in cardiac risk reduction—are just not enough. You may need drugs as an adjunctive therapy to better control certain markers. Of course, the information in this section does not replace consultations with your doctor, but it will give you a better understanding of your options and the right questions to ask.

Aspirin Therapy

AS NOTED EARLIER, THE RISK OF A HEART ATTACK INCREASES WITH the blood's propensity to clot and seal off a coronary artery. Clotting can also stop blood flow to the brain, causing a stroke. It is important, then, to reduce any tendency toward dangerous coagulation.

A landmark study, published in the *New England Journal of Medicine,* suggests that taking aspirin regularly is one of the best ways to reduce clotting risk. Aspirin's anticoagulant ability prevents platelets from sticking together, thereby lessening the chance of clots forming and blocking narrowed coronary arteries. As one researcher described it, "Aspirin is like the lumberjack who prevents logjams."

Three other major health benefits can be derived from aspirin therapy:

- Regular aspirin use may ease the severity of new heart problems. According to one report, hospitalized patients with chest pain were far less likely to have experienced a heart attack if they were on aspirin therapy at the time.

- Aspirin can help to minimize damage at the onset of a heart attack. Studies show that when taken during or immediately following a

SEE YOUR DOCTOR

It's important to talk to your doctor *before* taking any drug. But it's equally important to *keep* talking. Science changes; new drugs are developed; old drugs are made more powerful; and combinations of some drugs and/or food supplements may be dangerous. It's crucial to keep up.

CARRY UNCOATED ASPIRIN WITH YOU

Many doctors recommend carrying regular aspirin tablets with you to be used in a cardiac emergency. A study of more than 17,000 patients found a 23% reduction in the death rate and a 49% reduction in new or recurrent heart attacks when aspirin was taken within 24 hours of experiencing heart attack symptoms. As a result, doctors now advise that people who think they're having a heart attack should chew and swallow one regular uncoated adult aspirin (325 mg). It's estimated that this recommendation, if widely adopted, would save an additional 5,000 to 10,000 lives in the United States each year.

heart attack, aspirin reduces the risk of death immediately and during the first five weeks after the attack.

- Aspirin decreases coronary artery inflammation.

Both the FDA and the American Heart Association strongly recommend aspirin for "secondary" prevention. Clearly, an aspirin regimen can be beneficial for people who have suffered a heart attack or stroke, who have undergone coronary bypass surgery or balloon angioplasty or who have stable angina. The research results are unequivocal. Aspirin therapy can prevent heart attacks in people with a history of heart disease. Indeed, aspirin could reduce new heart problems by about 25% in patients with known cardiovascular disease.

A Cleveland Clinic study of 6,174 adults with heart disease found that regular aspirin users experienced a 33% lower mortality rate during a follow-up period of three years as compared with patients who didn't take aspirin.

Should everyone with known or suspected heart disease be on aspirin? Absolutely not. For people with certain heart rhythm irregularities (such as atrial fibrillation), other anticlotting medications may be more effective. Very rarely, aspirin has been linked to problems with nasal polyps and asthma; moreover, some diabetics shouldn't use it. Generally, aspirin is used with greater caution in elderly individuals, in patients with stomach ulcers, liver disease or known allergies, and in women considering pregnancy. Combining aspirin with some medications like Coumadin or anti-inflammatory drugs such as ibuprofen can lead to severe bleeding problems. There may also be other serious interactions between aspirin and other drugs a person may be taking.

Although there is good agreement on the use of aspirin in high-risk women (defined as those with known heart disease or with a greater than 20% risk of developing the disease over 10 years), recommendations for aspirin therapy in moderate- and lower-risk women are unclear and controversial. Uncontrolled high blood pressure is not uncommon in women, and aspirin therapy may increase the risk of stroke in this setting. Moreover, the risk of gastrointestinal bleeding and other adverse side effects may outweigh the potential benefits of aspirin in women at lower risk for cardiovascular disease. Consequently, contemporary guidelines suggest a conservative approach until the results of additional clinical trials are available.

However, for the vast majority of patients with heart disease, the benefits of aspirin therapy clearly outweigh the risks. With its proven cardioprotective benefits, aspirin is typically continued indefinitely, although other antiplatelet medications (e.g., clopidogrel) combined with it may be prescribed for shorter periods, especially after coronary angioplasty with stent placement. In the United States, the aspirin doses most frequently recommended are 80, 160 or 325 milligrams per day, but because it can cause major bleeding, the appropriate dose is the lowest dose that is effective in preventing both heart attack and stroke, because these two diseases have the same risk factors and frequently coexist.

In a review of major clinical trials conducted to date, Dr. James Dalen at the University of Arizona reported that the risk of major bleeding was extremely low and comparable for those taking 80 or 160 milligrams per day. What's the optimal cardioprotective aspirin dosage? Dr. Dalen concluded that the safest and most appropriate dose to prevent initial and recurrent cardiovascular events is 160 milligrams per day. Or you can take a 325-milligram tablet every other day. According to Dr. Edward Giovannucci, a researcher on the Harvard Nurses' Health Study, "Four to six regular-size aspirin tablets a week seem to provide the maximum benefit. Gobbling more tablets or higher doses will not help to further reduce risk and may increase side effects." Talk with your doctor to determine if aspirin therapy could be of benefit to you.

311

ASPIRIN ALONE?

A study of heart attack patients at 78 V.A. medical centers came to the surprising conclusion that giving heart attack survivors a low dose of the more expensive anticoagulant drug warfarin (Coumadin) in combination with low-dose aspirin did not prevent heart attacks or strokes better than aspirin alone. Patients began therapy within two weeks of suffering a heart attack and were followed for an average of nearly three years. Mortality rates, recurrent heart attacks, and strokes were virtually identical in the combined-therapy and aspirin-only groups. Said Dr. Louis Fiore, one of the principal researchers, "We had hoped the combined regimen might double the effectiveness of the drugs, but it didn't."

Cholesterol-Lowering Drugs

BECAUSE ELEVATED CHOLESTEROL IS A PREDICTIVE MARKER FOR heart disease and heart attack, levels need to be managed carefully to reduce cardiovascular risk. Most people can lower their cholesterol by 10% to 20% by adopting a low-fat diet, exercising and losing weight. But for some people lifestyle changes alone are not strong enough to combat "bad genes." That's why millions of Americans now use drug therapy to reach their cholesterol goals. Nonetheless, fewer than half of those who qualify for any kind of lipid-modifying treatment for cardiovascular risk reduction are receiving it. Moreover, only about 50% of the individuals who are prescribed a lipid-lowering drug are still taking it 6 months later; after 12 months, this figure falls to 30% to 40%.

A number of effective drugs are available to help control total cholesterol, LDL, HDL and triglycerides. Talk to your doctor to determine if drug therapy is appropriate for you.

Statin Drugs

Introduced in the late 1980s, statins are most doctors' drug of choice for lowering total and LDL cholesterol. Statins block cholesterol production in the liver; the body, which needs a certain amount of cholesterol to function, compensates by drawing on cholesterol found in the blood. This reduces the amount of cholesterol that could damage arteries. Depending on the drug and dosage, statins typically decrease total cholesterol by 22% to 42%, lower LDL cholesterol by 18% to 55%, increase HDL cholesterol by 5% to 15% and reduce triglycerides by 7% to 30%. As a general rule, when lower statin doses are doubled, total cholesterol and LDL cholesterol are reduced on average an additional 5% and 7%, respectively.

Taken in capsule form, statin drugs are the only lipid-lowering drugs that have been proven to reduce the risk of death from cardiovascular disease. They also have been shown to reduce the risk of first and second heart attacks. Commonly prescribed statins include:

DRUG	BRAND NAME
Pravastatin	Pravachol
Lovastatin	Mevacor
Simvastatin	Zocor
Atorvastatin	Lipitor
Fluvastatin	Lescol
Rosuvastatin	Crestor

Statin drugs are generally recommended for people with no or one risk factor whose LDL cholesterol is 190 milligrams per deciliter (mg/dl) or higher; those whose LDL is 130 to 160 mg/dl or higher and have at least two other risk factors for heart disease; or those whose LDL is 100 mg/dl or higher and who have known cardiovascular disease. However, a growing body of evidence suggests that using these criteria alone may result in the undertreatment of many persons who may benefit from an intensive lipid-lowering statin regimen. According to Dr. William Roberts, we simply cannot wait for a cardiovascular event to treat our LDL cholesterol levels. In his view, the goal for all populations—not just those with previous cardiovascular events—needs to be an LDL cholesterol below 100 mg/dl and ideally below 70. Others point out that statins may work in

---

BEFORE YOU START . . .

Before taking a statin drug, be sure to discuss with your doctor whether or not you meet the indications for therapy. A study of 29,000 primary-care patients drawn from Boston's Brigham and Women's Hospital found that fewer than one in three individuals taking statin drugs to prevent heart disease met National Cholesterol Education Program guidelines for who should take them. According to Dr. Susan Abookire, the study leader, a number of factors explain the results. "Doctors may not follow the guidelines or keep up with current research on statins," says Dr. Abookire. "To be on the safe side, some physicians may prescribe more medication rather than less. And finally, doctors are influenced by what their patients want, which is driven by advertising."

---

ways beyond LDL cholesterol lowering to reduce cardiovascular events. Recent studies have also demonstrated the benefits of statins in persons with "normal" LDL cholesterol but increased levels of C-reactive protein, an inflammatory marker that has been linked to heart attack and stroke.

Statin drugs are so effective that doctors are using them increasingly for people who have "normal" or only slightly elevated cholesterol levels. One study published in the *British Medical Journal* concluded that statins could reduce the risk of dying from a heart attack by 30% even among those with normal cholesterol levels and no signs of cardiovascular disease. That's because the non-cholesterol effects of statins, such as controlling clotting and inflammation, may be as important as the cholesterol effects. In the Air Force/Texas Coronary Atherosclerosis Study, researchers found that statin drugs also reduced levels of C-reactive protein. "Statins are turning out to be a real two-for-one," says Dr. Paul Ridker of Brigham and Women's Hospital. "They certainly reduce cholesterol. But they also reduce C-reactive protein, an independent predictor of heart disease."

In a recent *New England Journal of Medicine*, researchers reported data from nearly 18,000 individuals who, in simple blood tests, had normal LDL cholesterol (below 130) but elevated levels of C-reactive protein (2 or higher), a marker of inflammation that scientists have long suspected was part of the heart disease puzzle. The JUPITER Trial examined whether a statin, in this case rosuvastatin (Crestor), could reduce the risk of adverse cardiovascular events in a population that would not normally be considered "at risk" based on LDL cholesterol alone. Patients were divided into two groups, one given a placebo or dummy pill and the other rosuvastatin. After observing them for just under two years, researchers found that the statin reduced the risk of cardiovascular events by 44% as compared with those given placebos, and the study was prematurely stopped. According to Dr. Paul Ridker, these findings "reconfirm that individuals with elevated C-reactive protein are at high risk for heart attack and stroke, even when LDL cholesterol is low."

In addition, other studies suggest that statins may help to ward off Alzheimer's disease, osteoporosis and, in combination with aspirin, colon cancer. The efficacy of statins is reflected in the most current National Cholesterol Education Program Guidelines, which suggest that about 36 million Americans could benefit from drug therapy, up from a previous estimate of 15 million Americans. Says Dr. Antonio Gotto, former president of the American Heart Association, "I'm not recommending putting statins in the drinking water, but millions more people could benefit from their use."

NIX THE GRAPEFRUIT

Unlike other citrus fruits, grapefruit contains substances that disable certain enzymes in your body, sometimes for many hours. Without these enzymes, some statin drugs end up in the bloodstream at higher concentrations, which can put you at risk for serious muscle aches or weakness. Although an occasional small glass of grapefruit juice may be fine, experts recommend not drinking it at the same time you take the medication.

So, what's the downside? First, statins are costly. Next, you presumably have to be on these drugs for the rest of your life, but to date the effects of such long-term use are virtually undocumented. More significantly, in rare cases statins can cause elevations in some liver enzymes that could ultimately result in liver damage, so people using these drugs need regular blood testing. In addition, statins have been linked to very rare reports of a muscle weakness called rhabdomyolysis, a potentially life-threatening condition in which muscle cells are destroyed and released into the bloodstream, which can cause generalized muscle pain and discomfort and, in rare cases, kidney failure. Patients on statins should report any unusual muscle tenderness or soreness to their physician.

Ezetimibe

Ezetimibe (Zetia) is a cholesterol absorption inhibitor that is also available in combination with the statin drug simvastatin (sold together as Vytorin). Ezetimibe acts in the intestine to limit the absorption of dietary cholesterol and generally adds an extra 20% LDL cholesterol reduction to that seen with statins alone. On the other hand, it has little effect on triglycerides or HDL cholesterol.

Recently, the Ezetimibe and Simvastatin in Hypercholesterolemia Enhances Atherosclerosis Regression (ENHANCE) trial reported no added benefit of the combination of ezetimibe and simvastatin over simvastatin alone. Conducted in 720 patients with elevated cholesterol levels, the trial showed no significant change in carotid artery thickness (a commonly used clinical test to predict whether a drug will be effective in lowering cardiac events) with either drug regimen, despite significantly greater reductions in LDL cholesterol in the combined therapy group. These results were highly unexpected, leading some to even question the value of lowering cholesterol. Over a two-year follow up, there were also no differences in cardiovascular events between the two groups in the trial.

Unfortunately, because ENHANCE was a small-scale trial, the results are extremely difficult to interpret. And there were numerous other limitations to the study design. Some health care providers overstated the findings, whereas others were blindsided by the results. In addition, many in the medical community and the media misinterpreted the results, creating a great deal of confusion and raising more questions than answers for patients, physicians, pharmaceutical companies and health agencies. Moreover, the primary end point was arterial thickness, a rough indicator of disease progression, not "fatty plaque" as was misstated in some media reports.

Should one small-scale clinical trial diminish our confidence in the cardioprotective benefits of lowering total and LDL cholesterol via lifestyle modification, drug therapy, or both? Absolutely not! An overwhelming body of scientific evidence has now shown that whatever the total cholesterol level is, reduction of that level by approximately 40 mg/dl reduces the relative risk of an initial or recurrent cardiovascular event by half. Recent studies have also shown that more aggressive lowering of LDL cholesterol (from 100 to between 60 and 70 mg/dl) is associated with further reductions in cardiovascular and all-cause mortality.

Despite the disappointing ENHANCE outcomes, two therapeutic objectives remain warranted. First, strive to achieve targets for levels of cholesterol with the use of statins plus drugs that have shown clinical benefits when added to statins (e.g., resins, niacin, fibrates) and redouble efforts at dietary modification, regular exercise, and weight reduction, if appropriate. Second, consider combination therapy (including ezetimibe) for individuals in whom goal levels are not achieved. The trial designed to specifically determine whether or not ezetimibe in combination with

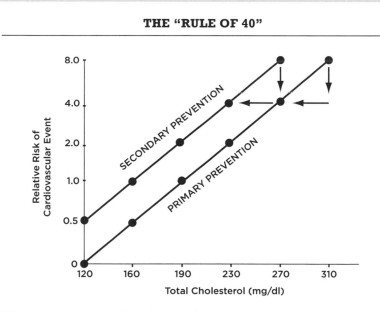

THE "RULE OF 40"

Effects of serum total cholesterol reduction on the risk of an initial (primary prevention) or recurrent (secondary prevention) cardiovascular event. Occurrence of an event shifts the "risk line" to the left. Each 40-mg/dl reduction in total cholesterol reduces the relative risk by half.

simvastatin further reduces clinical events, known as the IMPROVE-IT study, will not be available until approximately 2012. Until such data are available, patients taking ezetimibe should discuss its continued use with their physician.

Resins

Also called bile acid sequestrants, resins are considered the safest of the lipid-altering drugs and have been used successfully for nearly 30 years to reduce LDL cholesterol. Usually taken as a sandlike powder mixed with juice or water, they bind with bile salts in the intestines and flush them out of the system. To replenish the bile acid pool, the liver then draws cholesterol from the bloodstream, thereby reducing the blood's LDL concentration. In addition, resins promote cholesterol elimination in stools.

Resins are especially effective for people with high cholesterol who cannot tolerate statins. They're also less expensive than statins and have fewer potentially serious side effects. However, unless taken in significant amounts, resins usually do not produce the dramatic drop in cholesterol that statin drugs do. In addition, it's more of a hassle to take them, particularly when you're away from home. Furthermore, resins can raise the triglyceride level and have only very modest effects on raising HDL cholesterol.

Some of the most prevalent resins include cholestyramine (Questran), colestipol (Colestid) and colesevelam (WelChol). Questran and Colestid cannot be taken in combination with other medications, including statins; they may bind to and remove such drugs. WelChol does not have these drawbacks, which is why it's believed to be especially effective as adjunctive therapy for people already on statin drugs who need further cholesterol reduction.

Niacin

Also called nicotinic acid or vitamin B_3, niacin is an old standby for cholesterol control. Inexpensive and effective, it decreases total and LDL cholesterol, the latter by 5% to 25%. However, it does something that most other cholesterol drugs cannot do. Niacin lowers triglycerides

BE WARY OF OVER-THE-COUNTER CHOLESTEROL FIGHTERS

A number of over-the-counter products claim to lower cholesterol, but once again, some of these claims are hollow. Here's a quick rundown:

■ Soluble fiber in capsules and powders, often found in health food stores, is not effective in reducing cholesterol. Stick with foods that are rich in soluble fiber: oatmeal, oat bran, apples, oranges, beans and corn.

■ There is little evidence that garlic oil, garlic powder or garlic supplements lower cholesterol.

■ Fish oil capsules may not lower cholesterol levels, although they can help to reduce triglycerides.

■ Stay away from a dietary supplement of red yeast extract called Cholestin. It may be less of a supplement and more of an unapproved drug.

The bottom line: *Don't self-medicate.*

by 20% to 50% and increases HDL by 15% to 35%. Accordingly, niacin is the best HDL cholesterol raiser of the lipid-altering agents. In some cases, niacin is prescribed along with a statin drug to maximize the therapy.

Niacin is effective only in massive doses, usually one to three grams (1,000 to 3,000 mg) per day, or 50 to 100 times the USRDA. Unfortunately, large doses of niacin can have bothersome side effects, including flushing, hyperglycemia, hot flashes, itching, nausea, blurred vision and headache. Typically, side effects disappear as tolerance is gained. Sustained-release versions of niacin, taken once a day (instead of two or three times as with vitamin B_3), seem to help.

Since liver damage is a rare but more serious side effect, you should never take massive doses of niacin without first consulting your physician. Then, be sure to have your blood test checked for liver function. If you have liver disease, diabetes, gout, peptic ulcers or glaucoma, or if you're on a blood thinner, your doctor may not recommend niacin therapy for you.

Some of the most common brands of niacin include B_3-50, B_3-500-GR, Niacin SR, Niacor, Niaspan ER, Nico-400, Nicolar, Nicobid and Slo-Niacin.

Fibrates

These drugs, notably gemfibrozil (Lopid) and fenofibrate (Tricor), are used mainly to decrease triglycerides, usually by 20% to 50%. An additional benefit is that they can increase protective HDL by 10% to 20% and decrease harmful LDL by 5% to 20%. Gemfibrozil lowers the triglyceride level as well as or more effectively than any of the other lipid-lowering drugs, but it has only modest effects on LDL cholesterol levels. Also, it sometimes raises rather than lowers LDL cholesterol.

Side effects of these drugs include digestive problems, gallstones and muscle weakness.

Hormone Therapy

BECAUSE THE RISK OF HEART DISEASE INCREASES MARKEDLY AS women pass menopause, many scientists and doctors have thought that estrogen exerts a cardioprotective effect and that hormone therapy could reduce the rate of postmenopausal cardiac events. Surprisingly, however, the Heart and Estrogen/Progestin Replacement Study (HERS), the first large-scale randomized clinical trial to test this hypothesis, found that treatment with oral estrogen plus progestin did *not* reduce the overall rate of new heart attacks in postmenopausal women with known coronary disease. Several theories have been proposed to explain these disappointing results, including an inadequate follow-up duration (4.1 years). Yet two reports in the *Journal of the American Medical Association,* involving an extended follow-up (6.8 years) of the HERS subjects, and five subsequent trials came to a similar conclusion.

The results of the Women's Health Initiative trial, the largest study ever conducted in the United States of women's midlife health issues, reported an increased overall health risk in healthy postmenopausal women receiving combined hormone therapy as compared with women who were given a placebo. Between 1993 and 1998, 16,608 women aged 50 to 79 who had not had a hysterectomy were randomly assigned to two groups, one receiving Prempro (estrogen and progestin), the other a sugar pill. Although it was scheduled to run until 2005, the study was stopped prematurely because the women taking Prempro demonstrated a higher incidence of heart attack, stroke, breast cancer and blood clots.

More recently, the estrogen-alone component of the Women's Health Initiative reported that estrogen increases the risk of stroke and reduces the risk of hip and other fractures, but does not significantly affect the incidence of heart disease or overall mortality.

Prompted by these new studies, the American Heart Association has now updated its recommendations, suggesting that hormone therapy should not be used for the purpose of preventing a second heart attack or death among women with established heart disease. It also advises against starting or continuing estrogen therapy alone or combined therapy for the prevention of coronary heart disease.

In summary, estrogen alone or combined estrogen and progestin—treatments used by millions of women for relief of menopause symptoms as well as the prevention of other chronic diseases—should not be recommended to reduce the risk of cardiovascular events. Talk to your doctor about hormone therapy in light of these new findings and your personal and family health history. "The message is not that all women should stop hormones," says Dr. Margery Gass of the University of Cincinnati. "It's that each woman should consider why she's on hormone therapy—and how she might accomplish her health goals another way."

ACE Inhibitors

ANGIOTENSIN-CONVERTING ENZYME INHIBITORS, ALSO CALLED ACE inhibitors, belong to a class of cardiac drugs called antihypertensives, normally administered to patients with high blood pressure but also used to treat congestive heart failure or after major heart attacks where considerable heart damage has occurred. ACE inhibitors may be referred to either by their generic names, which commonly end in "il" (benazepril, captopril, enalapril, lisinopril, ramipril), or by their brand names: Lotensin, Capoten, Vasotec, Zestril or Prinivil and Altace. These medications are believed to block an enzyme that causes blood vessels to constrict. By relaxing or dilating blood vessels, they end up reducing blood pressure and increasing the supply of blood and oxygen to the heart muscle.

Angiotensin-receptor blockers (ARBs) are often prescribed for patients who are intolerant of ACE inhibitors. These antihypertensive drugs may especially benefit patients with heart failure, those who have had major heart attacks and individuals with diabetes and/or chronic kidney disease. ARBs are similar to ACE inhibitors in the way they lower blood pressure and inhibit sodium and water reabsorption in the kidneys.

The Survival and Ventricular Enlargement (SAVE) trial enrolled more than 2,200 major heart attack survivors and randomly assigned them to either a placebo or treatment with an ACE inhibitor. Patients were then followed for an average of three and a half years. Drug therapy reduced the risk of death by about 20%, recurrent hospitalizations by 22% and recurrent heart attacks by 25%, as well as the need for coronary bypass surgery or balloon angioplasty.

The Studies of Left Ventricular Dysfunction (SOLVD) trials also assessed the effects of ACE inhibitor therapy in patients with a history of heart failure and residual cardiac impairment. Follow-up averaged slightly more than three years. Overall, drug therapy reduced cardiovascular mortality, new heart attacks and recurrent anginal pain by about 20% each.

Although the results of these well-designed follow-up studies have consistently demonstrated fewer subsequent cardiovascular complications in patients assigned to ACE inhibitor therapy, it remained unclear whether a broader population of heart patients (those without major heart damage) would also benefit from such therapy. This question was resolved when the

SPEAKING FROM EXPERIENCE

Doctors today have an impressive array of pharmaceutical weapons to use in the fight against heart disease, but I sometimes worry about the downside. Many people think drugs are magic cures that will solve their cardiovascular problems without any lifestyle effort on their part. They forget that drugs are adjunctive therapies, meaning that they are used *in addition* to, not *instead of,* healthy lifestyle changes. Together, drug therapy and lifestyle changes provide independent and additive benefits.

Consider statins, for instance. These drugs are very effective in lowering LDL cholesterol, but that doesn't mean a person taking them can eat a high-fat diet. That's why drugs come *after* healthy lifestyle changes in our recommendations. **—J.P.**

Heart Outcomes Prevention Evaluation (HOPE) study was stopped before its scheduled conclusion because of overwhelming evidence that ramipril reduced the overall number of cardiovascular problems by a remarkable 22%. Moreover, investigators also found that drug-treated patients developed heart failure and diabetes less often and had fewer interventional procedures, such as coronary bypass surgery and balloon angioplasty.

Beta-Blockers

FORMALLY CALLED BETA-ADRENERGIC BLOCKING AGENTS, THESE drugs are used to treat high blood pressure, relieve angina, abolish heart rhythm irregularities and prevent recurrent heart attacks. Referred to by either their generic names, which commonly end in "ol" (atenolol, metoprolol, nadolol, propranolol, timolol), or their brand names (Tenormin, Lopressor or Toprol, Corgard, Inderal and Blocadren), they work by affecting the response to certain nerve impulses throughout the body. Consequently, they decrease the heart's blood and oxygen requirements by reducing its workload while helping it to maintain a normal rhythm.

Long-term administration of beta-blockers after a heart attack has been unequivocally shown to improve survival rate. In the Beta-Blocker in Heart Attack Trial (BHAT), nearly 4,000 heart attack survivors were followed for an average of 25 months. The first year, mortality for patients who were randomly assigned to receive beta-blocker therapy was reduced by 39%, as compared with mortality for those who received a placebo. However, among one-year survivors, benefit from continued treatment appeared to be largely restricted to those at the highest risk for new or recurrent heart attacks.

Another analysis of 16 major trials, involving more than 18,000 heart attack patients, demonstrated convincingly the therapeutic benefit of starting treatment soon after the cardiac event. Beta-blocker therapy reduced the risk of death by 20% and of recurrent heart attacks by 25%. These percentages were based on all patients, regardless of whether or not they faithfully adhered to their prescribed drug regimen. Accordingly, the benefits may be even greater for compliant and high-risk patients.

Several mechanisms may explain the reduced cardiovascular mortality with long-term beta-blocker therapy after a heart attack. A chief effect of beta-blockers in numerous studies appears to be a reduction in sudden cardiac death, supporting the belief that these drugs combat potentially lethal heart rhythms. Others suggest that the lowering of heart rate and blood pressure may be especially important in reducing the potential for cardiac ischemia (lack of blood to the heart), which has been linked to threatening heart rhythms. Beta-blockers may also lessen the workload of the heart muscle, which may decrease the severity of a heart attack if administered before or soon after the onset of symptoms and reduce the potential for blood clotting.

A recent analysis of numerous clinical trials found that the benefit of beta-blocker therapy after a heart attack is strongly related to the magnitude of reduction in resting heart rate. Each 10-beat-per-minute reduction was found to reduce the relative risk of cardiac death by about 30%.

In summary, beta-blocker therapy can be useful for preventing subsequent heart attacks and potentially fatal rhythm disturbances in heart attack survivors. Patients who may also benefit from these medications include the elderly, individuals with heart failure or lung disease and heart attack survivors who have not undergone coronary bypass surgery or balloon angioplasty.

Combination Drug Therapy

THE PAST DECADE HAS SEEN A NOTABLE INCREASE IN MEDICATIONS with proven effectiveness in reducing nonfatal and fatal cardiovascular events in patients with documented coronary artery disease. These drugs, including antiplatelet agents (e.g., aspirin), statins, beta-blockers and ACE inhibitors, are individually highly effective in reducing recurrent cardiovascular events. However, the impact of the combination of these prescribed medications has not been reported.

Recently, researchers examined the use of these four medications in nearly 1,400 consecutive patients with angina pectoris or acute myocardial infarction (heart attack) who were discharged from the same hospital system and followed for six months. Results indicated that patients taking the greatest number of these drugs generally demonstrated the lowest death rates—when cardioprotective drugs are prescribed together, they may have incremental and even synergistic benefits in appropriate patients. Nevertheless, these drugs continue to be underutilized.

Testing for Coronary Heart Disease

I F ANGINA OR OTHER SYMPTOMS have you worried about coronary heart disease, it makes sense to schedule a physical exam that will evaluate the condition of your heart and arteries. Your doctor will take your family history, listen to your heart, check your blood pressure and pulse, and probably assess your weight and body-fat distribution. You should also have a blood test for total cholesterol, LDL, HDL, triglycerides and glucose.

In addition, because of the latest research, many physicians are now evaluating levels of C-reactive protein and lipoprotein-associated phospholipase A_2 (indicators of arterial inflammation).

In the event that heart disease is suspected, a variety of diagnostic tests may be employed to help analyze your situation. Given the fact that sudden cardiac death is the first sign of heart disease for thousands of people each year, diagnostic tests are becoming increasingly important. Such tests are administered on a progressive basis and can usually be grouped into three levels of sophistication: basic, intermediate and advanced. Promising new tests are also in the works.

Basic Tests

ONE OF THE MOST COMMON DIAGNOSTIC TESTS IS THE CHEST X-RAY. By examining photographs of the chest's interior, the doctor can assess the size of the heart (which could be enlarged due to heart failure), discover certain structural abnormalities and detect fluid in the lungs.

An *electrocardiogram* (ECG) is part of most annual physicals and is recorded while the patient's heart is "at rest." Electrodes attached to the arms, legs and chest allow the doctor to evaluate the electronic impulses given off by the heart and look for evidence of rhythm irregularities, chamber enlargement, ischemia (insufficient blood supply via the coronary arteries) and heart attack. Sometimes ECG readings are taken continuously

For some men, impotence may indicate underlying heart disease. In one study, 50 men were referred to a medical center because the cause of their erectile dysfunction could not be determined. Although none of the men had symptoms, 20 of them had significant coronary artery blockages. Researchers may eventually categorize impotence as a "penile stress test" that can warn of serious heart problems.

over a 24-hour period using a Holter monitor hooked up to chest electrodes. Readings over a period of time can show heart rhythm irregularities and, to a lesser extent, evidence of insufficient blood supply to the heart.

Unfortunately, a resting ECG will not generally disclose a blockage until the artery channel is completely obstructed. When the heart is not under a heavy workload, the ECG results may be "normal" even when the channel is severely blocked, as long as the muscle is getting enough blood to meet its resting oxygen requirements. Only when an artery is severely obstructed and blood flow is impeded to the point where the heart has an insufficient oxygen supply does the ECG show an abnormality. Several years ago, for instance, the mayor of Chicago died of a heart attack as he was leaving his cardiologist's office after an examination in which his resting ECG was normal.

A simple test called the *ankle/brachial blood pressure index* (ABI) measures systolic blood pressure in the upper arm and ankle. If a pressure reading in the ankle is significantly lower than that in the arm, an increased risk of peripheral arterial disease (PAD), or atherosclerosis of the lower extremities, may be indicated. The normal range of ABI values is between 0.90 and 1.30. Progressively lower values are indicative of mild-to-severe PAD. This condition is frequently observed in people with diabetes and a history of cigarette smoking or coronary artery, carotid or renal disease.

Ultrasound tests are noninvasive evaluations that use high-frequency sound waves to create graphic images of the heart's structures, pumping action and blood flow. These tests may also be used to screen for varied cardiovascular abnormalities.

Stroke screening/carotid artery ultrasound. The carotid arteries are the main arteries in the neck that supply blood to the brain. This test screens for possible narrowing and blockages in these blood vessels, which is a major risk factor for stroke.

Abdominal aortic aneurysm ultrasound. An aneurysm is a bulge or weakness in a blood vessel, much like a bulge on an overinflated inner tube. This test screens the aorta, the major blood vessel in the abdomen, for a bulge or weakness—the abnormality that caused the death of actor John Ritter.

Intermediate Tests

IF THE BASIC TESTS SHOW A PROBLEM, OR IF YOUR DOCTOR NEEDS more information, one of the intermediate tests will likely be used. These may include an exercise stress test, pharmacologic (drug) stress or a diagnostic technique called echocardiography.

Exercise Stress Tests

Basically an ECG performed during exercise, usually on a treadmill or stationary bike, the standard exercise stress test evaluates the heart when it's beating more rapidly than when it's at rest. The intensity of the exercise increases as the test progresses, and blood pressure readings are taken at intervals to assess the heart's pumping power when the workload is increased. Often used to evaluate symptoms such as shortness of breath or chest pain, an exercise stress test is successful in detecting coronary heart disease in about 70% of individuals with the disease.

In some cases, it may be important to measure the patient's breathing responses during the exercise test. This methodology, which requires sophisticated equipment, a face mask or mouthpiece, and frequent calibration, may be helpful in differentiating pulmonary from cardiac limitations. It also provides an exact measure of cardiopulmonary fitness, expressed as metabolic equivalents (METs). When a person is at rest, significant blockage of the coronary arteries (generally considered to be 75% or more) may not be severe enough to result in an insufficient delivery of oxygen to the heart muscle. During exercise, however, an impaired blood supply to the heart may cause anginal chest pain, a change in the ECG pattern (called ST-segment depression), or both.

This test provides a very good diagnostic and prognostic tool, particularly for middle-aged men. Doctors have even found it to be effective in identifying men with silent cardiac ischemia, in which coronary arteries are narrowed and blood flow is diminished but no angina or other symptoms are present. Studies have found that men who have silent ischemia and other risk factors (such as high cholesterol, high blood pressure and smoking) have four to six times the risk of heart attack. By identifying the increased likelihood of disease with an exercise stress test, additional diagnostic studies (such as thallium or cardiolite stress testing and/or cardiac catheterization) can be used to clarify the location and extent of coronary blockages so that preventive action can be taken.

There is one note of caution, however. Exercise stress tests are not always predictive, especially for young men and women or for middle-aged women. These tests fail to detect slight coronary blockages, whereas most heart attacks are due to mild-to-moderate plaque rupture. Consequently, an exercise stress test with or without imaging can be normal despite the presence of coronary plaque that may rupture. More often, exercise tests suggest coronary heart disease when it does not exist; this is called a false-positive result and is associated with young women in particular. Nonetheless, these tests provide an enormously powerful prognostic tool, especially when taking fitness and non-ECG measures into account.

An exercise stress test with *myocardial perfusion imaging* permits doctors to observe the manner in which blood moves through the vessels and is taken up by the heart. A small amount of thallium or cardiolite is injected intravenously while the patient is near maximal exercise on a treadmill and the heart is being "stressed." Immediately after the test, an X-ray scan is taken and compared with another scan taken while the heart is at rest. This test can reveal inactive scar tissue (the result of a previous heart attack) and areas deprived of oxygen due to reduced blood flow. By examining these images, doctors can pinpoint potential sites of coronary artery blockages.

Patients who are limited in their ability to exercise may benefit from *pharmacologic stress testing,* which uses medication such as dobutamine to increase heart rate or persantine to dilate coronary arteries. This form of testing is associated with an accuracy of 85% to 90% in detecting significant coronary blockages.

Positron emission tomography (PET) scans use radioactive tracers to create three-dimensional pictures of the heart. This test can determine

RECOVERY HEART RATE:
A VALUABLE PROGNOSTIC INDICATOR

An exercise stress test is also a good way to give doctors a look at their patients' heart recovery rate, or how much the heartbeat slows after they have exercised to exhaustion and then recovered.

Normally the maximal heart rate drops between 15 and 25 beats soon after exhaustive exercise, but researchers discovered that for people whose heart rate falls 12 beats or less at one minute after exercising, the risk of dying within six years is four times greater.

whether there is adequate blood flow to the heart and the amount of damage to the heart after a heart attack. During a PET scan, an electrocardiogram is monitored continuously, and an intravenous (IV) line is inserted into a vein in the arm while the patient lies on an exam table under a camera. A radioactive tracer (rubidium) and a medication to cause the heart to react as if the patient were exercising (dipyridamole) are then injected into the IV, followed by a small additional amount of rubidium, to allow the physician to view the blood flow to the heart muscle while it is under stress.

Radionuclide ventriculography traces a nuclear isotope that has been injected into the patient's bloodstream. During exercise, the patient pedals a stationary bike in the supine, upright or semi-upright position while X-ray pictures are taken to determine how much of the isotope is being pumped out of the heart's ventricles during each beat. Taken at varied angles, the pictures can also measure chamber volume, evaluate the heart's pumping function and identify wall motion abnormalities. An advantage of this noninvasive technique is that it is highly accurate in detecting the presence of coronary artery disease. Moreover, it can be used serially to evaluate the effects of medication, balloon angioplasty and bypass surgery.

Echocardiography

Used more and more these days to provide additional diagnostic information, echocardiography relies on a recording sensor to bounce ultrasound waves off the heart to create an image of the muscle at work.

Echocardiography can show areas of the heart that have been damaged by a heart attack. It can also be combined with a stress test to reveal wall motion abnormalities, which can indicate areas of the heart that are not receiving enough blood.

An echocardiograph can also measure the ejection fraction—a key indicator in determining the health and function of the heart. Ejection fraction is the percentage of blood pumped out of the left ventricle, the heart's main pumping chamber, with each heartbeat. Normal values range from 50% to 66%, which means that over half of the blood that fills the left ventricle is pumped out to the body with each contraction. On the other hand, a major heart attack can reduce the ejection fraction to 35% or less.

Advanced Testing

CORONARY ANGIOGRAPHY, ALSO CALLED CARDIAC CATHETERIZATION, is the definitive "gold standard" test for coronary heart disease. First, a thin plastic tube called a catheter is inserted into an artery in the leg or arm and threaded into the heart. Then a dye is injected into the catheter. As the dye flows through the coronary arteries, each of which is only

---

SPEAKING FROM EXPERIENCE

I was apprehensive going in for my angiogram—after all, this was an invasive procedure—but the medical team explained what was happening step by step and that relaxed me. I was awake and alert the whole time. I expected some pain when the catheter was inserted, but all I felt was a slight pressure.

I really couldn't feel any of the catheter's movement as it was threaded into my heart. There was a feeling of sudden heat, like a hot flash, when the dye was released, but it lasted only a moment or two. What allowed me to keep my mind off the physical aspects of the procedure was the fact that I could watch what was happening on a monitor. I could identify the arteries, see when the dye was released and, unfortunately, pinpoint the place where the artery narrowed and I had a problem. It was this test that convinced me to have bypass surgery.   **—J.P.**

---

about the size of a strand of cooked spaghetti, the doctor can identify and assess narrow spots and blockages via X-ray imaging.

Its ability to show specific sites of narrowing makes angiography a key diagnostic technique when evaluating the need for balloon angioplasty or bypass surgery.

Newer Diagnostic/Screening Tests

COMPUTED TOMOGRAPHY (CT) IS ALSO BEING USED TO FIND EARLY coronary heart disease by detecting calcium in the coronary arteries. Calcium deposits, believed to be by-products of inflammation and precursors of artery blockages, are considered predictors of increased risk of heart disease and stroke, especially in persons with multiple risk factors. One study showed that patients whose calcium buildup increased 20% or more each year had an 18-fold greater chance of suffering a heart attack than those with less calcium in the heart. Thus if the CT scan shows a large amount of calcium, a narrowing of the coronary artery is suggested. However, because certain forms of heart disease (e.g., "vulnerable plaque" atherosclerosis) escape detection during this CT scan, the accuracy of this test in predicting your risk for life-threatening cardiac events, such as a heart attack, remains imperfect.

Another tomographic test, called *electron-beam computed tomography* (EBCT), is 10 times faster than the standard CT scan and therefore capable of producing a rapid evaluation of calcium deposits in the coronary arteries. Cardiac CT uses advanced technology with intravenous contrast dye to visualize the coronary arteries. During the test, the patient lies on a table that moves inside a doughnut-shaped scanner. In a study by Dr. Harvey Hecht, published in the *Journal of the American College of Cardiology,* 304 women underwent both cholesterol testing and EBCT scans. The results showed that cholesterol screening failed to identify nearly half the women over age 55 who exhibited scans showing calcified plaque; in women under 55, cholesterol screening failed about 40% of the time.

Several years ago, Dr. Paolo Raggi and associates studied 632 symptom-free patients with coronary risk factors who were screened by EBCT and followed for an average of 32 months for the development of cardiac events (heart attack or sudden cardiac death). Their results showed that calcium scores of zero were associated with an event rate of 0.1% per year; in contrast, the annualized event rate was 2.1% for scores of 1 to 99, 4.1% for scores of 100 to 400 and 4.8% for scores over 400. Interestingly, calcification scores above 100 were associated with cardiac event rates that were higher than those of patients with known coronary heart disease. The investigators concluded that the risk of subsequent cardiac problems is greatly increased in the presence of coronary artery calcification.

While CT and EBCT scans are reliable, most experts believe they are not for everyone. "Because calcium deposits do not automatically lead to heart disease in all cases, it is too soon to recommend widespread screening," says Dr. Carlos Iribarren, a researcher at Kaiser Permanente. Other authorities emphasize that coronary plaque with calcium is generally mature, more stable and not prone to rupture. In addition, coronary calcification is found in virtually all men older than 60 and women over 70. If you have two or more cardiac risk factors but no symptoms, the test may be useful in evaluating your condition. However, the benefit of routine screening for heart disease with EBCT remains unproven.

Computed tomography angiograms (coronary CTAs) help determine whether significant plaque deposits have built up in the coronary

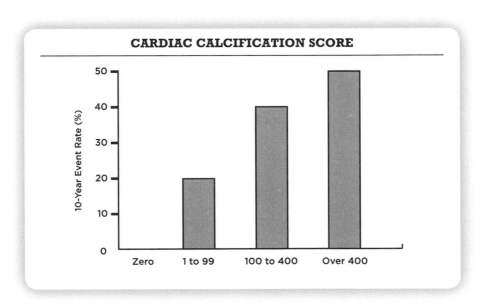

CARDIAC CALCIFICATION SCORE

arteries. A coronary CTA is derived from a special type of X-ray examination in which the patient receives an iodine-containing contrast dye via an intravenous line to ensure the sharpest images possible. Medications to slow or stabilize the patient's heart rate and rhythm may also be used for better imaging results. During the examination, which usually takes about 10 minutes, X-rays passing through the body are picked up by special detectors in the scanner. Typically, higher numbers of these detectors result in clearer final images, so coronary CTAs are often referred to as "multi-slice" CT scanning (e.g., 64-slice CT). These faster scanners are now able to take images of the coronary arteries that are nearly comparable to those taken during a heart catheterization.

This new technology has consistently shown the ability to detect not only significant coronary blockages but early subclinical coronary artery disease (e.g., nonobstructive plaques) that may potentially be treated with appropriate lifestyle changes and/or drug therapy. Recent studies also suggest that these evaluations may be helpful in clarifying the need for advanced diagnostic testing in patients presenting with chest pain at hospital emergency departments. Critics, however, point out that coronary CTAs are not quite as accurate in detecting disease in the smaller heart artery branches, and that certain patient subsets (those who are extremely overweight or who have abnormal heart rhythms) may not be suitable candidates for this test because imaging quality may be compromised. Others have expressed concerns regarding the associated radiation exposure. According to a just-published multicenter study, heart scans on average expose patients to radiation equivalent to getting 600 chest X-rays at once. The researchers cautioned that such levels could raise your cancer risk.

Finally, *intravascular ultrasound* (IVUS) is increasingly used to detect unstable coronary lesions, those most likely to rupture and clot. IVUS is similar to a cardiac catheterization in that a long, thin tube is threaded into the coronary arteries. However, the tube carries an ultrasound probe at its tip to take sonar pictures from inside the artery. The images show the amount of plaque, its shape and composition, and to what extent it has infiltrated the channel opening as well as the artery wall. Accordingly, IVUS allows the doctor to view the artery from the inside out; in other words, the doughnut itself, rather than just the hole in the doughnut.

Revascularization Treatments for Coronary Heart Disease

F HEART DISEASE IS DIAGNOSED, your doctor may recommend a number of options including medications (such as nitroglycerin to reduce angina, statin drugs to lower cholesterol or aspirin therapy), a low-fat diet, an exercise program, stress management techniques and smoking cessation. In addition, depending on your symptoms and/or the severity of the disease, you may be a candidate for coronary revascularization.

Balloon Angioplasty

THE MOST COMMON REVASCULARIZATION PROCEDURE IS BALLOON angioplasty, also called percutaneous transluminal coronary angioplasty (PTCA). In 2006, for example, according to data provided by the American Heart Association, 1.3 million coronary angioplasty procedures were performed. In this procedure, a small, flexible catheter is inserted in an artery of the leg or arm and then threaded through the arterial system into the coronary arteries. Using X-rays as a guide, the cardiologist can move the catheter into the narrowed spot.

Next, a second catheter with a tiny balloon on its tip goes through the first catheter. When this catheter reaches the clogged artery, its balloon is inflated. The balloon gently pushes the fatty plaque against the arterial wall, thus opening the artery so blood can flow more easily. At this point, the balloon and catheters are taken out. Angioplasty takes an hour or two and is done under local anesthesia. Not everyone is a candidate for this procedure; in some cases, blockages are so tortuous or severe that it cannot be performed.

In stretching the walls of the coronary arteries, the balloon catheter may cause slight arterial injuries. Unfortunately, such injuries can promote the formation of blood clots. In 4% to 12% of procedures, clot-related complications occur. To reduce this likelihood, anticoagulant drugs such as aspirin, heparin and clopidogrel (Plavix) are used during and after balloon angioplasty.

Early on, this procedure had a high failure rate and often had to be repeated. But in 1994 the Food and Drug Administration approved the use of the Palmaz-Schatz stent, a tiny, flexible cylinder designed to prevent the collapse of a vessel that has been opened. Made of stainless steel, the mesh-like stent provides support and serves as a kind of scaffolding to keep the artery open. Although they are now the workhorses in this cardiac procedure, scar tissue forms at the sites of up to 30% of these stents and the blood vessel clogs or narrows again, a condition known as restenosis.

Researchers such as Dr. Gregory Chapman at the University of Alabama at Birmingham believe that this Achilles' heel of angioplasty

REPEAT REVASCULARIZATIONS

In 2001, as Vice President Dick Cheney recuperated after doctors once again unblocked a coronary artery, questions resurfaced about high-tech treatments and their effectiveness. Cheney has had four heart attacks (the first three decades ago), a quadruple bypass operation and two balloon angioplasties, yet his cardiac history is not that unusual. About 1.3 million angioplasties are performed each year. Bypass surgery is done nearly 450,000 times annually. Many are repeats.

These numbers teach us a sobering lesson: The vessels used to bypass blocked coronary arteries may close, other coronary arteries can become clogged or scar tissue may form at a metal stent implanted to reopen an artery—as was the case with the vice president. Each of these can jeopardize the heart, causing symptoms or new events to occur.

Fortunately, aggressive medical treatment in combination with lifestyle changes can slow, halt and sometimes even reverse the progression of heart disease.

has been overcome by coating stents with sirolimus, a drug that prevents restenosis. Indeed numerous trials now support the value of drug-eluting stents. In one study of patients who had undergone drug-eluting stenting, tests after a period of four months revealed no restenosis; after eight months, none of the patients had suffered a heart attack or stroke and none needed a second angioplasty. Stents are now being used routinely in emergency situations to open up blocked coronary arteries during heart attacks.

Several studies have also shown that acute heart attack patients fare better with angioplasty, especially when it's followed by selected anticlotting drugs (clopidogrel and aspirin), than with clot-busting drugs known as thrombolytic therapy.

Angioplasty vs. Optimal Medical Therapy

Although coronary angioplasty is known to improve survival when done to restore blood flow during a heart attack, until recently no study had examined the ability of coronary angioplasty to improve outcomes over and above modern, optimal medical therapy in coronary patients with or without anginal symptoms. This question was addressed when the results of the Clinical Outcomes Utilizing Revascularization and Aggressive Drug Evaluation (COURAGE) were published in the *New England Journal of Medicine* (April 2007).

Researchers enrolled 2,287 patients with known heart disease at 50 hospitals in the United States and Canada, randomizing them to one of two treatment groups: angioplasty (to "fix" existing coronary blockages) plus optimal medical therapy or optimal medical therapy alone. Thus, both groups received aggressive medical therapy, which included an array of medications designed to reduce symptoms and achieve recommended cholesterol and blood pressure levels, as well as lifestyle programs such as smoking cessation, exercise, weight management and nutritional counseling. Enrolled patients had signs and/or symptoms of insufficient coronary blood flow and at least a 70% blockage of one or more coronary arteries.

Over a follow-up period averaging nearly five years, a total of 211 deaths or nonfatal heart attacks (the primary focus of COURAGE) occurred in the coronary angioplasty group (19%), compared with 202 in the medical therapy group (18.5%), a statistically nonsignificant difference. When stroke and hospitalizations for anginal symptoms were examined, again no differences were seen between groups. On the other hand, the angioplasty group reported fewer anginal symptoms during the trial. The investigators concluded that as an initial management strategy in patients with stable heart disease, elective coronary angioplasty did not reduce the risk of death, heart attack or other major cardiovascular events when added to optimal medical therapy.

Two recent separate analyses of the randomized trials conducted to date, comparing coronary angioplasty with medical management in patients who had stable coronary artery disease, came to differing conclusions. One found no significant differences between the two treatment strategies, whereas the other favored the angioplasty group. On the other hand, two just-published studies concluded that drugs and heart bypass surgery protected patients better than artery-opening angioplasty with stenting.

Late Angioplasty and Stenting

According to several recent major trials, coronary angioplasty plus stenting failed to further reduce major cardiovascular events or improve heart function in patients who had the intervention 3 to 28 days after a heart attack. These findings could lead to lower rates of unnecessary coronary procedures in stable patients, which could also result in substantial health care cost savings.

Early treatment of heart attacks remains a critically important therapy. *Remember:* Time is muscle.

Bypass Surgery

FOR MULTIPLE BLOCKAGES, TYPICAL IN PEOPLE SUFFERING FROM severe coronary heart disease, coronary artery bypass graft (CABG, pronounced "cabbage") may be recommended. Although bypass surgery is performed about a half-million times a year, it remains a major, expensive operation and is not without potential complications such as heart attack and stroke. The surgery involves cutting open the breastbone, prying apart the rib cage and stopping the exposed heart as the the blood vessels are reconfigured to reroute blood flow to the heart.

The bypass procedure typically takes three to six hours. The surgeon harvests a vein from the leg or an artery from the chest and attaches one end of the blood vessel to the aorta. The other end is attached to the coronary artery below the point where it is clogged. This creates a new arterial channel that will allow blood to flow freely to the heart. Literally bypassing the blocked area, the procedure has a high long-term success rate, especially when a chest artery is used.

SPEAKING FROM EXPERIENCE

Bypass surgery probably saved my life, but people considering this procedure should be aware of four things. To start with, it's designed to take away the pain of restricted blood flow, yet it does not take away the underlying cause—coronary heart disease—even though it may put you in a better position to bring about the lifestyle changes that are needed to stabilize and potentially reverse the disease.

Second, a bypass doesn't necessarily last forever. If you don't take care of it by adopting a healthy lifestyle, you might get just a few years out of it. Third, the physical recovery can be daunting. I had some complications, so it took me about six months to regain my strength and stamina. Others have done it sooner.

Finally, you have to be prepared for mental changes. According to a study at Duke University, about 42% of bypass patients experience a subtle change in personality and suffer an impairment of memory and cognitive abilities five years after surgery. At my seminars, I've had wives of bypass patients tell me, "This is not the man I married. His personality is different." Further studies are needed to determine the importance of such changes to real-world behavior. However, many physicians hypothesize that these results are more often found in patients who have undergone bypass surgery while on the heart-lung machine, particularly if the operation takes over four hours.   **—J.P.**

Minimally invasive direct coronary artery bypass surgery is a newer, gentler technique that allows for a less invasive approach to bypassing blocked coronary arteries. Instead of opening the chest and working on a heart that is stopped, the surgeon operates with fiberoptic scopes through small incisions between the ribs to work directly on the beating heart.

For this reason, the procedure is sometimes called keyhole surgery. No heart-lung machine is used. This procedure avoids the massive chest damage inflicted by open-heart surgery and reduces pain, recovery time and expense.

Emerging Interventional Techniques

A NUMBER OF INNOVATIVE PROCEDURES ARE BEING USED ON A limited basis. Although much more experience needs to be gained in the use of these techniques before they become as common as angioplasty and bypass surgery, many doctors believe them to be the wave of the future.

Radiation Therapy

One of the ongoing problems in coronary revascularization is that in a significant number of patients who undergo balloon angioplasty, the arteries close up again within six months after the procedure. Although the use of drug-eluting stents has helped, up to 30% of stented vessels are closed due to restenosis at the six-month mark. Many doctors feel that radiation therapy used as a complement to angioplasty may be the answer. That's because radiation inhibits cell growth (as it does with cancer).

In this procedure, tiny radioactive pellets are sent through a catheter to the blockage in the artery and then held in place for several minutes to deliver a dose of radiation before being retrieved. The radiation inhibits scar tissue that could result in subsequent restenosis. A pilot study involving 24 patients showed almost no narrowing of blood vessels six months after angioplasty. Broader studies have confirmed the technology, which is now being applied on a larger scale in the United States.

Off-Pump Coronary Artery Bypass

In conventional open-heart bypass surgery, doctors work on a heart that has been stopped. The job of circulating oxygen-rich blood throughout the body is performed by the heart-lung machine, which slightly raises the risk of complications such as mental impairment. Using the off-pump coronary artery bypass (OPCAB) technique, surgeons open the chest as in normal bypass surgery but operate on the beating heart without the use of the heart-lung machine. A special tool restrains the section of the heart being worked on. While potential complications may be minimized, OPCAB is more difficult to perform than conventional surgery.

The objective of OPCAB is to decrease the complications of conventional coronary artery bypass surgery, which uses a heart-lung machine to maintain circulation, while the surgeon operates on a heart that has stopped beating. Also of great interest is the possibility that the OPCAB may lessen the risk of adverse cognitive changes, including memory loss, with conventional heart surgery. A recent study conducted at the Cleveland Clinic concluded that both on- and off-pump surgery had very low rates of death, stroke and heart attack. However, the off-pump patients had fewer cognitive side effects, less kidney failure and fewer infections of chest incisions. The researchers concluded that patients at high risk for complications from bypass surgery may benefit the most from OPCAB.

Angiogenesis

The process called angiogenesis involves implanting tiny "growth factor" capsules in the walls of the heart to spur the growth of new blood vessels. While still in the experimental stage, several clinical trials are under way to assess its potential. Other recent studies have transplanted specialized bone marrow cells into hearts with inadequate blood and oxygen supply in an effort to stimulate angiogenesis. It could be particularly important for people with arteries so diseased that angioplasty and bypass surgery have been ruled out.

"We *can* grow new vessels," says Dr. Michael Simons at the Yale School of Medicine. "But at this stage we're still groping our way through, trying to figure out the biology."

Cardiac Rehabilitation Programs

WHETHER YOU'RE WORKING to prevent heart disease or facing treatment after a heart attack, bypass surgery or angioplasty, the approach is very similar. Both instances call for addressing the underlying causes of heart disease: hypertension, cigarette smoking, high-fat diets, obesity, diabetes, unbridled stress and a sedentary lifestyle. Current thinking holds that multifactoral risk factor modification using diet, drugs and exercise may slow, halt or even reverse the progression of heart disease.

Such modification is often fairly simple to achieve before a cardiac event takes place. There is no great pressure for immediate change, so you can gradually ease into an exercise program or trade your double burger for a healthier chicken sandwich. But it's not the same for those who have experienced a heart attack or who have been diagnosed with coronary heart disease. Making lifestyle changes is often very difficult. In addition to confusion over what to do and how to do it, as well as fear about future health, there often is an added burden: the belief that total change must take place immediately. This can produce such mental stress that the heart patient becomes immobilized and accomplishes nothing.

Cardiac rehabilitation programs can help. Designed to provide a mix of education and action in a supportive environment, they make it easier for patients to take charge of their lifestyle habits and achieve a better quality of life. Moreover, rehab staff members provide doctors with valuable ongoing surveillance data (e.g., unusual shortness of breath, heart rhythm irregularities and the development of new anginal symptoms), enabling them to better medically manage their patients. Most programs define themselves as being in the business of "helping patients to help themselves."

Rehabilitation Basics

THE OBJECTIVES OF CARDIAC REHABILITATION ARE TO INCREASE physical fitness, decrease symptoms, stop cigarette smoking, modify cholesterol and other lipids, decrease body weight and body fat, reduce blood pressure and generally improve psychosocial well-being. To those ends, contemporary programs offer a menu of services to meet individual needs. And in order to accomplish their objectives, structured programs are generally staffed by a mix of health professionals: doctors, cardiac nurse specialists, exercise physiologists, dietitians and behavior therapists. However, home-based rehabilitation guided by health professionals has been shown to be an effective alternative to group programs.

Cardiac rehabilitation programs are generally based on three to four phases:

- *Phase I*, called the inpatient phase, takes place while the patient is still hospitalized following a heart attack or bypass surgery and includes low-level walking, self-care activities and intermittent sitting or standing. Risk factors, post-hospital medical care, medications and limitations are discussed with the patient and his or her family as they receive support and insight into what the future holds for them.

- *Phase II* is the beginning of outpatient cardiac rehabilitation, usually lasting from 4 to 12 weeks. During this time, the patient starts a formal, ECG-monitored rehabilitation program under the direction of the cardiac rehabilitation medical team. Exercise conducted during this

---

SPEAKING FROM EXPERIENCE

When I had my bypass surgery in 1977, I didn't go to rehab. It wasn't available at the time, so I just went home and tried to make the best of it. My questions about which exercises I should do, how to change my diet or manage stress went unanswered—until I started investigating these topics on my own.

Cardiac patients and their families should not be in that situation. I tell patients to be proactive with their doctors about getting into a cardiac rehab program, where they'll receive information, instruction, exercise therapy, ongoing medical surveillance and support. **—J.P.**

phase (usually on a treadmill or an exercise bike) not only gets the patient moving again (albeit gently) but also provides the team with information for determining the patient's clinical status and establishing guidelines for further exercise.

- *Phase III* usually lasts three to six months. In addition to increased exercise, the patient receives counseling on risk factor modification, stress management and diet. Phase III rehabilitation normally involves the safe incremental progression of exercise together with other important lifestyle interventions. Patients usually participate in 50-to-60-minute exercise sessions up to three times a week. In addition, they are encouraged to increase physical activity in daily living. A pedometer can be helpful in achieving this objective.

- *Phase IV* consists of the exercise a patient will do for the rest of his or her life, either in a medically supervised setting or on an informal (i.e., home-based) basis. Specific exercises are up to the patient: treadmill, stair-climber, rowing machine, weight lifting, pool activities, aerobic dance or less standardized routines.

Issues Regarding Rehabilitation Effectiveness and Utilization

UNTIL RECENTLY, THE MOST COMPELLING EVIDENCE TO SUPPORT the benefits of cardiac rehabilitation came from analyses, using survey data from the 1980s, of heart attack survivors (primarily middle-aged men) who had undergone exercise-based rehabilitation programs. It has been suggested, however, that these results cannot necessarily be extrapolated to patients who have had bypass graft surgery, coronary angioplasty, or both. Another view holds that the availability of emergent coronary revascularization procedures and cardioprotective drugs unavailable at the time of these earlier trials may serve to diminish the impact of cardiac rehabilitation programs on modern-day patients.

To clarify these issues, Dr. Rod Taylor and his associates at the University of Birmingham in England conducted an analysis of 48 randomized trials of cardiac rehabilitation of six months or more. The study population included nearly 9,000 patients, including a significant number of women and older adults, and individuals who had undergone coronary revascularization procedures, as compared with the earlier analyses. Compared with usual care, cardiac rehabilitation reduced total and cardiac mortality by 20% and 26%, respectively, with no difference across a number of patient subgroups. Importantly, the beneficial effect of exercise-based cardiac rehabilitation on total mortality was independent of whether the trial was published before or after 1995, suggesting that the mortality benefits of cardiac rehabilitation persist in modern cardiology.

Despite these impressive outcomes, a recent report found low national utilization rates of cardiac rehabilitation. Overall, cardiac rehabilitation was used in only 14% of Medicare beneficiaries who survived a heart attack and in 31% of patients who underwent coronary artery bypass surgery. In an accompanying editorial, Dr. Randal Thomas wrote: "This study is a wake-up call to all providers of cardiovascular health care to find solutions to this problem to help our patients maneuver more safely through the whitewater rapids of the rehabilitative and preventive stages of post–coronary heart disease event care. We have been missing this boat for too long. It is time for us all to find better ways to help our patients climb aboard."

SPEAKING FROM EXPERIENCE

Several years ago, I counseled a new patient in our cardiac rehab program. Bill, a 48-year-old truck driver in good physical condition, had recently experienced a mild heart attack. His face was racked with anxiety and depression—he clearly thought his life was over and that he was on "borrowed time."

I reviewed his medical records and found that his ejection fraction after the heart attack was still within the normal range, at 50%. His fitness from a post–heart attack exercise stress test was 12.5 METs, high for a healthy man his age. Thus, two key prognostic indicators were in his favor! "If you take care of yourself, I think you've got another 30-plus years ahead of you," I told him.

Heart patients often assume the worst. We've got to do a better job in promoting hope and optimism. Today, many coronary patients live perfectly normal life spans. Others even exceed the longevity of friends and family members.   —B.F.

Sources, Credits and Websites

1. Selected Sources

Aboa-Eboulé, C., et al. "Job Strain and Risk of Acute Recurrent Coronary Heart Disease Events." *Journal of the American Medical Association* (October 2007).

Ades, P.A. "Cardiac Rehabilitation and Secondary Prevention of Coronary Heart Disease." *New England Journal of Medicine* (September 2001).

Albert, C.M., et al. "Effect of Folic Acid and B Vitamins on Risk of Cardiovascular Events and Total Mortality Among Women at High Risk for Cardiovascular Disease. A Randomized Trial." *Journal of the American Medical Association* (May 2008).

American Heart Association. "Revised Dietary Guidelines." *Circulation* (October 2000).

———— *Heart Disease and Stroke Statistics*, 2007 update.

Anderson, J.L., et al. "Plasma Homocysteine Predicts Mortality Independently of Traditional Risk Factors." *Circulation* (September 2000).

Andrews, T.O., et al. "Effect of Cholesterol Reduction on Myocardial Ischemia in Patients with Coronary Disease." *Circulation* (January 1997).

Appel, L.J., et al. "Dietary Approaches to Prevent and Treat Hypertension. A Scientific Statement from the American Heart Association." *Hypertension* (February 2006).

Armstrong, M.L., et al. "Regression of Coronary Atherosclerosis in Rhesus Monkeys." *Circulation Research* (1959).

Arruda-Olson, A.M., et al. "Cardiovascular Effects of Sildenafil During Exercise in Men with Known or Probable Coronary Artery Disease. A Randomized Crossover Trial." *Journal of the American Medical Association* (February 2002).

Ballantyne, C.M., et al. "Lipoprotein-Associated Phospholipase A_2, High-Sensitivity C-Reactive Protein, and Risk for Incident Coronary Heart Disease in Middle-Aged Men and Women in the Atherosclerosis Risk in Communities (ARIC) Study." *Circulation* (February 2004).

Barefoot, J.C., et al. "Symptoms of Depression, Acute Myocardial Infarction, and Total Mortality." *Circulation* (May 1996).

Barnard, R.J., et al. "Effects of Intensive Diet and Exercise Intervention in Patients Taking Cholesterol-Lowering Drugs." *American Journal of Cardiology* (April 1997).

Bassett, D.R., et al. "Physical Activity in an Old Order Amish Community." *Medicine and Science in Sports and Exercise* (January 2004).

Baylin, A., et al. "Adipose Tissue α-Linolenic Acid and Nonfatal Acute Myocardial Infarction in Costa Rica." *Circulation* (April 2003).

Blair, S.N., et al. "Influences of Cardiorespiratory Fitness and Other Precursors on Cardiovascular Disease and All-Cause Mortality in Men and Women." *Journal of the American Medical Association* (July 1996).

Blankenhorn, D., et al. "The Influence of Diet on the Appearance of New Lesions in Human Coronary Arteries." *Journal of the American Medical Association* (October 1990).

Blumenthal, J.A., et al. "Effects of Exercise and Stress Management Training on Markers of Cardiovascular Risk in Patients with Ischemic Heart Disease. A Randomized Controlled Trial." *Journal of the American Medical Association* (April 2005).

Boden, W.E., et al. "Optimal Medical Therapy with or without PCI for Stable Coronary Disease." *New England Journal of Medicine* (April 2007).

Bonaa, K.H., et al. "Homocysteine Lowering and Cardiovascular Events after Acute Myocardial Infarction." *New England Journal of Medicine* (April 2006).

Bonetti, P.O., et al. "Enhanced External Counterpulsation Improves Endothelial Function in Patients with Symptomatic Coronary Artery Disease." *Journal of the American College of Cardiology* (May 2003).

Bravata, D.M., et al. "Using Pedometers to Increase Physical Activity and Improve Health. A Systematic Review." *Journal of the American Medical Association* (November 2007).

Brown, A.G., et al. "Regression of Coronary Artery Disease as a Result of Intensive Lipid-Lowering Therapy in Men with High Levels of Apolipoprotein B." *New England Journal of Medicine* (March 1990).

Brown, L., et al. "Cholesterol-Lowering Effects of Dietary Fiber." *American Journal of Clinical Nutrition* (July 1999).

Campos, H., et al. "α-Linolenic Acid and Risk of Nonfatal Acute Myocardial Infarction." *Circulation* (July 2008).

Cannon, C.P., et al. "Intensive Versus Moderate Lipid Lowering with Statins After Acute Coronary Syndromes." *New England Journal of Medicine* (April 2004).

Case, R.B., et al. "Living Alone After Myocardial Infarction: Impact on Prognosis." *Journal of the American Medical Association* (January 1992).

Chiuve, S.E., et al. "Healthy Lifestyle Factors in the Primary Prevention of Coronary Heart Disease Among Men. Benefits Among Users and Nonusers of Lipid-Lowering and Antihypertensive Medications." *Circulation* (July 2006).

Cucherat, M. "Quantitative Relationship Between Resting Heart Rate Reduction and Magnitude of Clinical Benefits in Post-Myocardial Infarction: A Meta-Regression of Randomized Clinical Trials." *European Heart Journal* (December 2007).

Dalen, J.E. "Aspirin to Prevent Heart Attack and Stroke: What's the Right Dose?" *American Journal of Medicine* (March 2006).

Danesh, J., et al. "Association of Fibrinogen with Coronary Heart Disease." *Journal of the American Medical Association* (May 1998).

——— et al. "Low-Grade Inflammation and Coronary Heart Disease." *British Medical Journal* (July 2000).

——— et al. "Lipoprotein(a) and Risk of Myocardial Infarction." *Circulation* (September 2000).

Dansky, H.M., and Fisher, E.A. "High-Density Lipoprotein and Plaque Regression." *Circulation* (November 1999).

Davidson, M.H., Guest Editor. "Omega-3 Fatty Acids and Cardiovascular Disease Reduction." *American Journal of Cardiology* (August 2006).

———. "Advances in the Detection of Rupture-Prone Plaque: The Role of Lipoprotein-Associated Phospholipase A_2 in Cardiovascular Risk Assessment." *American Journal of Cardiology* (June 2008).

Daviglus, M.L., et al. "Fish Consumption and the 30-Year Risk of Fatal Myocardial Infarction." *New England Journal of Medicine* (April 1997).

De Feyter, P.J., and Van Pelt, N. "Spiral Computer Tomography Coronary Angiography. A New Diagnostic Tool Developing Its Role in Clinical Cardiology." *Journal of the American College of Cardiology* (February 2007).

Despres, J.P., et al. "Hyperinsulinemia as an Independent Risk Factor for Ischemic Heart Disease." *New England Journal of Medicine* (April 1996).

Dhingra, R., et al. "Soft Drink Consumption and Risk of Developing Cardiometabolic Risk Factors and the Metabolic Syndrome in Middle-Aged Adults in the Community." *Circulation* (July 2007).

Diabetes Prevention Program Research Group. "Reduction in the Incidence of Type 2 Diabetes with Lifestyle Intervention or Metformin." *New England Journal of Medicine* (February 2002).

Dimsdale, J.E. "Psychological Stress and Cardiovascular Disease." *Journal of the American College of Cardiology* (April 2008).

Doll, R., et al. "Mortality in Relation to Smoking: 50 Years' Observations on Male British Doctors." *British Medical Journal* (June 2004).

Dunn, A.L., et al. "Comparison of Lifestyle and Structured Interventions to Increase Physical Activity and Cardiorespiratory Fitness." *Journal of the American Medical Association* (January 1999).

Dupuis, J., et al. "Cholesterol Reduction Rapidly Improves Endothelial Function." *Circulation* (June 1999).

Dutcher, J.R., et al. "Comparison of Left Ventricular Ejection Fraction and Exercise Capacity as Predictors of Two- and Five-Year Mortality Following Acute Myocardial Infarction." *American Journal of Cardiology* (February 2007).

Džavík, V., et al. "Randomized Trial of Percutaneous Coronary Intervention for Subacute Infarct-Related Coronary Artery Occlusion to Achieve Long-Term Patency and Improve Ventricular Function. The Total Occlusion Study of Canada (TOSCA-2 Trial)." *Circulation* (December 2006).

Eckel, R.H., et al. "Understanding the Complexity of *Trans* Fatty Acid Reduction in the American Diet. American Heart Association *Trans* Fat Conference 2006. Report of the *Trans* Fat Conference Planning Group." *Circulation* (April 2007).

Enas, E.A. "Triglycerides and Small, Dense Low-Density Lipoprotein." *Journal of the American Medical Association* (December 1998).

Ford, E.S., et al. "Explaining the Decrease in U.S. Deaths from Coronary Disease, 1980–2000." *New England Journal of Medicine* (January 2007).

Forrester, J.S., and Prediman, K.S. "Lipid Lowering Versus Revascularization." *Circulation* (August 1997).

Franklin, B.A. "Psychosocial Considerations in Heart Disease." *Journal of the Hong Kong College of Cardiology* (February 2001).

———. "Coronary Revascularization and Medical Management of Coronary Artery Disease: Changing Paradigms and Perceptions." *European Journal of Cardiovascular Prevention and Rehabilitation* (October 2006).

Franklin, B.A., and Vanhecke, T.E. "Counseling Patients to Make Cardioprotective Lifestyle Changes: Strategies for Success." *Preventive Cardiology* (Winter 2008).

Franklin, B.A., and Gordon, N.F., *Contemporary Diagnosis and Management in Cardiovascular Exercise* (1st edition). Newtown, Pennsylvania: Handbooks in Health Care Company, January 2009.

Franklin, Barry A., et al. "Cardiac Demands of Heavy Snow Shoveling." *Journal of the American Medical Association* (March 1995).

———. "Avoiding Repeat Cardiac Events: The ABCDE's of Tertiary Prevention." *The Physician and Sportsmedicine* (September 2000).

———. "New Insights in Preventive Cardiology and Cardiac Rehabilitation." *Current Opinion in Cardiology* (September 2008).

Frasure-Smith, N., et al. "Social Support, Depression, and Mortality During the First Year After Myocardial Infarction." *Circulation* (April 2000).

Freemantle, N., et al. "Beta Blockade After Myocardial Infarction." *British Medical Journal* (June 1999).

Glagov, S., et al. "Compensatory Enlargement of Human Atherosclerotic Coronary Arteries." *New England Journal of Medicine* (May 1987).

Gotto, A.M. "Low High-Density Lipoprotein Cholesterol as a Risk Factor in Coronary Heart Disease." *Circulation* (May 2001).

Grady, D., et al. "Cardiovascular Disease Outcomes During 6.8 Years of Hormone Therapy. Heart and Estrogen/Progestin Replacement Study Follow-Up (HERS II)." *Journal of the American Medical Association* (July 2002).

Graudal, N.A., et al. "Effects of Sodium Restriction on Blood Pressure." *Journal of the American Medical Association* (May 2001).

Greenland, P., et al. "Major Risk Factors as Antecedents of Fatal and Nonfatal Coronary Heart Disease Events." *Journal of the American Medical Association* (August 2003).

———. "ACCF/AHA 2007 Clinical Expert Consensus Document on Coronary Artery Calcium Scoring by Computed Tomography in Global Cardiovascular Risk Assessment and in Evaluation of Patients with Chest Pain." *Journal of the American College of Cardiology* (January 2007).

Grundy, S.M., et al. "Diagnosis and Management of the Metabolic Syndrome. An American Heart Association/National Heart, Lung and Blood Institute Scientific Statement." *Circulation* (October 2005).

Gullette, E., et al. "Effects of Mental Stress on Myocardial Ischemia During Daily Life." *Journal of the American Medical Association* (May 1997).

Gussekloo, J., et al. "C-Reactive Protein, Stroke, and Cardiovascular Disease." *Arteriosclerosis, Thrombosis, and Vascular Biology* (April 2000).

Hambrecht, R., et al. "Various Intensities of Leisure-Time Physical Activity in Patients with Coronary Artery Disease: Effects on Cardiorespiratory Fitness and Progression of Coronary Atherosclerotic Lesions." *Journal of the American College of Cardiology* (August 1993).

———. "Effect of Exercise on Coronary Endothelial Function in Patients with Coronary Artery Disease." *New England Journal of Medicine* (February 2000).

———. "Percutaneous Coronary Angioplasty Compared with Exercise Training in Patients with Stable Coronary Artery Disease. A Randomized Trial." *Circulation* (March 2004).

Haskell, W.L., et al. "Physical Activity and Public Health. Updated Recommendation for Adults from the American College of Sports Medicine and the American Heart Association." *Circulation* (August 2007).

Heart Outcomes Prevention Evaluation Study Investigators. "Effects of an Angiotensin-Converting Enzyme Inhibitor, Ramipril, on Cardiovascular Events in High-Risk Patients." *New England Journal of Medicine* (January 2000).

———. "Vitamin E Supplementation and Cardiovascular Events in High-Risk Patients." *New England Journal of Medicine* (January 2000).

Heart Outcomes Prevention Evaluation (HOPE) 2 Investigators. "Homocysteine Lowering with Folic Acid and B Vitamins in Vascular Disease." *New England Journal of Medicine* (April 2006).

Heiss, C., et al. "Brief Secondhand Smoke Exposure Depresses Endothelial Progenitor Cells Activity and Endothelial Function." *Journal of the American College of Cardiology* (May 2008).

Heitzer, T., et al. "Antioxidant Vitamin C Has Beneficial Effect on Artery Lining." *Circulation* (July 1996).

Hennekens, C.H. "Update on Aspirin in the Treatment and Prevention of Cardiovascular Disease." *American Heart Journal* (April 1999).

Hippisley-Cox, J., et al. "Depression as a Risk Factor for Ischemic Heart Disease in Men." *British Medical Journal* (June 1998).

Hochman, J.S., et al. "Coronary Intervention for Persistent Occlusion After Myocardial Infarction." *New England Journal of Medicine* (December 2006).

HOPE and HOPE-TOO Trial Investigators. "Effects of Long-Term Vitamin E Supplementation on Cardiovascular Events and Cancer. A Randomized Controlled Trial." *Journal of the American Medical Association* (March 2005).

Howard, B.V., and Kritchevsky, D. "Phytochemicals and Cardiovascular Disease." *Circulation* (June 1997).

Hu, F.B., et al. "Prospective Study of Major Dietary Patterns and Risk of Coronary Heart Disease in Men." *American Journal of Clinical Nutrition* (October 2000).

Hulley, S., et al. "Randomized Trial of Estrogen Plus Progestin for Secondary Prevention of Coronary Heart Disease in Postmenopausal Women." *Journal of the American Medical Association* (August 1998).

Iestra, J.A., et al. "Effect Size Estimates of Lifestyle and Dietary Changes on All-Cause Mortality in Coronary Artery Disease Patients." *Circulation* (August 2005).

Ironson, G., et al. "Effects of Anger on Left Ventricular Ejection Fraction in Coronary Artery Disease." *American Journal of Cardiology* (August 1992).

Jenkins, D.J.A., et al. "Effects of a Dietary Portfolio of Cholesterol-Lowering Foods vs. Lovastatin on Serum Lipids and C-Reactive Protein." *Journal of the American Medical Association* (July 2003).

Jensen, M.K., et al. "Obesity, Behavioral Lifestyle Factors, and Risk of Acute Coronary Events." *Circulation* (June 2008).

Jiang, E., et al. "Mental Stress–Induced Myocardial Ischemia and Cardiac Events." *Journal of the American Medical Association* (June 1996).

Katritsis, D.G., and Joannidis, J.P.A. "Percutaneous Coronary Intervention Versus Conservative Therapy in Nonacute Coronary Artery Disease. A Meta-Analysis." *Circulation* (June 2005).

Kavanagh, T., et al. "Prediction of Long-Term Prognosis in 12,169 Men Referred for Cardiac Rehabilitation." *Circulation* (August 2002).

———. "Peak Oxygen Intake and Cardiac Mortality in Women Referred for Cardiac Rehabilitation." *Journal of the American College of Cardiology* (December 2003).

———. "Usefulness of Improvement in Walking Distance Versus Peak Oxygen Uptake in Predicting Prognosis After Myocardial Infarction and/or Coronary Artery Bypass Grafting in Men." *American Journal of Cardiology* (May 2008).

Khot, U.N., et al. "Prevalence of Conventional Risk Factors in Patients with Coronary Heart Disease." *Journal of the American Medical Association* (August 2003).

Knudtson, M.L., et al. "Chelation Therapy for Ischemic Heart Disease." *Journal of the American Medical Association* (January 2002).

Koenig, W., et al. "Lipoprotein-Associated Phospholipase A_2 Adds to Risk Prediction of Incident Coronary Events by C-Reactive Protein in Apparently Healthy Middle-Aged Men from the General Population. Results from the 14-Year Follow-Up of a Large Cohort from Southern Germany." *Circulation* (October 2004).

Kokkinos, P., et al. "Exercise Capacity and Mortality in Black and White Men." *Circulation* (February 2008).

Krantz, D.S., et al. "Effects of Mental Stress in Patients with Coronary Artery Disease." *Journal of the American Medical Association* (April 2000).

Kraus, W.E., et al. "Effects of the Amount and Intensity of Exercise on Plasma Lipoproteins." *New England Journal of Medicine* (November 2002).

Lagrand, W.K., et al. "C-Reactive Protein as a Cardiovascular Risk Factor." *Circulation* (July 1999).

Leon, A.S., et al. "Cardiac Rehabilitation and Secondary Prevention of Coronary Heart Disease. An American Heart Association Scientific Statement from the Council on Clinical Cardiology (Subcommittee on Exercise, Cardiac Rehabilitation, and Prevention) and the Council on Nutrition, Physical Activity, and Metabolism (Subcommittee on Physical Activity), in Collaboration with the American Association of Cardiovascular and Pulmonary Rehabilitation." *Circulation* (January 2005).

Leor, J., et al. "Sudden Cardiac Death Triggered by an Earthquake." *New England Journal of Medicine* (February 1996).

Libby, P. "Atherosclerosis: The New View." *Scientific American* (May 2002).

Lichtenstein, A.H., et al. "Diet and Lifestyle Recommendations Revision, 2006. A Scientific Statement from the American Heart Association Nutrition Committee." *Circulation* (July 2006).

Little, W.C., et al. "Can Coronary Angiography Predict the Site of a Subsequent Myocardial Infarction in Patients with Mild to Moderate Coronary Artery Disease?" *Circulation* (November 1988).

Liu, S., et al. "Whole-Grain Consumption and Risk of Coronary Heart Disease: Results from the Nurses' Health Study. *American Journal of Clinical Nutrition* (September 1999).

———. "Fruit and Vegetable Intake and Risk of Cardiovascular Disease." *American Journal of Clinical Nutrition* (October 2000).

Lopez-Garcia, E., et al. "Consumption of *Trans* Fatty Acids Is Related to Plasma Biomarkers of Inflammation and Endothelial Dysfunction." *Journal of Nutrition* (March 2005).

Lotufo, P.A., et al. "Male Pattern Baldness and Coronary Heart Disease: The Physicians' Health Study." *Archives of Internal Medicine* (January 2000).

Madala, M.C., et al. "Obesity and Age of First Non-ST-Segment Elevation Myocardial Infarction." *Journal of the American College of Cardiology* (September 2008).

Manson, J.E., et al. "A Prospective Study of Walking as Compared with Vigorous Exercise in the Prevention of Coronary Heart Disease in Women." *New England Journal of Medicine* (August 1999).

Mittleman, M.A. "Air Pollution, Exercise, and Cardiovascular Risk." *New England Journal of Medicine* (September 2007).

Mosca, L., et al. "Evidence-Based Guidelines for Cardiovascular Disease Prevention in Women." *Circulation* (February 2004).

Moussavi, S., et al. "Depression, Chronic Diseases, and Decrements in Health: Results from the World Health Surveys." *Lancet* (September 2007).

Mozaffarian, D., et al. "Trans Fatty Acids and Cardiovascular Disease." *New England Journal of Medicine* (April 2006).

Mukherjee, D., et al. "Impact of Combination Evidence-Based Medical Therapy on Mortality in Patients with Acute Coronary Syndromes." *Circulation* (February 2004).

Myers, J., et al. "Exercise Capacity and Mortality Among Men Referred for Exercise Testing." *New England Journal of Medicine* (March 2002).

Nissen, S.E., et al. "Effect of Intensive Compared with Moderate Lipid-Lowering Therapy on Progression of Coronary Atherosclerosis. A Randomized Controlled Trial." *Journal of the American Medical Association* (March 2004).

Oberman, A. "Emerging Cardiovascular Risk Factors." *Clinical Reviews* (Spring 2000).

Ochoa, A.B., and Franklin, B.A. "Enhanced External Counterpulsation Therapy: A Noninvasive Approach to Treating Heart Disease." *American Journal of Medicine and Sports* (May/June 2003).

Ornish, D., et al. "Effects of Stress Management Training and Dietary Changes in Treating Ischemic Heart Disease." *Journal of the American Medical Association* (January 1983).

———. "Can Lifestyle Changes Reverse Coronary Heart Disease?" *Lancet* (July 1990).

Packard, C.J., et al. "Lipoprotein-Associated Phospholipase A_2 as an Independent Predictor of Coronary Heart Disease." *New England Journal of Medicine* (October 2000).

Pearson, T.A., et al. "Most Patients Do Not Achieve Target LDL Cholesterol Levels." *Archives of Internal Medicine* (February 2000).

———. "Markers of Inflammation and Cardiovascular Disease. Application to Clinical and Public Health Practice: A Statement for Healthcare Professionals from the Centers for Disease Control and Prevention and the American Heart Association." *Circulation* (January 2003).

Piscatella, J.C. *Don't Eat Your Heart Out Cookbook*. New York: Workman Publishing, 1994.

———. *The Fat-Gram Guide to Restaurant Food*. New York: Workman Publishing, 1997.

———. *The Road to a Healthy Heart Runs Through the Kitchen*. New York: Workman Publishing, 2005.

Piscatella, J.C., and Piscatella, B., *The Healthy Heart Cookbook*. New York: Black Dog and Leventhal Publishers, 2004.

Piscatella, J.C., et al. *Fat-Proof Your Child*. New York: Workman Publishing, 1997.

Pitt, B., et al. "Aggressive Lipid-Lowering Therapy Compared with Angioplasty in Stable Coronary Artery Disease." *New England Journal of Medicine* (July 1999).

Pope, C.A., III, et al. "Lung Cancer, Cardiopulmonary Mortality, and Long-Term Exposure to Fine Particulate Air Pollution." *Journal of the American Medical Association* (March 2002).

Preventive Cardiovascular Nurses Association. *National Guidelines and Tools for Cardiovascular Risk Reduction*, Revised Edition. New York: Philips Healthcare Communications, Inc., 2007.

Psota, T.L., et al. "Dietary Omega-3 Fatty Acid Intake and Cardiovascular Risk." *American Journal of Cardiology* (August 2006).

Rader, D.J. "Inflammatory Markers of Coronary Risk." *New England Journal of Medicine* (October 2000).

———. and Brewer, H.D. "Lipoprotein(a): Clinical Approach to a Unique Atherogenic Lipoprotein." *Journal of the American Medical Association* (February 1992).

Raggi, P., et al. "Identification of Patients at Increased Risk of First Unheralded Acute Myocardial Infarction by Electron-Beam Computer Tomography." *Circulation* (February 2000).

Reaven, G.M. "Insulin Resistance, Its Consequences, and Coronary Heart Disease." *Circulation* (May 1996).

Rehman, J., et al. "Exercise Acutely Increases Circulating Endothelial Progenitor Cells and Monocyte-/Macrophage-Derived Angiogenic Cells." *Journal of the American College of Cardiology* (June 2004).

Ribiero, J.P., et al. "The Effectiveness of a Low-Lipid Diet and Exercise in the Management of Coronary Artery Disease." *American Heart Journal* (February 1984).

Ridker, P.M. "High-Sensitivity C-Reactive Protein." *Circulation* (April 2001).

Ridker, P.M, et al. "C-Reactive Protein and Other Markers of Inflammation in the Prediction of Cardiovascular Disease in Women." *New England Journal of Medicine* (March 2000).

———. "Rosuvastatin to Prevent Vascular Events in Men and Women with Elevated C-Reactive Protein." *New England Journal of Medicine* (November 2008).

Rimm, E.B., et al. "Vegetable, Fruit, and Cereal Fiber Intake and Risk of Coronary Heart Disease Among Men." *Journal of the American Medical Association* (February 1996).

Roberts, W.C. "Preventing and Arresting Coronary Atherosclerosis." *American Heart Journal* (September 1995).

———. "The Underused Miracle Drugs: The Statin Drugs Are to Atherosclerosis What Penicillin Was to Infectious Disease." *American Journal of Cardiology* (August 1996).

———. "Shifting from Decreasing to Actually Preventing and Arresting Atherosclerosis." *American Journal of Cardiology* (March 1999).

———. "Atherosclerosis: Its Cause and Its Prevention." *American Journal of Cardiology* (December 2006).

Rutherford, J.D., et al. "Effects of Captopril on Ischemic Events After Myocardial Infarction: Results of the Survival and Ventricular Enlargement Trial." *Circulation* (October 1994).

Sacks, F.M., et al. "Effects on Blood Pressure of Reduced Dietary Sodium and the Dietary Approaches to Stop Hypertension (DASH) Diet." *New England Journal of Medicine* (January 2001).

Sandkamp, M., et al. "Lipoprotein(a) Is an Independent Risk Factor for Myocardial Infarction at a Young Age." *Clinical Chemistry* (January 1990).

Schömig, A., et al. "A Meta-Analysis of 17 Randomized Trials of a Percutaneous Coronary Intervention-Based Strategy in Patients with Stable Coronary Artery Disease." *Journal of the American College of Cardiology* (September 2008).

Sdringola, S., et al. "Combined Intense Lifestyle and Pharmacologic Lipid Treatment Further Reduce Coronary Events and Myocardial Perfusion Abnormalities Compared with Usual-Care Cholesterol-Lowering Drugs in Coronary Artery Disease." *Journal of the American College of Cardiology* (January 2003).

Sesso, H.D., et al. "Physical Activity and Coronary Heart Disease in Men: The Harvard Alumni Health Study." *Circulation* (August 2000).

Shen, B-J., et al. "Anxiety Characteristics Independently and Prospectively Predict Myocardial Infarction in Men. The Unique Contribution of Anxiety Among Psychologic Factors." *Journal of the American College of Cardiology* (January 2008).

Smith, S.C., Jr., "Risk Reduction Therapy: The Challenge to Change." *Circulation* (June 1996).

Smith, S.C., Jr., et al. "AHA/ACC Guidelines for Secondary Prevention for Patients with Coronary and Other Atherosclerotic Vascular Disease: 2006 Update." *Circulation* (May 2006).

Stampfer, M.J., et al. "Primary Prevention of Coronary Disease in Women Through Diet and Lifestyle." *New England Journal of Medicine* (July 2000).

Suaya, J.A., et al. "Use of Cardiac Rehabilitation by Medicare Beneficiaries After Myocardial Infarction or Coronary Bypass Surgery." *Circulation* (October 2007).

Sui, X., et al. "Cardiorespiratory Fitness and Adiposity as Mortality Predictors in Older Adults." *Journal of the American Medical Association* (December 2007).

Tankó, L.B., et al. "Enlarged Waist Combined with Elevated Triglycerides Is a Strong Predictor of Accelerated Atherogenesis and Related Cardiovascular Mortality in Postmenopausal Women." *Circulation* (April 2005).

Taylor, R.S., et al. "Exercise-Based Rehabilitation for Patients with Coronary Heart Disease: Systematic Review and Meta-Analysis of Randomized Controlled Trials." *American Journal of Medicine* (May 2004).

———. "Mortality Reductions in Patients Receiving Exercise-Based Cardiac Rehabilitation: How Much Can Be Attributed to Cardiovascular Risk Factor Improvements?" *European Journal of Cardiovascular Prevention and Rehabilitation* (June 2006).

Third Report of the National Cholesterol Education Program (NCEP) Expert Panel on Detection, Evaluation, and Treatment of High Blood Cholesterol in Adults (Adult Treatment Panel III). National Cholesterol Education Program, National Heart, Lung and Blood Institute, National Institutes of Health, 2001.

Thomas, R.J., et al. "AACVPR/ACC/AHA 2007 Performance Measures on Cardiac Rehabilitation for Referral to and Delivery of Cardiac Rehabilitation/Secondary Prevention Services." *Circulation* (October 2007).

Thompson, P.D., et al. "Exercise and Acute Cardiovascular Events. Placing the Risks into Perspective. A Scientific Statement from the American Heart Association Council on Nutrition, Physical Activity, and Metabolism and the Council on Clinical Cardiology." *Circulation* (May 2007).

Tonstad, S., et al. "Effect of Maintenance Therapy with Varenicline on Smoking Cessation. A Randomized Controlled Trial." *Journal of the American Medical Association* (July 2006).

Tu, J.V., et al. "Use of Cardiac Procedures and Outcomes in Elderly Patients with Myocardial Infarction in the United States and Canada." *New England Journal of Medicine* (May 1997).

Tuomilehto, J., et al. "Prevention of Type 2 Diabetes Mellitus by Changes in Lifestyle Among Subjects with Impaired Glucose Tolerance." *New England Journal of Medicine* (May 2001).

Urano, H., et al. "Enhanced External Counter-Pulsation Improves Exercise Tolerance, Reduces Exercise-Induced Myocardial Ischemia and Improves Left Ventricular Diastolic Filling in Patients with Coronary Artery Disease." *Journal of the American College of Cardiology* (January 2001).

Vakkailainen, J., et al. "Endothelial Dysfunction in Men with Small LDL Particles." *Circulation* (August 2000).

Vanhees, L., et al. "Prognostic Significance of Peak Exercise Capacity in Patients with Coronary Artery Disease." *Journal of the American College of Cardiology* (February 1994).

Vita, A.J., et al. "Aging, Health Risks, and Cumulative Disability." *New England Journal of Medicine* (April 1998).

Wenger, N.J. "Current Status of Cardiac Rehabilitation." *Journal of the American College of Cardiology* (April 2008).

Wilbert-Lampen, U., et al. "Cardiovascular Events During World Cup Soccer." *New England Journal of Medicine* (January 2008).

Williams, J.E., et al. "Anger Proneness Predicts Coronary Heart Disease Risk." *Circulation* (May 2000).

Williams, M.A., et al. "Resistance Exercise in Individuals with and without Cardiovascular Disease, 2007 Update. A Scientific Statement from the American Heart Association Council on Clinical Cardiology and Council on Nutrition, Physical Activity, and Metabolism." *Circulation* (July 2007).

Williams, R.B., et al. "Prognostic Importance of Social and Economic Resources Among Medically Treated Patients with Angiographically Documented Coronary Artery Disease." *Journal of the American Medical Association* (January 1992).

Women's Health Initiative Steering Committee. "Effects of Conjugated Equine Estrogen in Postmenopausal Women with Hysterectomy. The Women's Health Initiative Randomized Controlled Trial." *Journal of the American Medical Association* (April 2004).

Writing Group for the Women's Health Initiative Investigators. "Risks and Benefits of Estrogen Plus Progestin in Healthy Postmenopausal Women. Principal Results from the Women's Health Initiative Randomized Controlled Trial." *Journal of the American Medical Association* (July 2002).

Writing Group of the PREMIER Collaborative Research Group. "Effects of Comprehensive Lifestyle Modification on Blood Pressure Control. Main Results of the PREMIER Clinical Trial." *Journal of the American Medical Association* (April 2003).

2. Credits

Pages 34–35: Body Mass Index Table. Adapted from *Clinical Guidelines on the Identification, Evaluation and Treatment of Overweight and Obesity in Adults: The Evidence Report. NIH, September 1998.*

Page 53: Duke Activity Status Report. *American Journal of Cardiology,* Vol. 64, pp. 651–54, 1989, Hlatky et al., "A Brief Self-Administered Questionnaire . . . ," with permission of Excerpta Medica Inc.

Pages 60–61: Type A Behavior Test. From *60 Second Stress Management* by Dr. Andrew Goliszek. Reprinted with permission from New Horizon Press, Far Hills, New Jersey. Copyright © 1992 by Dr. Andrew Goliszek.

Pages 66–67: Anger and Hostility Profile. Arnst Ogden Medical Center, Elmira, New York. Used with permission.

Page 70: Depression Screening Test, adapted from HANDS (Harvard Department of Psychiatry/National Depression Screening Day Scale). Copyright © 1998 by President and Fellows of Harvard College and Screening for Mental Health.

Pages 106–108: Life Events Scale. Reprinted from *Journal of Psychosomatic Research,* Vol. 11: 213–18, 1967, T.H. Holmes and R.H. Rahe, "The Social Readjustment Scale," with permission from Elsevier Science.

Page 128: Resiliency Test. Adapted from *The Survivor Personality* by Al Siebert, Ph.D. (New York: Perigee Books, 1996).

Page 154: Energy Intake/Expenditure. Published in *Medicine and Science in Sports and Exercise,* Vol. 31, No. 11, 1999. J.O. Hill and E.L. Melanson, "Overview of the determinants of overweight and obesity." Used with permission from Lippincott Williams & Wilkins.

Page 160: Activity Pyramid. Copyright © 2002 Park Nicollet *Health Source.* Park Nicollet Institute. Reprinted by permission.

Page 166: Borg RPE Scale. For correct usage, instruction and administration, see *Borg's Perceived Exertion and Pain Scales* by Gunnar Borg, Ph.D. (Champaign, Illinois: Human Kinetics, 1998).

Page 239: Body-Fat Percentage. Adapted, by permission, from J.H. Wilmore, *Sensible Fitness.* (Champaign, Illinois: Human Kinetics, 1986), pp. 30–31.

Page 305: "One at a Time." From *Chicken Soup for the Soul* by Jack Canfield and Mark V. Hansen (Deerfield Beach, Florida: HCI Books, 1993), pp. 22–23.

3. Recommended Websites

American Association of Cardiovascular and Pulmonary Rehabilitation	www.aacvpr.org
American College of Cardiology	www.acc.org
American College of Sports Medicine	www.acsm.org
American Council on Exercise	www.acefitness.org
American Diabetes Association	www.diabetes.org
American Dietetic Association	www.eatright.org
American Heart Association	www.americanheart.org
Federal Trade Commission Consumer Line	www.ftc.gov
Institute for Fitness & Health	www.joepiscatella.com
National Academy of Sports Medicine	www.nasm.org
National Strength and Conditioning Association	www.nsca-lift.org
Nutrition Action	www.cspinet.org
Shape Up America	www.shapeup.org
Tufts Health & Nutrition Newsletter	tuftshealthletter.com

Index

A

Abdominal aortic aneurysm ultrasound, 327
Abdominal fat, xxiii, 31–32
  metabolic syndrome and, 46–48
  stress and, 103
  waist circumference and, xxiii, 32, 58, 76
ACE inhibitors, 90, 321–23, 324
Activity Pyramid, 160–61
Acute alarm, 103
Addiction, 121
Adrenaline, xxi, 102
Aerobic capacity:
  as cardiac marker, 48–54, 77
  low, fatigue and, 187
  as predictor of mortality, 49–51
  quantifying in METs, 49, 51–52
  reclaiming past level of, 171
  simpler techniques for measurement of,
    51–54
Aerobic dancing, 150, 161, 162, 195–96
Aerobic exercise, 10, 11, 48, 156, 159,
  161–68, 177
  activities for, 161–62
  brisk walking as, 150, 161, 163, 168,
    181–83
  cycling, 155, 161, 162, 172, 189–91, 194
  frequency of, 162
  health benefits of, 150, 152, 156
  intensity of, xxiv–xxv, 150, 162–67, 169, 197
  mood disorders and, 123
  running or jogging, 150, 152, 155, 156,
    161, 168, 169, 172, 181, 194, 196
  step aerobics, 195
  talk test and, 163
  time factor and, 167–68
  triglycerides and, 84
  Type A behavior and, 123
African-Americans, 42, 43, 147
Aggression, 64, 103, 121, 136
Aging:
  exercise and, xxiii, 157–58, 178
  reducing stiffness of, 170, 171, 178
Air pollution, xx–xxi
Alcohol, 72, 84, 132, 203
  blood pressure and, 90
  coronary inflammation and, 28, 227–28, 288
  excessive consumption of, 227
  HDL and, 83, 227
  health benefits of, 227–28

  healthy eating and, 88, 210, 227–28, 235,
    288–89, 301
  moderate consumption of, 210, 227–28,
    235, 288–89
  quick answers to questions about, xxxvii
  sexual activity and, xxvii
  sleep habits and, 125
  stress and, 109, 112
Alcoholism, 100
Allen, Woody, 116
Alzheimer's disease, 10, 315
Androgens, 109
Aneurysms, 327
Anger and hostility, 59, 64–68, 114–15
  assessing tendency toward, 66–68, 79
  controlling, 141, 142–43
  dangers of, 142
  heart attacks and, xxi–xxii, 65–66
  in women, 65
Angina, xxiii, 68, 310, 322, 323, 327, 328, 337
  quick answers to questions about, xviii–xix,
    xxxiii
Angiogenesis, 340
Angiography, coronary (cardiac
  catheterization), xxxix, xl, 328, 330–31
Angioplasty. See Balloon angioplasty
Angiotensin-receptor blockers (ARBs),
  321–22
Ankle/brachial blood pressure index (ABI),
  326
Antibiotics, 27
Antihypertensives, 40, 92, 321–23
Antioxidants, 82, 213, 229–31, 235
  in alcoholic beverages, 227
  flavonoids, 282, 283
  foods high in, 284–86
  in supplement form, 229–30, 231
Anxiety, 69, 114–15, 122, 125
  see also Stress
Apnea, obstructive sleep, xxi, xxxv
Apolipoprotein B (Apo B), 17–18
Appetite, 214, 216
Arby's, 298
Arm ergometers, 194
Arteries. See Coronary arteries
Arthritis, 31
Asian diets, 213
Aspirin therapy, xv, xxxv–xxxvi, 28, 85, 86,
  282, 304, 309–12, 315, 324, 335, 336

About the Authors

JOSEPH C. PISCATELLA is one of the country's most respected experts on how to live a healthy lifestyle in the real world. He is a visionary who has improved the lives of millions of people through his books, live presentations and PBS television shows.

Mr. Piscatella has written and coauthored numerous books enthusiastically endorsed by health professionals: *Don't Eat Your Heart Out Cookbook, Choices for a Healthy Heart, Controlling Your Fat Tooth, Fat-Proof Your Child, The Fat-Gram Guide to Restaurant Food, Take a Load off Your Heart, The Healthy Heart Cookbook, The Road to a Healthy Heart Runs Through the Kitchen* and *Positive Mind, Healthy Heart*. Over 5,500 hospitals use his books in cardiac rehabilitation, weight loss and prevention programs.

President of the Institute for Fitness and Health in Gig Harbor, Washington, he lectures frequently on lifestyle management skills; over two million people have attended his programs. He has hosted three PBS television programs on heart health (one on the health of children is in preproduction) and is a frequent guest on *Today,* CNN and *Good Morning America.*

Joe Piscatella knows the science of healthy living but he understands its practical application as well. He went through coronary bypass surgery at age 32. The prognosis was not good, with doctors predicting he would not live to be 40. But Joe's philosophy was that "You can't change the cards you were dealt, but you can change they way you play those cards." And he did. How has it worked? Joe recently celebrated the 33rd anniversary of that surgery. Says Dr. William C. Roberts of *The American Journal of Cardiology,* "Joe Piscatella knows more about healthy living than anyone I know."

Please visit www.joepiscatella.com and www.facebook.com/JoePiscatella for more information on Joe and his work.

BARRY A. FRANKLIN, PH.D., is director of Cardiac Rehabilitation and Exercise Laboratories at William Beaumont Hospital. He holds adjunct faculty appointments at Oakland University, Wayne State University School of Medicine and the University of Michigan Medical School. During his tenure at William Beaumont Hospital since 1985, the cardiac rehabilitation program and stress testing laboratories have achieved national and international recognition in the treatment and evaluation of coronary artery disease. Pursuing his interest in combining exercise physiology with cardiology, Dr. Franklin and his associates have studied the physiologic responses to numerous occupational and leisure-time activities, including snow shoveling, lawn mowing and stair-climbing. Other areas of research interest include the primary and secondary prevention of heart disease, comprehensive cardiovascular risk reduction, obesity and metabolism, exercise testing and prescription, and lipids/lipoproteins.

Over the years, Dr. Franklin's professional accomplishments have been recognized through a number of honors and awards, including: Award of Excellence and Pollock Established Investigator Award (American Association of Cardiovascular and Pulmonary Rehabilitation); Citation Award and Honor Award (American College of Sports Medicine); Award of Meritorious Achievement (American Heart Association); Outstanding Medical Research Award: "Seeker of the Truth" (William Beaumont Hospital, Royal Oak).

He has served as president of the American Association of Cardiovascular and Pulmonary Rehabilitation and of the American College of Sports Medicine. He is immediate past chair of the American Heart Association Council on Nutrition, Physical Activity and Metabolism. Currently, he serves as chair, AHA Advocacy Coordinating Committee, and sits on the national AHA board of trustees. He is a past editor in chief of the *Journal of Cardiopulmonary Rehabilitation* and he holds formal editorial board appointments with 17 other scientific and clinical journals.

Dr. Franklin has written or edited more than 500 scientific and clinical publications, including 27 books. He is a coauthor of the AHA text entitled *The No-Fad Diet*. Since 1976, he has given over 800 invited presentations to state, national and international, medical and lay audiences.